Randomized Controlled Trials in Evidence-Based Dentistry

Richie Kohli • Harjit S. Sehgal
Peter Milgrom
Editors

Randomized Controlled Trials in Evidence-Based Dentistry

Springer

Editors
Richie Kohli
Division of Dental Public Health,
School of Dentistry
Oregon Health & Science University
Portland, OR, USA

Harjit S. Sehgal
Division of Periodontology, Department
of Regenerative and Reconstructive
Sciences
Oregon Health & Science University
Portland, OR, USA

Peter Milgrom
University of Washington
Seattle, WA, USA

ISBN 978-3-031-47650-1 ISBN 978-3-031-47651-8 (eBook)
https://doi.org/10.1007/978-3-031-47651-8

This Springer imprint is published by the registered company Springer Nature Switzerland AG
The registered company address is: Gewerbestrasse 11, 6330 Cham, Switzerland

Paper in this product is recyclable.

To our Mentors, Colleagues, Friends

To our Families

And the Almighty

Foreword

Evidence-based medicine represents a considerable epistemic change in clinical reasoning that can rightly be considered a Kuhnian paradigm shift. This change is in large part the result of the culmination of progress made over the last century in clinical research methodology designed to inform clinicians of "what works" in patient care. For centuries, medical care relied on traditional practices passed down through expert opinion often mired in pseudoscientific beliefs about the causes and cures of disease. When improvements in clinical practice did occur, it was often the result of simple (i.e., non-experimental) trial and error, a process that was often valid only when effect sizes were dramatic (e.g., antibiotics for pneumonia). If the therapeutic benefit was small or occurred after a long latency, its value in treating a disease could easily be missed. Thus, trial and error approaches to finding and testing new therapies suffered from both false negatives and, in the absence of the use of placebo or control groups, false positives. As scientific thinking matured, tradition-based medicine began to be replaced by new approaches to treatment informed by case reports or mechanistic reasoning derived from principles from the basic pathophysiological sciences. These too were fraught with errors that led, often for decades, to the use of ineffective or in some cases harmful treatments.

By the early twentieth century, important advances in scientific methodology began to emerge through the efforts of such luminaries as R.A. Fisher and Sir Austin Bradford Hill, among others. Fisher championed inductive approaches, meaning that therapeutic efficacy needed to be determined through the application of probabilistic reasoning based on strong quantitative methods. Hill, along with Fisher, understood the need for controlling the potential for bias inherent in observational research studies. The remedies that they helped to develop included experimental research designs that emphasized such features as random assignment, allocation concealment, and the use of a placebo. In so doing, they laid the foundation for what is now a fundamental tool of clinical research, the randomized controlled trial (RCT). By the end of the twentieth century, RCTs were accepted as a minimally biased research design given their superiority in identifying effective therapies coupled with advances in information technology allowing for bedside access to relevant clinical literature. This provided the impetus that led to what is now known as evidence-based medicine (EBM). As significant as RCTs have become to clinical practice, it is important to note that it would be a misrepresentation of EBM principles to abandon the role of clinical expertise and mechanistic reasoning, as these too play an important role in ensuring high-quality patient care.

The exponential growth of RCTs reported in the medical literature over the prior 50 years was at once validating their importance for informing clinical practice while also leading to concern that the sheer volume of published studies would overwhelm busy clinicians' efforts to remain current. The EBM response to this deluge of information was the development of the systematic review, a process that relied heavily (but not exclusively) on RCTs to answer well-focused clinical questions. Thus clinicians, through accessing only one publication, could quickly understand the current evidence on a specific clinical topic. Moreover, as clinical expertise from seasoned clinicians and patient values and preferences were still valued as vital in understanding how, when, and for whom evidence from clinical research should best be applied, the clinical practice guideline (CPG) emerged as a logical outgrowth from the knowledge created from systematic reviews.

Given the foundational importance of RCTs for informing clinical practice, especially through their role in SRs and CPGs, a conscientious clinician would be well served by a thorough grounding in RCT methodology. This textbook provides such a comprehensive guide crafted to empower dental professionals with the essential knowledge and skills required to engage in and critically appraise clinical trials. Its pages provide a journey through the intricacies of research methodology, ethical considerations, and the practical nuances of conducting and interpreting clinical trials specific to dentistry.

Through these chapters, the reader will understand the transformative impact clinical trials can have on the landscape of oral healthcare. The EBM paradigm acknowledges that dentistry has been deeply rooted in empirical knowledge passed down through generations and this experiential wisdom is invaluable. However, through the integration of rigorous scientific inquiry derived from clinical trials the profession is propelled into a new era—one where decisions are not just based on tradition, but on a foundation of evidence meticulously constructed through systematic investigation judiciously tempered by expert clinical judgment.

This textbook was conceived to advance an understanding of and to increase the application of RCTs in clinical care. It is organized in two parts. Part I delves into the fundamental principles of clinical trial design and methodology. Here the fundamental philosophy underlying the use of RCTs is explained along with the nuances of formulating research questions, selecting appropriate study designs, and implementing robust methodologies to ensure the validity and reliability of findings. Understanding the intricacies of randomization, blinding, and control groups is essential for designing trials that withstand the scrutiny of scientific evaluation. This section serves as the cornerstone for any dental professional aspiring to understand the value of this ever-expanding body of evidence in oral healthcare.

Part II of the textbook explores the practical aspects of conducting clinical trials within the context of various dental specialties. From recruiting participants and obtaining informed consent to managing data and navigating regulatory requirements, these chapters serve as a comprehensive guide for dental researchers and clinicians alike. Real-world examples illustrate the application of theoretical concepts, providing readers with a practical roadmap to guide them in their own research endeavors. The importance of an often-overlooked aspect of clinical research, effective communication of research findings, is also emphasized as is the need to ensure that attention is paid to patient-relevant outcomes such as treatment cost and quality of life as important elements of the research design.

This textbook is not merely a compendium of facts and figures; it is a call to action for every dental professional to embrace the role of a lifelong learner and a critical thinker. The journey through clinical trials is both challenging and rewarding, demanding dedication, perseverance, and a commitment to the highest standards of scientific inquiry and ethical clinical practice. For clinicians wishing to deepen their understanding of the scientific rationale for clinical practice, this textbook serves as a guiding light, illuminating the path toward a future where dentistry is grounded in evidence, compassion, and excellence.

University of Pittsburgh
Pittsburgh, PA, USA
Robert Weyant

Preface

We, as educators and researchers, have dedicated our diverse careers to advancing oral health through evidence-based dentistry. We have authored pivotal chapters and enlisted seasoned colleagues to contribute, representing various dental specialties. Some chapters required extended periods due to the necessity of sourcing experienced authors and navigating the extensive literature base.

This book serves as a primer on the application of rigorously tested methods in conducting randomized trials within dentistry. It not only elucidates existing methodologies and areas for enhancement but also identifies gaps in the research landscape. Our citation choices were necessarily discerning, yet we believe the chapters are current as of early 2023 when the manuscript was finalized. This work addresses a void in dental literature particularly pertinent to graduate students and early-stage investigators, although clinicians will find many chapters of interest.

The impetus behind our writing and editing endeavors stems from the profound significance of good oral health. We assert that dental care professionals should have access to and employ the most contemporary and validated treatments. We sincerely hope that you, esteemed reader, will discern value in our work. Please feel free to share your comments and suggestions at kohli@ohsu.edu.

Portland, OR, USA — Richie Kohli
Portland, OR, USA — Harjit S. Sehgal
Seattle, WA, USA — Peter Milgrom

Contents

Part I

Dentistry and Randomized Controlled Trials

The Role of Randomized Controlled Trials in Clinical Dentistry and Future Directions

1

Alonso Carrasco-Labra, Jamie Spomer, Marcelo W. B. Araujo, Richie Kohli, and Peter Milgrom

Randomized clinical trials (RCTs) are an essential step in the often long and tortuous path of translating "benchtop" successes into safe and effective advances in patient care. Studies conducted in Medicine suggest that the path typically takes anywhere between 17 and 20 years [1, 2]. Even the recent rapid development and implementation of SARS-2 vaccines was based on many years of preliminary work in immunology [3] and other fields. Previously clinicians' choices were limited to case reports and observational studies that had huge limitations in terms of rigor and generalizability. Today, RCTs may focus on the prevention of disease or the diagnosis, control, or treatment of oral conditions overcoming these limitations. Primary outcomes may be clinical, patient-reported, or behavioral. Secondary outcomes may be surrogates or markers of disease progression [4]. Often RCTs, especially those that test drugs and devices, include measures of adverse effects or harms. Pre-clinical scientific discoveries may transition into any number of clinical trials as the body of evidence evolves. This is a process and rarely does a single trial answer all clinical questions. Indeed, RCTs require the investigator to narrow and focus the question to be studied a priori. They are not exploratory. The quality of the resulting evidence depends largely on the clarity and rigorous study design and execution. Experts across various disciplines of medicine have developed a system for Grading of Recommendations Assessment, Development and Evaluation (GRADE) system (Table 1.1) [5]. This system is helpful to clinicians because the higher the category of the certainty of the evidence (i.e., high, moderate, low, and very low certainty), the greater certainty of the evidence and the more significant are the clinical applications. At the aggregate level, systematic reviews and meta-analyses allow then for the synthesis of the results of multiple RCTs, which

A. Carrasco-Labra (✉)
Department for Preventive and Restorative Sciences, Center for Integrative Global Oral Health, School of Dental Medicine, University of Pennsylvania, Philadelphia, PA, USA
e-mail: carrascl@upenn.edu

J. Spomer
Research and Laboratories, American Dental Association Science & Research Institute, LLC, Chicago, IL, USA
e-mail: Spomerj@ada.org

M. W. B. Araujo
American Dental Association Science & Research Institute, LLC, Chicago, IL, USA
e-mail: Araujom@ada.org

R. Kohli
Division of Dental Public Health, School of Dentistry, Oregon Health & Science University, Portland, OR, USA
e-mail: kohli@ohsu.edu

P. Milgrom
Oral Health Sciences, University of Washington, Seattle, WA, USA
e-mail: dfrc@uw.edu

R. Kohli et al. (eds.), *Randomized Controlled Trials in Evidence-Based Dentistry*,
https://doi.org/10.1007/978-3-031-47651-8_1

Table 1.1 Certainty of evidence and its significance in the GRADE approach

Certainty of evidence level	Definition
High	We are very confident that the true effect lies close to that of the estimate of the effect
Moderate	We are moderately confident in the effect estimate. The true effect is likely to be close to the estimate of the effect, but there is a possibility that is substantially different
Low	Our confidence in the effect estimate is limited: The true effect may be substantially different from the estimate of the effect
Very low	We have very little confidence in the effect estimate: The true effect is likely to be substantially different from the estimate of effect

Adapted from H. Balshem et al. GRADE guidelines: 3. Rating the quality of evidence. Journal of Clinical Epidemiology 64 (2011) 401–406

are an essential element for producing evidence-based clinical practice guidelines [6]. The American Dental Association Department of Evidence Synthesis and Translation Research and the ADA's Council of Scientific Affairs, as well as organizations like the Cochrane Collaboration have been active in disseminating and encouraging the adoption of such guidance. Nevertheless, clinicians' awareness of the evidence, acceptability of the findings from research, ability to apply the intervention of interest, and the patients' ability and willingness to accept science-based interventions are some additional barriers that need to be addressed. These areas are the subject of much needed research but beyond the scope of this textbook.

The purpose of this chapter is to discuss why clinical trials are important in clinical dentistry and identify important factors that influence their usefulness and validity. The areas addressed in this chapter are the following: framing the problem so it has potential clinical application; methodological/design issues that increase or decrease the validity and clinical relevance of the RCTs; key regulatory and ethical dilemmas which could be faced by novice researchers while planning and conducting randomized controlled trials; and special issues about the future of randomized controlled trials.

1.1 Framing the Problem So It Has Potential Clinical Application

Evidence-based medicine, and its application to clinical disciplines including Dentistry is defined as "the conscientious, explicit, and judicious use of current best evidence in making decisions about the care of individual patients […] integrating individual clinical expertise with the best available external clinical evidence from systematic research […] and compassionate use of individual patients' predicaments, rights, and preferences in making clinical decisions about their care" [7]. Patients, clinicians, insurers, policymakers, patient partner organizations, and academicians use this evidence to inform healthcare decisions and determine the best approaches to prevent, diagnose, treat, and define a condition's prognosis.

The nature of the underlying evidence is either experimental or observational. Experimental studies involve the explicit and intentional administration of an intervention to a group of participants to compare their outcome to another group, which serves as a control. In observational studies, the investigator plays a different role, not intervening in how an experimental treatment is administered but merely documenting its use and consequences. Observational studies, such as those that use cohort designs, also include a comparison group. This feature of observational studies allows them to become a suitable alternative to answer clinical research questions that, in many cases, are not possible using RCTs. For example, to study the effects (i.e., desirable and undesirable effects) of opioids compared to non-opioid analgesics (e.g., nonsteroidal anti-inflammatory drug or acetaminophen) for managing acute dental pain, many RCTs have been conducted. They primarily provide information regarding short-term beneficial outcomes (e.g., pain relief, rescue medication, and global assessment of pain control up to 8 h follow up). These trials may also address short-term harm outcomes (e.g., gastrointestinal adverse effects, central nervous system adverse effects up to 8 h follow up) [8]. However, other highly relevant adverse effects that require a longer follow-up to occur, like long-term opioid abuse, drug dependence, or mortality. For efficiency, these outcomes are not always informed by RCTs but rather by long-term cohort studies or large cross-sectional studies conducted using pre-existing databases such as hospital records [9, 10]. Other study reports like clinical case series have an integral role in describing clinicians' experience with new treatments in settings where other study designs may be ethically inappropriate or practically difficult, for example, because the condition of interest is infrequently observed (e.g., disease with an extremely low prevalence). Such studies have limitations that can include small sample sizes, lack of comparison groups, selection bias, and other problems. A recent example of a useful clinical case series study was conducted to determine the arrest of root surface caries lesions in older adults when teeth were treated topically with 38% silver diamine fluoride (SDF). In the report, the authors identify some of the limitations [11].

RCTs are the preferable approach to determine the effect (i.e., benefits and harms) of intervention in health outcomes. RCTs' superiority over observational studies is based on the argument that the treatment choice and subsequent allocation of participants to an experimental or control arm are determined by chance and not by a clinician or an investigator, minimizing the effect of bias. Thus, randomization helps to create treatment arms balanced regarding known and unknown factors prognostic for the outcomes of interest, minimizing the effect of bias ("Systematic deviation of results or inferences from the truth" [12]) and confounding ("The distortion of a measure of the effect of an exposure on an outcome due to the association of the exposure with other factors that influence the occurrence of the outcome" [12]), and leaving two similar groups with only one difference: the experimental intervention under assessment. For example, investigators conducted an RCT to study the effect of using chlorhexidine gel compared to chlorhexidine rinse for preventing alveolar osteitis after the extraction of mandibular third molars. Participants ($n = 73$) were appropriately randomized, and the randomization scheme was concealed. However, when exploring the extent to which prognostic factors were equally distributed, there were some between-group differences in the proportion of male participants (14 in the gel group versus 5 in the rinse group) and smokers (16 in the gel group versus 10 in the rinse group) [13]. In this example, the small sample size could be responsible for the prognostic imbalances in the face of proper randomization and allocation concealment.

The advantages that RCTs exhibit also come with an unavoidable limitation. Not all potential participants are willing to be randomized and investigators cannot study speculative or even potentially harmful treatments because ethical principles prevent them from deliberately exposing those participants to potentially harmful interventions. Other study designs—such as observational studies—may be appropriate. For example, studying the effect of dental radiographs on the incidence of meningiomas, a benign brain tumor, can only be addressed using observational studies [14]. It would be unethical to recruit participants for an RCT where one of the groups would receive a large dose of radiation from dental radiographs to compare that arm with another one receiving a lower dose from radiographs.

RCTs often provide the most trustworthy evidence of causality between an intervention and a health outcome [15]. They measure the clinical effects of an intervention compared to a control or comparator, which may be a currently accepted intervention (e.g., head-to-head comparison, usual care) or no intervention (e.g., no treatment, placebo-controlled comparison). The choice of the comparator often depends on whether there is an existing treatment that is well accepted and the ethics of withholding such a treatment from the participants. Other chapters in this text provide reference to the guidance of the International Council for Harmonization of Technical Requirements for Pharmaceuticals for Human Use and Good Clinical Practice Guidelines and advice to investigators of the US Food and Drug Administration or regulations of other countries. Following this guidance leads to trials designed to properly assess the *efficacy* and safety of an intervention. A collection of evidence, such as a series of RCTs, must occur for an efficacious intervention to be *effective* in the real-world conditions of clinical practice [16]. While efficacy refers to “the extent to which a specific intervention, procedure, regimen, or service produces a beneficial result under ideal conditions” [12]; effectiveness is verified when an intervention is “deployed in usual circumstances of living and practice, and does what is intended to do for a specific population” [12].

1.2 Methodological/Design Issues That Increase or Decrease the Validity and Clinical Relevance of RCTs

Randomization plays an essential role in balancing known and unknown prognostic factors between the study arms, allowing investigators to obtain an unbiased assessment of the treatment effect. In other words, when randomization is appropriately implemented, and an effect is found, the most likely explanation for that effect is the administration of the experimental intervention. Here is a brief description of some relevant strategies and practical examples:

1. Methodological strategies before the trial starts
   (a) Random sequence generation: Researchers should generate a sequence that will guide the process of allocating participants to the study arms. Such a sequence randomly defines which arm each participant will be assigned to at enrollment. This element of chance and the sequence itself are often computer-generated using statistical packages, which is preferable to other less reliable methods, like the day of the week, area code of the phone number, or simply alternating assignment of patients to either arm (pseudorandomization methods) [17]. A good example is provided from this study in orthodontics: “Random sequence generation was performed with a computerized random 1:1 allocation using block sizes of 2. Randomization was performed on a computer with SPSS Statistics Ver 27.0 (IBM, Tokyo, Japan) by Y.S. No changes were made to the protocol after the trial commencement. After screening, the groups were created and locked before the start of the study. Patients were randomly allocated to the fluoride application group as a control (Group 1) or the tooth surface disinfection group as a test (Group 2)” [18].
   (b) Allocation concealment: Even if the random sequence to assign participants to study arms was generated using valid methods, the prognostic balance may be altered if participants or research workers learn the treatment arm assignments. Investigators can implement allocation concealment, for example, by using remote web-based 24-h central telephone randomization services offered by a third-party sources. Often investigators place assignments in opaque, sealed envelopes that are opened at the time of the treatment intervention. However, the use of envelopes represents a greater threat to the appropriate concealment of the sequence and should not be the first method of choice [19]. An example is provided from the following study: an RCT assessing the effect of applying 25% silver nitrate solution ($AgNO_3$) plus 5% sodium fluoride (NaF) varnish with functionalized tricalcium phosphate (fTCP) compared to 25% silver nitrate solution ($AgNO_3$) plus 5% sodium fluoride (NaF) varnish (without fTCP) to arrest dentin caries lesions in primary teeth allocated 3-year-old children to each study arm in the following fashion: “Allocation numbers were sealed in a pile of opaque envelopes, and a field assistant implemented the treatment allocation” [20]. The study did not describe how they developed and monitored the allocation process to preserve concealment. A good example of extended criteria providing additional assurance is “Envelopes were sequentially numbered and opened sequentially only after participant details were written

on the envelope. Pressure-sensitive or carbon paper inside the envelope transferred the participant's details to the assignment card. Cardboard or aluminium foil inside the envelope rendered the envelope impermeable to intense light. Envelopes were sealed using tamper-proof security tape" [21].

2. Methodological strategy as the study is being conducted
   (a) Blinding: After participants are enrolled in the study and the intervention(s) of interest is(are) administered, the research personnel (e.g.., researchers, clinicians, data collectors, outcome adjudicators, and statisticians), patients, and their caregivers must remain unaware of the arm assignment. This is achieved by using a methodological strategy called blinding. The use of placebo, double-dummy approaches, and codes are some of the most common strategies in pharmacological/medical trials. In dental trials aiming to determine the effect of a procedure; however, the implementation of blinding for the clinicians performing the procedure under investigation is not always possible [19]. Instead those who evaluate the outcomes are blinded. Some have proposed using sham procedures, yet the use of sham treatments often creates methodological and ethical challenges [22]. When blinding strategies fail, the placebo effect, as an explanation of apparently promising results, cannot be excluded. It is also possible that participants and researchers in the trial may consciously or unconsciously deviate from the intended intervention protocol, biasing the effect estimate. Often training and fidelity checks are included in clinical research protocols to address such problems. The nature of the outcome of interest (subjective versus objective measure) and the ability to adjudicate the outcome in a blinded fashion are factors that influence the extent to which one can overcome the challenges of conducting trials assessing surgical as opposed to pharmacological interventions [19]. For example, an RCT was conducted to determine the effect of 10% polyvinylpyrrolidone–iodine (PVP-I; povidone–iodine) plus 5% sodium fluoride (NaF) topical varnish compared to applying 5% sodium fluoride topical varnish alone for the prevention of dental caries lesions in children reported that "all study personnel and participants were blinded to treatment assignment. This study is an example of how to manage blinding when the intervention may be easy to figure out by the investigators. This trial takes advantage of the use of a dedicated investigator not applying the intervention but focused only on outcome adjudication. To maintain blinding, caries scoring examinations preceded the application of varnishes. Staff members applying varnishes did not perform the caries scoring examinations to eliminate examiner bias and ensure blinding" [23].
3. Methodological strategies after the study is completed
   (a) Missing participant data: Even if all of the methodological strategies listed above were successfully implemented, a trial could still be at risk of bias due to missing participant measurements when conducting the analysis. Although more than 18 different types of missing data have been described, the risk of bias is of particular concern when there is an imbalance or difference in the proportion of missing outcome data in the intervention arm compared to the control [24]. This can often be linked to known side effects or unexpected adverse effects or simply the participant burden of the experimental intervention. In such situations, participants with a greater burden will drop out, which may make the treatment under investigation looking more favorable or providing misguided or biased results. Guidance for the appropriate analysis and reporting of missing data has been published elsewhere [25].
   (b) Intention-to-treat analysis (ITT): ITT ensures that all participants allocated to

each intervention arm are analyzed "as intended" or according to the allocation initially defined by the randomization sequence. Conducting the analysis of RCTs in this manner allows investigators to maintain the prognostic balance initially achieved by the randomization sequence and determine the robustness of the results to the protocol violations and cross-contamination between study arms. The intention-to-treat analysis is, by nature, pragmatic, generalizable, conservative and avoids an overestimation of the treatment effect [12]. On the other hand, per-protocol analysis excludes the results of the participants who dropout or cannot be followed up and or those whose treatment involved protocol variations (e.g., got the wrong treatment or were followed up outside the pre-established time frame for outcome measurement). Per-protocol analysis leads to distortion of "true" study results. An ITT analysis was used by Weintraub et al. in a fluoride efficacy study in which there were protocol deviations [26]. In this study, "All families received counseling, and children were randomized to the following groups: no fluoride varnish, fluoride varnish once/year, or fluoride varnish twice/year. A protocol deviation resulted in some children receiving less active fluoride varnish than assigned. Nevertheless, ITT analyses showed a fluoride varnish protective effect in caries incidence. Analyzing the number of actual, active fluoride varnish applications in a supplementary per protocol analysis received resulted in a dose-response effect" [26].

1.3 Types of RCTs

1. According to phases of the development of an intervention

   The process from the first concept of an intervention until its release to the market is long and often measured in years or even a decade. This process is designed to help investigators answer three essential research questions. (a) Does the treatment work at all in participants? (b) Is the treatment reasonably safe (does the benefits outweigh the potential harms)? And, (c) is the treatment better or as good as the current standard of care or what is currently used? At every step of this process, an increasing number of people are enrolled to increase generalizability and to minimize the exposure of a large number of patients un unknown harms at the early stages [27] (Table 1.2).

2. According to the study purpose

   RCTs have been broadly categorized into two main types depending on their primary goal: Explanatory or pragmatic. Explanatory or "efficacy" trials are driven by a research question that focuses on the intervention's biological mechanisms. They provide evidence of whether the treatment under investigation works when prescribed or provided by an expert or specialist to patients with high-level compliance under the most favorable conditions possible. In other words, explanatory trials answer the question, "can the treatment produce more good than harm under ideal circumstances?" [28]. Pragmatic trials, on the other hand, focus on the clinical or community-level application of an intervention and provide evidence as to whether the treatment of interest works when prescribed or applied by a variety of clinicians to participants that may or may not be fully adherent to the protocol under conditions that better mimic a clinical setting. Pragmatic trials answer the question, "can the treatment produce more good than harm under conditions similar to clinical practice?" [28]. For example, a comparison of how patients value and respond to information on risk given in three different consent forms during dental check-ups: the PREFER randomized controlled trial [29].

   Although these definitions are widely available in the literature, they have been criticized by some as oversimplistic. Instead, trials exhibit a pragmatic-explanatory continuum depending on the specifications of the study design and conduct. The PRECIS tool provides a representation of the different elements to consider when defining the purpose

Table 1.2 Phases in the development of randomized controlled trials according to objective and sample size

	Objective and examples	Sample size (participants)
Phase I	Exploratory study to determine potential toxicity, tolerability of a drug, and potential adverse events E.g. Phase 1 clinical trial of peptide therapeutic product, C16G2 for dental caries management (C3J Therapeutics, unpublished data [NTCs: NCT02509845, NCT03004365, and NCT03052842]) Phase 1 Study of Clinical and Radiographic Success of Antibacterial Cement in Infected Dentin of Deciduous Teeth [47]	10–20
Phase II	Study intended to obtain initial evidence of potential therapeutic efficacy with the evaluation of beneficial outcomes and assessment against potential risks E.g. Efficacy and safety of a novel mucoadhesive clobetasol patch for treatment of erosive oral lichen planus: a phase 2 randomized clinical trial [48]	30–60
Phase III	Study intended to determine the extent to which the new therapy is efficacious when compared with the currently available standard therapy, or with placebo in the absence of such a therapy E.g. A phase III randomized, double-blind, placebo- and active-comparator-controlled multiple-dose clinical trial to study the efficacy and safety of MK0663/etoricoxib 90 and 120 mg, ibuprofen 600 mg, and acetaminophen 600 mg/codeine 60 mg in the treatment of patients with postoperative dental pain [49]	100–1000s
Phase IV	Post-marketing surveillance intended to monitor in a large-scale and long-term fashion in the presence of adverse events E.g. Amoxicillin/clavulanic acid for the treatment of odontogenic infections: a randomized study comparing efficacy and tolerability versus clindamycin [50]	Hundreds of thousands

Table 1.3 Scores in the PRECIS tool for the randomized controlled trial: biodentine application as an apical plug on the healing of apical lesions on immature permanent molars

Eligibility	Recruitment	Setting	Organization	Flexibility: delivery	Flexibility: adherence	Follow-up	Primary outcome	Primary analysis
3	5	2	5	2	2	2	3	5

of a trial across ten domains [30]. This tool was improved and validated to create PRECIS-2 [31], which graphically is a 9-spoked "wheel" with nine domains based on trial design decisions.

(a) Eligibility criteria—Who is selected to participate in the trial?
(b) Recruitment—How are participants recruited into the trial?
(c) Setting—Where is the trial being done?
(d) Organization—What expertise and resources are needed to deliver the intervention?
(e) Flexibility delivery—How should the intervention be delivered?
(f) Flexibility adherence—What measures are in place to make sure participants adhere to the intervention?
(g) Follow up—How closely are participants followed-up?
(h) Primary outcome—How relevant it is to participants?
(i) Primary analysis—To what extent are all data included?

These nine domains are each scored on a 5-point Likert continuum (from 1 = very explanatory "ideal conditions" to 5 = very pragmatic "usual care conditions") with the goal that trialists, clinicians, and policymakers can more easily consider whether design decisions. For example, Tolibah et al. [32] randomized controlled clinical and radiographic trials to study the effect of Biodentine application as an apical plug on the healing of apical lesions on immature permanent molars, the scores in the PRECIS tool are presented in Table 1.3. The setting domain was scored as 2 as this study was conducted in the pediatric department, College of Dentistry, Damascus University from March

2020 and July 2021, but the conclusion. The most extremely pragmatic approach to setting (score 5) would be to do the trial in an identical setting to which the authors intend the results to be applied.

1.4 Key Regulatory and Ethical Dilemmas Which Could Be Faced by Novice Researchers While Planning and Conducting RCTs

While planning and conducting RCTs, sponsors, investigators, and review boards must adhere to Good Clinical Practice (GCP) and applicable local regulations to ensure human subject protections and the implementation of good study design and protocols.

The International Council for Harmonisation (ICH) Guideline for Good Clinical Practice is an international ethical and scientific quality standard regarding the design, conduct, record, and report of trials that involve human subjects [33]. The principles of ICH GCP are rooted in the World Medical Association's Declaration of Helsinki of 1964, which defines the responsibility of investigators and the basic principles for all medical research [34]. The principles provide the basis for conducting clinical studies in a manner that protects participants' safety and well-being, and the resulting evidence is credible and accurate.

The Principles of Good Clinical Practice [33]

1. Clinical trials should be conducted following the ethical principles that have their origin in the Declaration of Helsinki, consistent with GCP and the applicable regulatory requirement(s). Some relevant examples are the following:
   (a) Off-label drugs: Fluoride varnish has never been approved as a drug in the United States and is used off label. It may be impossible to use a placebo in a trial of a new varnish, requiring the comparator to be an established varnish.
   (b) Use of placebo or placing patients on a placebo when an effective treatment exists: Some industrial studies especially in developing countries have been criticized because they included a placebo arm in their new arginine toothpaste trial rather than providing the current gold standard therapy, e.g. fluoridated toothpaste for comparison [35]. If a new agent is tested only against a placebo, there is no certainty that it is more effective, or equally effective as an existing agent. Under these circumstances, new drugs should be tested against an active agent.
2. Before a trial is initiated, foreseeable risks and inconveniences should be weighed against the anticipated benefit for the individual trial participant and society. A trial should be initiated and continued only if the anticipated benefits justify the risks.
3. The rights, safety, and well-being of the trial participants are the most important considerations and should prevail over science and society's interests.
4. The available nonclinical and clinical information on an investigational product should adequately support the proposed clinical trial.
5. Clinical trials should be scientifically sound and described in a clear, detailed protocol. The study outcome measures should be predefined so it does not result in bias due to the preference of choosing one outcome measure over another after reviewing the data. Examples include periodontal studies where pocket depth measurements are one of the clinical outcome measures. It should be clear if the pocket depth outcome is defined at the patient level or tooth level, and average or range of pocket depths.
6. A trial should be conducted in compliance with the protocol that has received prior institutional review board (IRB)/independent ethics committee (IEC) approval/favorable opinion.
7. The medical care given to and medical decisions made on behalf of participants should always be the responsibility of a qualified physician or, when appropriate, of a qualified dentist.

8. Each individual involved in conducting a trial should be qualified by education, training, and experience to perform their respective task(s).
9. Freely given informed consent should be obtained from every participants before clinical trial participation. Today with online journals and online supplements it is possible for investigators to publish the scripts used in obtaining consent and the actual consent forms. Effective and ethically sound informed consent should ensure that the risks and benefits of research participation are consistent with a participant's values and preferences [36]. An example is that most participants who enroll in clinical pain research expect some improvement in their pain control. In cases where there is no direct benefit to the participant, e.g., conducting surveys, studying medication pharmacokinetics, etc. the informed consent process must take on additional burdens to ensure that participants who consent to research that will not benefit them personally truly understand that the benefit of the research is only on the societal level [36].
10. All clinical trial information should be recorded, handled, and stored in a way that allows accurate reporting, interpretation, and verification. Many journals now have the requirements to make the datasets publicly available and require data storage in supplementary materials or specific databases. The researchers should thus store data in an understandable format for future sharing. Researchers should also be motivated to release their data with benefits such as recognition, or possibly bonus points in grant and job applications [37]. Data management costs should also be included in funding research.
11. The confidentiality of records that could identify participant should be protected, respecting the privacy and confidentiality rules following the applicable regulatory requirement(s).
12. Investigational products should be manufactured, handled, and stored following applicable good manufacturing practice (GMP). They should be used in accordance with the approved protocol. In many device trials in dentistry, a manufacturer provides materials and they are generally not independently tested for assurance of the ingredients but probably should be. There may also be trade secrets that prevent the investigator from knowing what a product is but this does not excuse the obligation of the researcher to verify that an agent is, for example, biologically active. Especially with devices, there is rarely any collection of data on harms, largely because such data collection complicates or lengthens already poorly funded industry studies.
13. Studies should include procedures that assure the quality of every aspect of the trial that is to be implemented. Good studies have detailed procedure manuals in addition to the protocol.

The RCT sponsor is the institution, organization, company, or individual who manages and funds clinical research. The ultimate role of the sponsor is to uphold the quality and integrity of the trial. Sponsor responsibilities include, but are not limited to, the protocol design, securing approval/favorable opinion of the ethics review board, the manufacturing, labeling, coding, and supplying investigational products for the study, quality and risk management, adverse event reporting, and continuous monitoring of the trial [33]. The trial protocol and design indicate how the study will take place, and the data are managed and analyzed. The design includes measures to minimize or avoid bias, inclusion and exclusion criteria for subject selection, methods and timing for assessing, recording, and analyzing safety and efficacy parameters, statistical methods to be utilized, and data and records management strategies. Throughout the implementation of the study protocols, the sponsor must maintain communication with all concerned investigators and institutions, as well as the appropriate regulatory authorities, to provide prompt notification of any research findings that could adversely affect the safety of subjects, impact the conduct of the trial, or alter the ethics review board approval to continue the trial [33]. Trial monitoring is also a significant responsibility of the sponsor. Monitoring verifies the welfare of the study participants, compliance with GCP, and the accuracy and integrity of the trial data. While the trial sponsor may also be the investigator in some cases, the sponsor is most often responsible for selecting an experienced and capable investigator to implement the study design and protocols.

Investigators may also play a role in a practice-based research network (PBRN). PBRNs are usually comprised of practicing clinicians interested in clinical research and a desire to advance patient care and health outcomes in the "real world." PBRNs are often affiliated with academic institutions and have strong relationships with community stakeholders. The diversity in location, expertise, and experience, along with the wealth of knowledge that a PBRN can contribute to a clinical trial, is often offset by its inability to establish and maintain well-controlled, GCP-compliant research conditions required for RCTs. For these reasons, we believe that PBRNs are best designed and uniquely positioned to contribute evidence that will lead to the most effective outcomes. Contributions of observational and other non-randomized clinical studies, together with RCTs, will build a rich body of evidence to expedite the translation of research outcomes into safe and effective advances in clinical dentistry outcomes.

1.5 The Future of Randomized Controlled Trials

Recently, the use of large databases of patient-level data, including their clinical records, has been proposed as an alternative approach to the standard parameters of causality and the classic RCT when determining the efficacy and safety of experimental interventions [38]. This approach, referred to as "real-world evidence," promises to take advantage of pre-existing data collected over thousands or millions of patients during the provision of care that reflects clinical decisions implemented by clinicians and patients in real-world clinical settings. The US Food and Drug Administration (FDA) defines real-world data as "…data relating to patient health status and/or the delivery of health care routinely collected from a variety of sources" [39]. Using such a type of data has several advantages: (1) it provides a broad platform of patients with a favorable profile toward a high level of generalizability and applicability of knowledge to practice; (2) it serves as a valuable source to identify rare adverse events, often challenging to find out from classic RCTs; and (3) it offers an inexpensive and convenient source of data, otherwise collected for other purposes than research. It becomes apparent from the advantages described above that "real-world evidence" is simply a recent label for data that remains observational in nature, which carries well-documented limitations, including bias and confounding related to the allocation of patients to specific therapies. When occurring in clinical settings, such an allocation is highly influenced by the clinician's ability to establish a prognosis and decide the best potential course of action. This favorable and desirable approach that clinicians apply to maximize the chance of clinical success, on the other hand, makes treatment effects calculated using these data unavoidably affected by bias and confounding [40].

The previous arguments are not to say that electronic health records, claims and billing data, patient-generated data from wearables and mobile devices, data warehouse construction, and repositories are of no value, and only data from RCTs are meant to inform practice and policy. Instead, the future entails amalgamating the fundamental principles of causal inference from RCTs with large sample sizes, high generalizability, and logistical convenience of real-world data. This has opened the door to the conduct of registry-based RCTs, a type of pragmatic trial emerging as a new approach in comparative effectiveness research [41]. Although no registry-based RCTs have been conducted or published in dentistry, there are several examples in the medical literature [42]. For example, the TASTE trial is a large-scale RCT using a registry-based approach. Briefly, the investigators used the Swedish Coronary Angiography and Angioplasty Registry (SCAAR) to evaluate the use of intracoronary thrombus aspiration plus primary percutaneous coronary intervention (PCI) compared with PCI alone and its effect on 30-day mortality in patients with ST-segment elevation myocardial infarction [43]. Due to the presence of a registry, patient recruitment occurred at a fast pace ($n = 7244$), no patients were lost to follow-up, and the cost per participant recruited in the trial was only US $50, 98% cheaper than the cost of enrolling a patient in a traditional RCT [41].

When compared with conventional RCTs, registry-based RCTs are advantageous as they have the potential to accelerate the volume and pace of participant enrollment, reduce the chance of missing participant data, enhance the study findings' generalizability, and dramatically reduce the cost of participant recruitment. The amalgamation of registries and RCT methodologies also carries challenges and barriers to overcome. The quality of the data in the trial is directly related to the accuracy of the information collected by the registries. Ethical issues, like patients' privacy or the timing for implementing informed concern, the ability to cross-link databases of different sources and nature, and ascertain the treatment outcomes using data gathered from clinical records can also be cited as issues that clinical trialists using this design need to address [41].

1.6 Case Scenario Exercise

1.6.1 Case Scenario

A parallel-arm, blinded, RCT of 1-year duration in patients with metabolic syndrome (MetS) and periodontitis was conducted [44, 45]. Participants were randomized to an experimental treatment group (ETG) ($n = 82$) that received plaque control and root planning plus amoxicillin and metronidazole or to a control treatment group (CTG) ($n = 83$) that received plaque control instructions, supragingival scaling, and two placebos. Computer-generated randomization was used for the first eight participants enrolled, and the minimization method for the following participants, then allocated participants using opaque envelopes with cardboard inside so they were impermeable to light. The authors did not perform randomization according to the protocol, but changed the method during the trial. The allocation sequence was generated by a statistician without clinical involvement in the study, who also assigned the participants to study groups. The examiner, the patients, and the technician who performed the laboratory analyses were all blinded to group assignment. The active periodontal therapy was performed by three periodontists (AQ, CI, and PC) and was completed within 3–4 weeks of the baseline visit. Patients in the CTG received treatment consisting of plaque control, supragingival scaling, and two placebo tablets. Periodontal parameters were reassessed at 3, 6, 9, and 12 months after completion of therapy. The primary and secondary outcomes were changes in C-reactive protein (CRP) and fibrinogen levels, respectively. There were 3% of participants who lost to follow-up and were excluded from the analysis. Periodontal parameters significantly improved in both groups 3 months after therapy ($p = 0.0001$) and remained lower than baseline up to 12 months. The improvement of periodontal status was significantly greater in the ETG ($p = 0.0001$). A multiple linear regression analysis, controlled for sex, smoking, hypertension, and extent of periodontitis showed that CRP levels decreased with time and that this reduction was significant at 9 ($p = 0.024$) and 12 ($p = 0.001$) months in both groups, without difference between the groups. Fibrinogen levels significantly decreased in the ETG at 6 and 12 months but not in the CTG. The authors concluded that periodontal inflammation either with root planning and systemic antibiotics or with plaque control and subgingival scaling significantly reduces CRP levels after 9 months in patients with MetS.

Questions

1. What is the risk of bias related to the sequence generation in this study?
2. What is the risk of bias for allocation concealment?
3. Why do you think control group also received periodontal treatment and was not a trueuntreated control group?

Answers

1. It is unclear risk of bias for sequence generation as the authors did not perform randomization according to the protocol, but changed the method during the trial [46].
2. It is low as: (a) after randomization, participants were allocated using opaque envelopes with cardboard inside so they were impermeable to light, and (b) the allocation sequence was generated by a statistician without clinical involvement in the study, who also assigned the participants to study groups.
3. For ethical reasons, control patients of the current study were not a true untreated control group as used in conventional randomized clinical trials because of the acceptability and availability of the standard of care treatment for periodontitis.

References

1. Balas EA, Weingarten S, Garb CT, Blumenthal D, Boren SA, Brown GD, et al. Improving preventive care by prompting physicians. Arch Intern Med. 2000;160(3):301–8. ISSN: 0003-9926 (Print).
2. Ho K, Chockalingam A, Best A, Walsh G. Technology-enabled knowledge translation: building a framework for collaboration. CMAJ. 2003;168(6):710–1. ISSN: 0820-3946 (Print).
3. Wilson IA, Stanfield RL. 50 Years of structural immunology. J Biol Chem. 2021;296:100745.
4. Council on Dental Research. Guidelines for the use of human subjects in dental research. J Am Dent Assoc. 1979;98(1):86–8.
5. Balshem H, Helfand M, Schünemann HJ, Oxman AD, Kunz R, Brozek J, et al. GRADE guidelines: 3. Rating the quality of evidence. J Clin Epidemiol. 2011;64(4):401–6.
6. Glasziou P, Haynes B. The paths from research to improved health outcomes. Evid Based Nurs. 2005;8(2):36–8. ISSN: 1367-6539 (Print).
7. Sackett DL, Rosenberg WM, Gray JA, Haynes RB, Richardson WS. Evidence based medicine: what it is and what it isn't. BMJ. 1996;312(7023):71–2. ISSN: 0959-8138 (Print).
8. Moore PA, Ziegler KM, Lipman RD, Aminoshariae A, Carrasco-Labra A, Mariotti A. Benefits and harms associated with analgesic medications used in the management of acute dental pain: an overview of systematic reviews. J Am Dent Assoc. 2018;149(4):256–265.e3. ISSN: 1943-4723 (Electronic).
9. Harbaugh CM, Nalliah RP, Hu HM, Englesbe MJ, Waljee JF, Brummett CM, et al. Persistent opioid use after wisdom tooth extraction. JAMA. 2018;320(5):504–6. ISSN: 1538-3598 (Electronic).
10. Mojtabai R, Amin-Esmaeili M, Nejat E, Olfson M. Misuse of prescribed opioids in the United States. Pharmacoepidemiol Drug Saf. 2019;28(3):345–53. ISSN: 1099-1557 (Electronic).
11. Mitchell C, Gross AJ, Milgrom P, Mancl L, Prince DB. Silver diamine fluoride treatment of active root caries lesions in older adults: a case series. J Dent. 2021;105:103561.
12. Porta M, International Epidemiological Association. A dictionary of epidemiology. 6th ed. New York: Oxford University Press; 2014.
13. Hita-Iglesias P, Torres-Lagares D, Flores-Ruiz R, Magallanes-Abad N, Basallote-Gonzalez M, Gutierrez-Perez J-L. Effectiveness of chlorhexidine gel versus chlorhexidine rinse in reducing alveolar osteitis in mandibular third molar surgery. J Oral Maxillofac Surg. 2008;66(3):441–5. ISSN: 1531-5053 (Electronic).
14. Claus EB, Calvocoressi L, Bondy ML, Schildkraut JM, Wiemels JL, Wrensch M. Dental X-rays and risk of meningioma. Cancer. 2012;118(18):4530–7. ISSN: 1097-0142 (Electronic).
15. Devereaux PJ, Yusuf S. The evolution of the randomized controlled trial and its role in evidence-based decision making. J Intern Med. 2003;254(2):105–13.
16. Singal AG, Higgins PD, Waljee AK. A primer on effectiveness and efficacy trials. Clin Transl Gastroenterol. 2014;5(1):e45.
17. Higgins JPT, Savović J, Page MJ, Elbers RG, Sterne JAC. Chapter 8: Assessing risk of bias in a randomized trial. In: Higgins JPT, Thomas J, Chandler J, Cumpston M, Li T, Page M, et al., editors. Cochrane handbook for systematic reviews of interventions version 61 (updated Sept 2020). Cochrane; 2020. Available from www.trainingcochrane.org/handbook2020.
18. Shimpo Y, Nomura Y, Sekiya T, Arai C, Okada A, Sogabe K, et al. Effects of the dental caries preventive procedure on the white spot lesions during orthodontic treatment-an open label randomized controlled trial. J Clin Med. 2022;11(3):854.
19. Evaniew N, Carrasco-Labra A, Devereaux PJ, Tikkinen KA, Fei Y, Bhandari M, et al. How to use a randomized clinical trial addressing a surgical procedure: users' guide to the medical literature. JAMA Surg. 2016;151(7):657–62.

20. Chen KJ, Gao SS, Duangthip D, Lo EA-O, Chu CA-O. Randomized clinical trial on sodium fluoride with tricalcium phosphate. J Dent Res. 2021;100(1):66–73. ISSN: 1544-0591 (Electronic).
21. Higgins JPT, Savović J, Page MJ, Elbers RG, Sterne JAC. Chapter 8: Assessing risk of bias in a randomized trial. In: Higgins JPT, Thomas J, Chandler J, Cumpston M, Li T, Page MJ, Welch VA, editors. Cochrane handbook for systematic reviews of interventions version 6.3 (updated Feb 2022). Cochrane; 2022. Available from www.training.cochrane.org/handbook.
22. Angelos P. Sham surgery in research: a surgeon's view. Am J Bioeth. 2003;3(4):65–6.
23. Milgrom P, Tut O, Rothen M, Mancl L, Gallen M, Tanzer JM. Addition of povidone-iodine to fluoride varnish for dental caries: a randomized clinical trial. JDR Clin Trans Res. 2021;6(2):195–204. ISSN: 2380-0852 (Electronic).
24. Kahale LA, Guyatt GH, Agoritsas T, Briel M, Busse JW, Carrasco-Labra A, et al. A guidance was developed to identify participants with missing outcome data in randomized controlled trials. J Clin Epidemiol. 2019;115:55–63.
25. Akl EA, Shawwa K, Kahale LA, Agoritsas T, Brignardello-Petersen R, Busse JW, et al. Reporting missing participant data in randomised trials: systematic survey of the methodological literature and a proposed guide. BMJ Open. 2015;5(12):e008431.
26. Weintraub JA, Ramos-Gomez F, Jue B, Shain S, Hoover CI, Featherstone JD, et al. Fluoride varnish efficacy in preventing early childhood caries. J Dent Res. 2006;85(2):172–6.
27. Stanley K. Design of randomized controlled trials. Circulation. 2007;115(9):1164–9.
28. Haynes RB, Sackett DL, Guyatt GH, Tugwell P. Clinical epidemiology: how to do clinical practice research. 3rd ed. Philadelphia: Lippincott Williams & Wilkins; 2006.
29. Harris R, Lowers V, Laverty L, Vernazza C, Burnside G, Brown S, et al. Comparing how patients value and respond to information on risk given in three different forms during dental check-ups: the PREFER randomised controlled trial. Trials. 2020;21(1):21.
30. Thorpe KE, Zwarenstein M, Oxman AD, Treweek S, Furberg CD, Altman DG, et al. A pragmatic-explanatory continuum indicator summary (PRECIS): a tool to help trial designers. J Clin Epidemiol. 2009;62(5):464–75.
31. Loudon K, Treweek S, Sullivan F, Donnan P, Thorpe KE, Zwarenstein M. The PRECIS-2 tool: designing trials that are fit for purpose. BMJ. 2015;350:h2147.
32. Tolibah YA, Kouchaji C, Lazkani T, Ahmad IA, Baghdadi ZD. Comparison of MTA versus biodentine in apexification procedure for nonvital immature first permanent molars: a randomized clinical trial. Children (Basel). 2022;9(3):410.
33. International Council for Harmonisation of Technical Requirements for Pharmaceuticals for Human Use. Integrated addendum to ICH E6(R1): guideline for good clinical practice E6(R2). Current step 4 version. 2016.
34. Ripley EBD, Macrina FL. Chapter 2: Ethics in oral health research. In: Giannobile WV, Burt BA, Genco RJ, editors. Clinical research in oral health. 1st ed. Ames: Wiley-Blackwell; 2010.
35. Shaw D, Naimi-Akbar A, Astvaldsdottir A. The tribulations of toothpaste trials: unethical arginine dentifrice research. Br Dent J. 2015;219(12):567–9.
36. Casarett DJ, Karlawish J. Beyond informed consent: the ethical design of pain research. Pain Med. 2001;2(2):138–46.
37. Tedersoo L, Küngas R, Oras E, Köster K, Eenmaa H, Leijen Ä, et al. Data sharing practices and data availability upon request differ across scientific disciplines. Sci Data. 2021;8(1):192.
38. Collins R, Bowman L, Landray M, Peto R. The magic of randomization versus the myth of real-world evidence. N Engl J Med. 2020;382(7):674–8.
39. U.S. Food & Drug Administration (FDA). Real-world evidence. 2020. Available from: https://www.fda.gov/science-research/science-and-research-special-topics/real-world-evidence.
40. Gerstein HC, McMurray J, Holman RR. Real-world studies no substitute for RCTs in establishing efficacy. Lancet. 2019;393(10168):210–1.
41. Li G, Sajobi TT, Menon BK, Korngut L, Lowerison M, James M, et al. Registry-based randomized controlled trials—what are the advantages, challenges, and areas for future research? J Clin Epidemiol. 2016;80:16–24.
42. Fitzpatrick T, Perrier L, Shakik S, Cairncross Z, Tricco AC, Lix L, et al. Assessment of long-term follow-up of randomized trial participants by linkage to routinely collected data: a scoping review and analysis. JAMA Netw Open. 2018;1(8):e186019. ISSN: 2574-3805 (Electronic).
43. Fröbert O, Lagerqvist B, Olivecrona GK, Omerovic E, Gudnason T, Maeng M, Aasa M, et al. Thrombus aspiration during ST-segment elevation myocardial infarction. N Engl J Med. 2013;369(17):1587–97. ISSN: 1533-4406 (Electronic).
44. López NJ, Quintero A, Casanova PA, Ibieta CI, Baelum V, López R. Effects of periodontal therapy on systemic markers of inflammation in patients with metabolic syndrome: a controlled clinical trial. J Periodontol. 2012;83(3):267–78.
45. Lopez NJ, Quintero A, Ibieta CI, Valenzuela CY, Jara L, Llancaqueo M. Effects of periodontal therapy on markers of systemic inflammation in subjects at cardiovascular disease risk (effects of periodontal therapy on systemic inflammation). clinicaltrials.gov/ct2/show/NCT01046435. First posted 12 Jan 2010. Last visited 4 May 2022.
46. Liu W, Cao Y, Dong L, Zhu Y, Wu Y, Lv Z, et al. Periodontal therapy for primary or secondary prevention of cardiovascular disease in people with periodontitis. Cochrane Database Syst Rev. 2019;(12):CD009197. https://doi.org/10.1002/14651858.CD009197.pub4.
47. Ferreira JM, Pinheiro SL, Sampaio FC, Menezes VA. Use of glass ionomer cement containing antibiotics to seal off infected dentin: a randomized clinical trial. Braz Dent J. 2013;24(1):68–73.

48. Brennan MT, Madsen LS, Saunders DP, Napenas JJ, McCreary C, Ni Riordain R, et al. Efficacy and safety of a novel mucoadhesive clobetasol patch for treatment of erosive oral lichen planus: a phase 2 randomized clinical trial. J Oral Pathol Med. 2022;51(1):86–97.
49. Brown JD, Daniels SE, Bandy DP, Ko AT, Gammaitoni A, Mehta A, et al. Evaluation of multiday analgesia with etoricoxib in a double-blind, randomized controlled trial using the postoperative third-molar extraction dental pain model. Clin J Pain. 2013;29(6):492–8.
50. Tancawan AL, Pato MN, Abidin KZ, Asari AS, Thong TX, Kochhar P, et al. Amoxicillin/clavulanic acid for the treatment of odontogenic infections: a randomised study comparing efficacy and tolerability versus clindamycin. Int J Dent. 2015;2015:472470.

2 How to Conduct a Clinical Trial: Overview

Peter Milgrom and Donald L. Chi

2.1 Conception and Planning of a Clinical Trial

Theoretical model of the problem
Specific objectives/hypotheses
Theoretical model of the intervention
Scientific rationale

Clinical trials are conducted in order to answer specific questions about the efficacy, effectiveness, or safety of a clinical intervention. The intervention might be a new medical device, a drug, or a behavioral approach. Typically, trials are conducted in order to support or modify the standard of care. The results of randomized trials are considered the important level of evidence in developing practice guidelines and for the approval of medical devices and drugs. The levels of evidence and their importance are shown in Table 2.1. Efficacy questions address whether an intervention is able to produce the intended result. Often efficacy studies (often called phase 2 studies) are conducted in a single setting under the control of researchers and the participants are not fully representative of the intended population [1]. Effectiveness, on the other hand, in clinical trials parlance refers to whether an intervention is efficacious in the broad range of "real world" settings in which it is intended to be used and with a more representative group of participants. These are often called phase 3 studies or definitive trials. Normally, efficacy studies are conducted before a decision to carry out an effectiveness study. Nearly all clinical trials also address safety (sometimes called harms in the clinical trials literature) [2].

Table 2.1 Levels of evidence in descending order of strength by source of evidence[a]

Level	Source of evidence
1a	Systematic review of multiple high-quality randomized clinical trials
1b	Single high-quality randomized clinical trial
2a	Systematic review of multiple high-quality cohort studies
2b	Single cohort study; lower-quality randomized clinical trials
3a	Systematic review of high-quality case–control studies
3b	Single case–control study
4	Case series; poor quality cohort or case–control studies
5	Expert opinion

[a] http://www.cebm.net/2009/06/oxford-centre-evidence-based-medicine-levels-evidence-march-2009/

Clinical trials are focused efforts and depend on the investigator having a clear model of the clinical problem being tackled. The need for an intervention should stem from a careful review of the literature regarding the disease, condition, or problem. Similarly, the choice of an intervention to trial should logically flow from

P. Milgrom (✉) · D. L. Chi
University of Washington, Seattle, WA, USA
e-mail: dfrc@uw.edu; dchi@uw.edu

R. Kohli et al. (eds.), *Randomized Controlled Trials in Evidence-Based Dentistry*,
https://doi.org/10.1007/978-3-031-47651-8_2

the gaps or deficiencies in present interventions. Usually smaller scale formal studies (often called phase 1 studies or proof of principle studies) studies are carried out first to help clarify the need for and safety of a larger study [3]. Most importantly, the early studies allow for testing of procedures and measurement tools needed for a more advanced trial. They may also contribute to knowledge needed for defining a hypothesized effect size, and for conducting a power analysis and determining sample size. Note, these studies cannot be ad hoc or poorly conceived or documented.

The key elements of any clinical trial protocol are the specific objective and hypotheses. These are stated a priori. An example from one of the author's work [4] is below:

Primary objective

- To determine if the test varnish containing fluoride and iodine is superior to a control varnish containing only fluoride in the prevention of new caries lesions.

Secondary objectives

- To establish that the response of child participants to the test varnish was not inferior to the control varnish.
- To document the safety of the varnish.

The hypotheses were that the test varnish is superior to an active control varnish containing only fluoride in the prevention of new caries lesions and that the child participants experienced no more anxiety during the application of the test varnish than when the control varnish is applied, and to document the safety of the varnish.

2.1.1 Assembling Interdisciplinary Teams

Conducting a clinical trial is not a solo effort but does require a leader, often called the principal investigator (PI). It is the job of the PI to lead the team and to coordinate and assemble the results of the efforts of the individual team members. PIs typically have final responsibility for all aspects of a clinical trial. A successful trial requires the collaboration of a team, with the duties and responsibilities of all members carefully delineated in the protocol and manual of operations. A clinical trial may require multiple sites to facilitate participant recruitment. A typical organization chart for a clinical trial is shown in Fig. 2.1. Many teams include expert clinicians, methodologists with expertise in measurement and instrument design, trainers, bio-

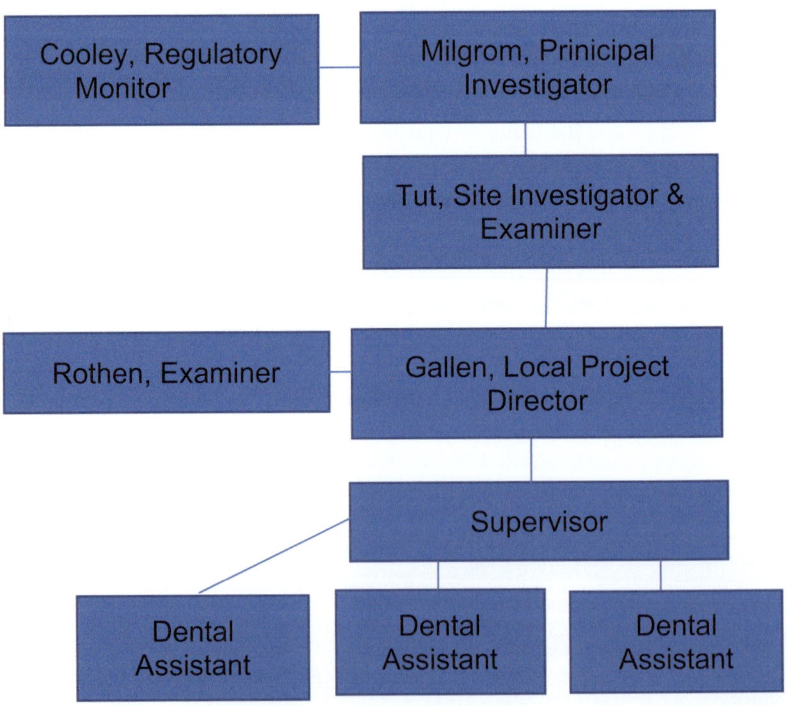

Fig. 2.1 Organization chart for a recent clinical trial by one of the authors (PM)

statisticians, data managers, and analysts. In situations where teams are incomplete, there are often gaps in the quality of the protocol or manual of operations, problems with measurement, or incomplete analyses. The process of team science is an emerging topic of scholarly interest [5, 6].

2.1.2 Study Timeline

Clinical trials are lengthy. The study timeline includes (1) defining the objective and hypotheses; (2) gaining access to a study population and setting; (3) writing the protocol and manual of operations; (4) gaining ethical and regulatory approvals; (5) budgeting; (6) hiring and training staff; (7) accrual of the participant population; (8) carrying out the trial; (9) entering and checking trial data; (10) analysis; and (11) dissemination of the results.

An example of a trial timeline for a single site phase 2 trial one of us conducted of a new dental varnish is given in Fig. 2.2.

2.1.3 Advisory Groups

Historically, investigators used and abused the populations from which participants were drawn

Task	9/16	10/16	11/16	1/17	2/17	3/17	5/17	9/17	12/17	2/18	5/18	9/18	12/18	3/19	6/1/19	7/1/19	9/1/19
Government Site Approval Letter	X																
IRB approval		X															
Contracts			X														
Equipment ordered		X															
Equipment delivered				X													
Drugs ordered			X														
Drugs delivered				X													
Regulatory Site visits				X										X			
Staff hires & training				X	X	X											
Recruitment						X											
Exams						X				X				X			
Treatments							X	X	X	X	X	X	X	X			
Data Entry															X		
Analysis																X	
Reporting																	X

Fig. 2.2 Trial timeline for single site phase 2 study by one of the authors (PM)

[7]. They are often described as "parachutists" who dropped in to conduct research and left without ever sharing the results of their work. This behavior engendered disbelief and anger and made carrying out clinical research in the same setting afterwards difficult. Today ethical researchers often have advisory groups drawn from the communities in which they are working, whether that be a clinic population or the population at large [8]. Indeed, some funders (e.g., the Patient-Centered Outcomes Research Institute in the United States) require formal community engagement plans and most granting agencies and foundations require dissemination plans (to be discussed later in this chapter). The individuals selected for advisory groups, who are typically paid for their time and service, can advise on the study from its conception through the actual interpretation and dissemination of the study results. Advisory groups need a structure and a formal job description. Members need leadership and need to know their obligations. The following is a typical charge to such an advisory group: providing community context on how the intervention might be perceived locally, identifying the most relevant outcomes that should be studied, helping to develop a participant recruitment strategy and problem solve during the trial, and playing a role in disseminating the research findings to local stakeholders.

2.1.4 Choosing Sites

Choosing a site or sites for a trial is one of the most important elements in planning. Successful clinical trialists have long-established bonds with the communities where they work. The communities are often underserved and have high rates of untreated dental diseases. We recommend to prospective researchers that they provide services in these communities for several years, to establish strong ties and friendships, prior to approaching community leaders or public health officials about conducting a trial in their community. Funders always request documentation of community acceptance prior to providing funding. Planning to gain community buy-in is always necessary.

There are many questions to ask oneself. Does the population have a high rate of the disease or condition I plan to study? Both of us have worked extensively in Alaska and the US-affiliated states in Micronesia [9, 10]. Tooth decay rates in these communities are high. Is the population accessible—how difficult and time consuming will be it to recruit the study participants? One of us previously planned a study on the Navajo Reservation in New Mexico. The study center was to be in Gallup (a small city) but the population was spread over a 60 mile radius and included many tiny rural communities. This made planning difficult. Is the population large enough? Many of Alaska Native communities have populations of less than 1000. This makes the prospect of recruiting a sample very tough. Is the potential participant population typical of those who have the disease generally? We will discuss the importance of this element further later in this chapter. How transitory is the population—do they move a lot? How difficult will it be to find the participants when it is time to do follow-up exams or interviews, for example? How much loss to follow-up can be expected? A review of trials in major journals showed that 21% failed to achieve adequate numbers at randomization and 48% failed to achieve adequate numbers at outcome assessment [11]. Achieving the planned enrollment in a trial requires realistic planning, time and personnel, sufficient budget, and potential loss of participants requires inflating planned sample sizes. Failure to achieve planned sample sizes reduces statistical power to detect differences in study conditions and loss to follow-up diminishes the validity of the findings.

2.1.5 Budgeting and Funding

Budget periods for clinical trial research may include preliminary work and site preparation, the active research period, data entry and quality control, and dissemination. In our experience, most studies are under budgeted and the investigators run out of money at the dissemination stage. Also, complicated trials—especially those in the community—experience participant accrual rates below predictions—and often have to spend more time and money to successfully recruit the required population. Low accrual rates sink clinical trials, reducing their statistical power and excluding generalizability. Typical budget categories for clinical trials research include: personnel, consulting fees (including for advisory committees or a Data Safety and Monitoring Board [DSMB]), supplies and materials (including study drugs), incentives for participants, travel, and dissemination. Most institutions have formal written policies about how budgets are constructed and approved. Nevertheless, rarely has any functionary in the budget department ever directed a clinical trial so the accurate estimation of costs is the responsibility of the PI and the research team.

2.1.6 Funding

Clinical trials can be very expensive. Large multicenter trials in the United States or within the European Community can cost millions of dollars. Trials of dental caries preventive agents or treatments for periodontal diseases can last 3 or more years. Public funders might include states (e.g., in 2019 California allocated millions of dollars to public health work from the Tobacco Settlement program) or the national government. The National Institutes of Health, the Centers for Disease Control and Prevention, the Food and Drug Administration, the Defense Advanced Research Projects Agency, the Health Services and Resources Administration, and other parts of the US government award grant funding for clinical research. A quasi-governmental agency, PCORI—the Patient Centered Outcomes Research Institute, gives funds for clinical trials. Parallel institutions exist in most countries, including the European Union and European countries, Japan, Hong Kong, Singapore, and the large states in Oceana, Australia, and New Zealand.

Private companies, particularly those that produce dental materials, and foundations also give grants to support research. Typically, however, the grants are small and support in vitro research. Very few pay the full cost of trials. Also, universities may place restrictions on commercial funding to assure the independence of the investigators and avoid actual or apparent conflicts of interest.

Reports of the outcomes of all clinical trials are required to include information on how the trial was financed and the role, if any, of the funders in the actual process of the research or interpretation of the findings. Historically, reporting of conflicts of interest in pharmacologic treatment trials was incomplete [12]. In academic institutions, investigators are required to file annual disclosures regarding potential conflicts of interest when trials are funded. The institutions may develop conflict management plans that specify what a conflicted investigator may or may not do within the research process.

2.1.7 Clinical Trial Insurance

Investigators working for large academic or public health institutions generally have insurance provided by their home organization. It is important, however, for the prospective investigator to understand the nature and extent of the coverage and, under what circumstances, the investigator themselves might be responsible for unforeseen damages. The home institution may also self-insure. It may be useful to contact the risk management office or official within the institution. Information about liability insurance will certainly be required for constructing consent forms and gaining ethical approval. Funders, such as foundations or government agencies, may also require proof of insurance.

Trials sponsored by industry or otherwise privately funded may require commercial insurance for liability or errors and omissions. They typically cover claims related to participant injury, adverse effects, and errors by trial employees. Such insurance may also cover work-related injuries of employees. Working in remote areas, as we have, sponsors may require evacuation insurance to insure study employees can be transported should they have a serious accident on the job. Examples requiring evacuation might include a serious road accident on a remote island site in the Pacific or a snowmobile accident when a study employee was visiting a village site to see participants in rural Alaska in winter. This kind of insurance may be needed to supplement personal insurance that is provided as part of general employment contracts. In a tooth decay study, one of us completed in a rural area involving about 300 children over 2 years. The commercial insurance costs alone exceeded US $5000 (2019 dollars) per year.

2.1.8 IRB (Ethics) Approval

Worldwide there are ethical rules governing the involvement of human subjects in clinical research [13]. The principles are articulated in the World Medical Association Declaration of Helsinki in 1964 and augmented periodically until today. They build on the International Code of Medical Ethics. The principles make clear that "considerations related to the well-being of the human subject should take precedence over the interests of science and society." Moreover, in most countries, these principles are codified in laws and regulations regarding all aspects of clinical research. All reputable scientific journals require evidence that the protocols of published clinical trials adhered to the Helsinki Declaration principles and no trials can be published without such evidence.

In the United States, the policy for protection of human subjects is called the "Common Rule." It was first published in 1991 and is codified in section 45 CFR part 46 of the Code of Federal Regulations. The parts include rules for the protection of all subjects in research as well as special protections for pregnant women, human fetuses, and neonates, prisoners, and children. Universities in the United States are charged with assuring that academic scholars follow these regulations. They do this by mandating training for investigators and by hosting federally licensed Institutional Review Boards (IRB) that carefully scrutinize research protocols before approval and monitor on-going research to assure the protection and welfare of research participants.

Institutions can provide required human subjects protection training or they can provide access to subscription-based national training resources. The not-for-profit Collaborative Institutional Training Initiative (CITI Program, URL: citiprogram.org) provides comprehensive human subjects training and is widely used by the major US academic institutions as well as industry. Courses are largely on-line and cover both medical device, pharmaceutical, and behavioral research as well subjects such as biosafety and biosecurity, conflicts of interest, and Good Clinical Practice (GCP). CITI also offers frequent webinars on related topics. Training is generally required for any investigator or staff member who will have contact with human subjects or will be handling protected information.

Employees of academic and research institutions in the United States generally apply to their own institution's IRB for approval of research. Approval is not required at the stage where an individual is seeking funding but rather when funding is secured. Government agencies in the United States will not release funds for research without documentation of IRB approval. Very often the institutions provide training for investigators to aid them in completing the process. When more than one institution is involved in clinical trial research, such as in a multi-center trial, a single institution takes the lead in reviewing and supervising the trial. Institutions generally have agreements that govern the collaborations. Also, there are independent IRBs that focus strictly on industry-supported clinical trials. Investigators at academic institutions should consult with their own IRB as well as sponsors in determining the appropriate IRB of record.

Research conducted outside the United States is also subject to review. Principal investigators should plan far in advance to determine the nature of and comply with local review policies while also recognizing that their home institution generally must approve their work.

2.1.9 FDA or Other Regulatory Issues Including Trial Monitoring like DSMB or CRO

Phase 3 clinical trials have a Data and Safety Monitoring Board (DSMB) [14]. Phase 1 or 2 studies may have a DSMB depending on the potential risks involved to participants. The DSMB consists of researchers, ethics experts, and statisticians outside of the study team and may be appointed by the investigator or the sponsor. In the case of studies sponsored by the National Institutes of Health, the DSMB is appointed by the PI with the concurrence of the program official. DSMBs are usually empaneled before the study commences and serve until the data are analyzed and reported. The DSMB receives annual reports on the progress of the study and has access to blinded reports on outcomes and adverse events. DSMBs will have a written charter specifying the duties of the members. The primary focus is participant safety. Recommendations are made to the Sponsor and Principal Investigator. A DSMB may recommend a study be halted prematurely. The DSMB is separate from the IRB, which maintains oversight.

In clinical trials under the purview of the FDA and similar governmental organizations throughout the world, the Sponsor will provide the agency with a copy of the DSMB charter.

Contract Research Organizations (CRO) are commercial companies that provide support to researchers and the industry on a contract basis. In the context of a clinical trial, the CRO may aid the investigator in organizing, managing and securing trial data, and in auditing the data quality. CROs typically make visits prior to study initiation, send staff to audit the completeness of records, and conduct monitoring visits. CROs issue formal reports that become part of the trial record. National Institutes of Health contracts with CRO organizations for this function. Similarly, a commercial sponsor may contract with a CRO to manage a trial but in this case, the CRO may also be advising on the overall management of a new drug or medical device application before the FDA or similar organizations in other countries. CROs vary considerably in size and scope of work.

DSMB members are typically compensated for their time and receive allowances for travel and other expenses in carrying out their duties. A PI must plan for the expenses of a DSMB within the study budget. In most cases, the Sponsor is responsible for the cost of using a CRO but how this is handled varies.

2.1.10 Registration of Trial

Virtually all scholarly journals today require that reports they publish represent clinical trials that were registered in advance of enrollment of participants. There are two key reasons. First, this protects against what is called publication bias. In this situation, authors—particularly those testing commercial products—only publish positive results and inflate the effectiveness of medical devices and drugs. Or, they may hide adverse effects. Without registration, the negative trials are in the shadows. Second, the registration of the study objectives, methods, and analysis plan establishes an a priori commitment to the outcome measure. Otherwise, there is a tendency of investigators to pick and choose among outcomes to report, after they have analyzed the data. Reporting quality continues to be low even after registration requirement policy implementation at journals [15].

Internationally, the World Health Organization International Clinical Trials Registry Platform (ICTRP) is a network of prospective trial registries [16]. Trials registered at ICTRP site receive a Universal Trial Number (UTN) which is then

Table 2.2 Elements of the World Health Organization Trial Registration Data Set[a]

1. Primary Registry and Trial Identifying Number
2. Date of Registration in Primary Registry
3. Secondary Identifying Numbers
4. Source(s) of Monetary or Material Support
5. Primary Sponsor
6. Secondary Sponsor(s)
7. Contact for Public Queries
8. Contact for Scientific Queries
9. Public Title
10. Scientific Title
11. Countries of Recruitment
12. Health Condition(s) or Problem(s) Studied
13. Intervention(s)
14. Key Inclusion and Exclusion Criteria
15. Study Type
16. Date of First Enrollment
17. Sample Size
18. Recruitment Status
19. Primary Outcome(s)
20. Key Secondary Outcomes
21. Ethics Review
22. Completion Date
23. Summary Results
24. Individual Clinical Trial Participant-Level Data Sharing Statement

[a] http://www.who.int/ictrp/network/trds/en/

included in publications from the trial. Table 2.2 describes the 24 elements of the Trial Registration Data Set [17]. Many individual countries have registries that partner with the ICTRP.

In the United States, clinical trials are registered with ClinicalTrials.Gov [18] administered by the US National Library of Medicine, part of the National Institutes of Health. Section 801 of the Food and Drug Administration Amendments Act of 2007, known at FDAAA 801, requires registration of clinical trials and their results where the studies involve medical devices, drug, and biologics. Data element definitions, templates, and checklists are available on the clinicaltrials.gov website. The required data is similar to that of ICTRP.

Registries do not charge a fee and are searchable electronically.

2.1.11 Staff Training and Certification Including Calibration and Fidelity

A critical part of trial planning and execution is formal staff training [19]. This is true whether the objectives of a trial involve testing a medical device or drug or a behavioral intervention. The protocol will outline the training objectives and general approach to training. The Manual of Procedures will contain the specific instruction that is carried out. During the recruitment phase, research staff members may be screening participants and obtaining informed consent. Often investigators prepare scripts for staff members to learn and follow. These scripts become part of the official trial record. They are designed to be sure that informed consent procedures approved by the IRB are adhered to. This is particularly important in behavioral trials where staff members may influence the outcome of the trial by what they say.

In large or complex trials, the PI may ask staff members to complete an examination regarding study procedures including documentation and data entry requirements. Others, particularly in behavioral studies, will have staff members practice procedures under supervision and use checklists to evaluate and guide the correction of behaviors. These activities result in formal certification that the staff members are prepared to carry out the study, strictly following the protocol. Longer studies include periodic retraining.

In clinical trials where the outcome to be measured is a clinical oral health measure such as the Periodontal Index, the International Caries Detection and Assessment System (ICDAS) or reading the results of a dental radiograph, training, calibration and assessment of examiner agreement or reliability is required. The training usually includes required reading and memorization of codes, practice with a skilled examiner, and then a calibration exercise in which the results of examinations are compared with a gold standard examiner. The exercise needs to include sufficient numbers of participants that are typical of the population to be recruited. Ten to 20 participants are needed. In this exercise, both the trainee examiner and the gold standard examiner assess the same participants. The study biostatistician will then calculate measures of examiner agreement. This may be an Interclass Correlation Coefficient (ICC) when the measure is continuous or Cohen's or Fleiss' kappa when the measure is ordinal or nominal. The method chosen may also depend on the number of examiners. The large statistical packages used in science today include programs for assessing agreement. Most studies have initial training immediately before baseline data collection and then have refresher training and calibration before follow-up. Reports of clinical trials are required to include the results of the examiner agreement.

If recorders are to write down scores vocalized by examiners, the recorders should be trained and should be used in the calibration exercise as they would be used in the actual trial data collection. Examiners should review the written results to be sure the recorder is collecting the data accurately. Studies where data are entered onto a tablet computer or similar electronic device also require training and testing. These devices are often programmed so that out of range or inappropriate codes cannot be entered.

2.1.12 Flow Chart

It is helpful in planning a trial and conveying to potential funders or regulatory reviewers how the trial will be carried out to construct a flow chart. Figure 2.3 is an example of a participant flow chart. The flow chart schematically shows the visits a participant will make and the procedures, treatments, or assessments to be carried out. The IRB may use the information in the flow chart to assess participant burden and determine whether it is reasonable and justified. Similarly, the flow chart is helpful in assessing staffing needs and planning the budget. Flaws in a protocol can oftentimes be recognized after reviewing a flow chart. Templates for constructing flow charts are widely available.

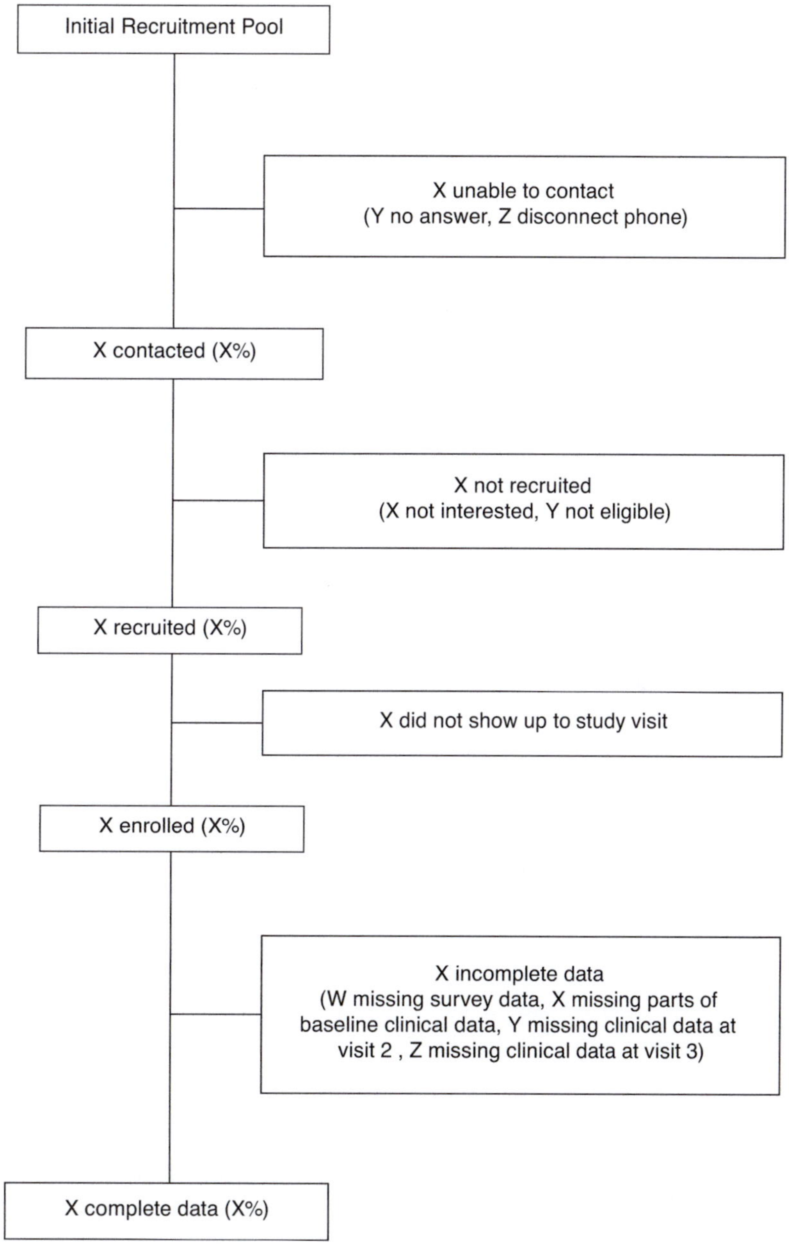

Fig. 2.3 Sample trial flow chart

2.2 Trial Design Including Allocation Ratio

Many trial designs are possible and the choice of a design depends on the study objective and hypothesis. A typical example of the statement of a design might be "This is a single center randomized, double-blind, placebo-controlled, parallel-group trial." A common element in studies of dental caries in children is a cluster-randomized design. In this case, children are clustered in schools and the schools become the unit of randomization. A design such as this might be chosen to avoid carryover effects or because it is more efficient to do only one treatment at a given school. Cluster randomization may be less efficient than simple randomization because the analysis has to take into consideration within cluster correlation.

The statement of the design should also include the allocation ratio of participants between the active treatment and the placebo. Most often the allocation ratio is 1:1 because it is statistically most efficient. It requires the fewest participants to power the trial. Unequal allocation may be used in an initial safety evaluation of a drug or device to maximize knowledge gained about adverse effects. Investigators may choose unequal allocation because they perceive that more participants will join a trial if they have a good chance of getting the active treatment. There is little evidence that this helps recruitment and can result in bias. If there is genuine uncertainty about what treatment is better, called equipoise, then there is no good scientific or ethical reason to have unequal allocation. To obtain the same power, a trial with unequal allocation requires 12% more participants if the ratio is 2:1 and 33% more participants if the ratio is 3:1. Reports of trials must include a statement of why unequal allocation was chosen. Regulators are likely to require justification for trials with unequal allocation ratios.

2.3 Participants

2.3.1 Eligibility

The protocol for any trial includes a formal statement of participant eligibility. This may include age, sex, language spoken or read, level of education, health status, dental condition, or other similar information. The protocol will specify exactly how each element is to be measured, how it is collected (for example, in person or over the phone), and who will collect it.

2.3.2 Exclusion Criteria

Similarly, the protocol will specify who and why a potential participant is to be excluded. This might be because someone is participating in another study currently, because they might move and be unavailable for follow-up, because they are allergic to a study medicine, or because they have a medical or dental condition that complicates their participation such as when individuals are receiving chronic antibiotic treatment that would complicate interpretation of effects from dental caries or periodontal disease treatments.

Effective trialists record the number of contacts with potential participants and the number and rate of inclusions and exclusions.

2.3.3 Settings and Locations Where Data Are to Be Collected

The trial protocol should specify the settings and locations where data are to be collected. When working with clinics, schools, or in other similar settings—particularly those away from the investigator's home institution, funders, and the IRB typically expect to see a formal letter indicating that those who control access to the site have reviewed the purposes of the study and have given permission for their site to be included. Potential investigators need to plan ahead of time for obtaining such letters as each individual site will have its own procedures for giving consent. In a clinic system, this might be reviewed and approved by a research committee. In a school system, teachers, principals, and the school's legal counsel might weigh in. In other settings, approval by a community advisory committee may be required.

2.4 Recruitment Including Dates

2.4.1 Planning for Accrual Problems

Inadequate and slow accrual or enrollment of participants is the primary reason that trials fail. Falling short may mean that a trial is underpowered. A DSMB or funder may halt a trial if accrual is inadequate. Planning for a trial often includes pilot work to provide evidence that the recruitment procedures and schedule are workable. For example, if a trial is to be carried out in a school and consent forms are sent home with the students, what rate of return of signed consent forms is anticipated? Will it be adequate? Is there a sufficient number of individuals that meet the recruitment inclusion criteria? Slow accrual is a budget buster. A back-up plan is always needed. Are there additional sites available? Will an advertising program help?

Trialists always record the beginning and end dates of recruitment. They often plot accrual rates and have regular meetings with research staff to review the progress of recruitment. If recruitment is problematic, they initiate backup plans before it is too late and they run out of funds, time, or review groups or the sponsor cancels the study.

2.5 Preventing Attrition, Documenting Attrition

Loss to follow-up, also called drop-out or attrition, is another leading cause of trial failure. Sample sizes are usually inflated to anticipate a certain rate of loss to follow-up. This may because, for example, older adults die before being able to complete a study or because children change schools and cannot be found. Annual rates of attrition in US studies can exceed 10% or 15%. See, for example, a Cochrane review of clinical studies comparing the effectiveness of Atraumatic Restorative Treatment versus conventional restorative treatment where multiple studies found to have loss to follow-up of 20% or more [20]. Because studies are powered to detect a treatment effect, loss to follow-up can result in an underpowered study where it is not possible to reach definitive conclusions about the efficacy or effectiveness of the study drug, device, or intervention. Note, the standard for trial analysis is "intention to treat." This means that data for each subject enrolled are included in the analysis, even if the participant dropped out. It is generally not permissible to report out trials where only data on those who finished a trial are included in the analysis as this result will be biased.

In reporting a trial, researchers need to document drop-outs or lost participants including when and why attrition occurred. Flow chart templates are available as part of the CONSORT Statement [21]. Many scientific journals expect that such a flow chart is submitted as part of the report of a trial. Similarly, the IRB, DSMB, and regulators will want to see this documentation.

2.6 Interventions

How and when administered
Details that can be replicated

Trial protocols specify the detailed nature of the treatment arms, whether they are devices, drugs, behavioral interventions, or placebos. They are described in sufficient detail so that the treatment could be replicated. The protocol will specify how and when the treatments are to be administered and who will carry them out.

2.7 Outcomes

The trial outcomes are clearly specified a priori. That means the investigator has a hypothesis and that the study has been powered to detect the effect that this outcome represents. The time point at which the outcomes are measured is also specified a priori. This is especially important in blinded clinical trials because choosing the outcome after one sees the results can result in bias. Sometimes this is called the trial endpoint.

2.7.1 Primary

The primary outcome is collected to test the main hypothesis of the clinical trial. Examples of primary outcomes in caries studies might be the ICDAS category, the number of newly decayed teeth, or periodontal attachment or pocket depth. It also could be the presence or absence of an intraoral lesion or pain. It is possible to have more than one primary outcome but not a long list. Some studies have both a clinical outcome and a patient-centered or patient-reported outcome. Examples of patient-centered measures are pain reports, satisfaction, and quality of life.

2.7.2 Secondary

Studies sometimes have secondary measures. Often the study is not powered strongly to detect changes in the secondary measures but they be helpful in understanding the main trial outcome or may allow for exploratory hypothesis testing that will be followed up in future studies.

2.8 Advanced Data Collection

2.8.1 What Is Important to Collect and Why, Generalizability, and Mechanisms of Action

For trials designed to detect changes in disease prevalence or health behaviors, it makes sense to collect such data at baseline and again at the end of the intervention. This allows investigators to test the main research hypothesis—does the new medication prevent tooth decay or did the behavioral intervention help to improve the frequency of toothbrushing? However, there are opportunities to collect data at other time points to answer questions related to the main hypothesis. For instance, trials may require multiple years of participation and follow up, which could turn away some potential participants. In these instances, there is value in collecting pre-baseline data before a team recruits for the intervention (e.g., tooth decay). After recruitment is complete, having pre-baseline data would allow the team to assess the degree of selection bias, interpret the main study findings, and determine generalizability.

Additional data can also be collected at other time points. If there is interest in identifying possible mechanisms driving an intervention, then interim data collection could be collected to measure these potential mechanisms (also called mediators) [22]. For instance, self-efficacy may be the hypothesized mechanism of a behavioral intervention [23]. Measuring self-efficacy at baseline and several time points during the intervention would result in longitudinal data to help test this mechanism hypothesis. When an intervention ends, there is the possibility of collecting data from participants to understand what went well and what parts of the intervention could be improved. Having these post-intervention data on hand could help the research team refine interventions for future testing.

Data collection plans require careful a priori attention to the conceptual model of the intervention as well as an understanding the effects of collecting additional data, like higher rates of participant dropout because of increased burden, extra staff time to collect the data, and costs of processing the data in the lab.

2.9 Sample Size

In planning a trial, investigators estimate the sample size needed to determine the difference between treatment arms. Trials may be superiority trials (e.g., the test drug is more effective than the comparison drug or a placebo) or equivalence trials (there is no difference between the arms). In superiority trials, the biostatistician uses pilot data or work from published studies to calculate the power, that is, the probability that a test of significance will pick detect a treatment effect that is present, that is, the probability of rejecting the null hypothesis. Power ranges from 0 to 1 and most clinical trials have sample sizes for testing the primary hypothesis with a power of at least 80%. Obviously, the better and more relevant the pilot data or data from other studies, the more likely the study will be large enough to find the treatment effect. Power calculations are specific to the type of analysis that is planned. Many studies are underpowered for assessing secondary outcomes. Power is reduced when there are interim analyses, such as when the primary outcome is at 2 years but the investigator also assesses the measure at 1 year.

Studies may have built-in stopping rules. Typically, this happens when the biostatistician finds that a treatment is particularly effective in an interim analysis and the DSMB finds that ethically the treatment should be available to all the participants. However, stopping a study early tends to over-estimate the effectiveness of the treatment being evaluated.

2.10 Randomization

2.10.1 Method

For most trials, simple randomization is sufficient. The study biostatistician can use any number of statistical programs to develop the randomization scheme. As discussed earlier in this chapter, the participant should have a known, usually equal, chance of being assigned to any of the treatment arms. Successful randomization requires that treatment assignments cannot be predicted in advance.

In practical terms, the biostatistician places the coded treatment choices in sequentially numbered closed envelopes, which are opened by the treating clinician only at the time of treatment. Or, in a study of school children, all of the children's ID numbers are assembled in a file and are assigned randomly to the treatment arm. Then, class lists are prepared with child's ID and treatment code. The children may be given color-coded cards or slips of paper that identify which treatment they are assigned to.

2.10.2 Type (e.g., Blocking, Stratification)

It is common that randomization is done in blocks. For example, a study conducted in schools may have assignments done separately for each school. The idea behind this is to make sure that bias is not inadvertently introduced into the study by having extremely unbalanced arms. Another example is where participants are first stratified by baseline dental caries score and then assigned to treatments within the strata.

2.10.3 Allocation Concealment (How Random Allocation Is Implemented)

In random assignment, allocation concealment prevents investigators from choosing treatment allocations for particular participants. Imagine, for example, a clinical trial being conducted in doctor's offices. A participant who is enrolled in the trial may want to receive the new treatment. This kind of assignment would create bias and decrease the validity of the trial results and must be avoided. Allocation concealment involves not disclosing to participants and those involved in recruiting trial participants the allocation sequence before random allocation occurs.

2.10.4 Implementation (Who Will Generate the Random Allocation, Who Will Enroll, Who Will Assign Condition)

The trial protocol will specify exactly how the assignment of participants to conditions will be carried out. That includes, as we discussed earlier, the generation of random allocation, as well as who will enroll participants and who will actually implement the assignment.

2.11 Blinding

Blinding is the practice of not telling participants in a clinical trial whether they are receiving a placebo or comparison treatment. In an experiment, if the subjects in the control group know that they are receiving a placebo, the placebo effect will be reduced or eliminated and the placebo will not serve its intended purpose. Similarly, examiners and others working directly with participants or evaluating outcomes are kept blind. A double-blinded design means that neither the participant nor the investigative team are aware of whether the treatment received or being administered is the test device or agent or a placebo. In a pharmaceutical study with two treatment arms, the treatments might be labeled A and B. The definition of the codes is kept in a secure place by someone not involved in working with participants. Often the biostatistician is the keeper of the code. And, codes are typically not broken or treatments revealed until after the data are analyzed.

Behavioral studies may not allow blinding of participants or staff members administering the interventions. In this case, examiners are not informed of the assignments and collect outcome data in a blind fashion. As with drug or device studies, data may be analyzed before the codes are opened.

2.12 Statistical Methods

The biostatistician is a critical member of the investigative team. This individual participates in the design of the study and writing of the protocol as well as in the analyses of the data. Experienced investigators know that bringing in the statistician after a study is poorly designed is a big mistake. Generally, sponsors or funders expect that the team will include a biostatistician and country regulators, such as the FDA, are unlikely to accept studies done without such a person on the investigative team.

We advise new investigators to create mock data sets and attempt the planned analyses before any participant is enrolled or any data are collected. This allows the novice investigator to carefully assess whether the planned analysis approach will yield the intended test of the hypothesis.

2.12.1 Intention to Treat Versus Per Protocol

Primary tests of hypotheses in clinical trials follow the "intention to treat" principle. This means that every participant who is enrolled and for whom there are some data is included. Drop-outs and participants lost to follow-up are included. Reputable scientific journals will not publish the results of trials that do not follow this principle. In contrast, one can find many older studies—especially commercially sponsored studies—where the data were analyzed "per protocol." This means that only the data from subjects with complete records are included in the analysis of results. This biases upwardly the effects of the study agent. Sometimes, per protocol analyses are conducted secondarily to explore possible treatment effects when studies are underpowered.

It is beyond the scope of this chapter to address in detail the statistical approaches to analyzing clinical trial data. Nevertheless, clinical trials ask relatively straightforward questions and the first test of a hypothesis should be simple and unadjusted. The biostatistician will check the impact of randomization on the balance of the levels of moderators that might impact the strength of the effect of the treatment. Examples of moderators are age and sex. Within a caries study in children, for example, age may impact the number of teeth at risk or the length of time the teeth have been in the mouth and at risk. The randomization process aims to balance these factors within the groups. Randomization in caries studies is often stratified by the number of carious lesions at baseline to avoid imbalance. Additional analyses may adjust for such factors. Also, regression models have been developed that account for the often skewed distribution of dental caries where many teeth or people have none or very low numbers of lesions. Models that include effect modifiers are useful secondary analyses to generate hypotheses for future research.

2.13 Data Security

It is the responsibility of the PI to maintain the security of clinical trial data. The security of personally identifiable data in the United States is governed by the Health Insurance Portability and Accountability Act of 1996 (HIPAA). IRBs review plans for data security. Data forms and computer files contain identification numbers instead of participant names and the list of names and codes is stored separately. Paper forms are in locked cabinets and rooms accessible only to authorized investigators. Computer files are password protected. Studies regulated under the US FDA and many other government organizations must use data management systems. The standards are contained in Chapter 21 CFR Part 11 of the Code of Federal Regulations. FDA employs auditors who review the trial documentation to determine at the project level if a study is compliant. Data security and confidentiality are included in the training required of investigators and research staff members.

2.14 Harms

Study drugs or other interventions have the potential to cause harm. These unexpected outcomes are called Adverse Effects (AE) in formal parlance. AEs are different than known side effects. Table 2.3 describes the typical AEs that are collected in sophisticated clinical trials. Most AEs are unrelated to the study but are nonetheless captured in a consistent way. For submission of trials to country regulators such as the FDA, 24–48 h in-person post-treatment checks for all participants are desired. In other studies, participants may be sampled or follow-up may be done

Table 2.3 Examples of adverse effects within clinical trials[a]

Adverse event	Mild	Moderate	Severe
Oral mucositis by exam (e.g., erythema, ulceration)	Asymptomatic or mild symptoms; intervention not indicated	Moderate pain; not interfering with oral intake; modified diet indicated	Severe pain; interfering with oral intake
Allergic reaction (e.g., difficulty swallowing or breathing, swelling around the lips or skin of the face, itchiness around the lips or skin of the face, hives, or rash)	Transient flushing or rash, drug fever <38 °C (<100.4 °F); intervention not indicated	Intervention or infusion interruption indicated; responds promptly to symptomatic treatment (e.g., antihistamines, NSAIDS, narcotics); prophylactic medications indicated for ≤24 h	Prolonged (e.g., not rapidly responsive to symptomatic medication and/or brief interruption of infusion); recurrence of symptoms following initial improvement; hospitalization indicated for clinical sequelae (e.g., renal impairment, pulmonary infiltrates) Life-threatening consequences; urgent intervention indicated or death
Anaphylaxis	–	–	Symptomatic bronchospasm, with or without urticarial; parenteral intervention indicated; allergy-related edema/angioedema; hypotension Life-threatening consequences; urgent intervention indicated or death
Vomiting	1–2 episodes (separated by 5 min) in 24 h	3–5 episodes (separated by 5 min) in 24 h	≥6 episodes (separated by 5 min) in 24 h; hospitalization
Gastrointestinal pain (e.g., stomachache)	Mild pain	Moderate pain; limiting instrumental ADL	Severe pain; limiting self-care ADL
Diarrhea	Increase of <4 stools per day over baseline	Increase of 4–6 stools per day over baseline	Increase of ≥7 stools per day over baseline; incontinence; hospitalization
Nausea	Loss of appetite without alteration in eating habits	Oral intake decreased without significant weight loss, dehydration, or malnutrition	Inadequate oral caloric or fluid intake; tube feeding, TPN, or hospitalization

[a] Adapted from Advantage Protocol 2019-10-19 Phase 2 Efficacy & Safety Evaluation of Advantage Anti-Caries Varnish for Primary Prevention with permission. Sponsor Contact: Peter Milgrom, DDS

by telephone. Investigators are asked to assess the degree to which an AE is related to the study device or drug. Major trials have a medical monitor who reviews AE reports. The FDA and many other country regulators have strict requirements for reporting severe AEs in a timely way. Mild or moderate AEs are normally reported in annual reports to the regulator.

AEs are reported by organ systems and are internationally standardized. Coding is done by the investigator using the Medical Dictionary for Regulatory Activities (MedDRA) based on the AE reports after they have been reviewed by the study Medical Monitor [24]. Training is available on the MedDRA website and through courses and webinars offered to investigators and study staff. MedDRA are both downloadable and available online. MedDRA is under the direction of the International Council for Harmonisation of Technical Requirements for Pharmaceuticals for Human Use (ICH). MedDRA is available upon subscription. The summary report of AEs should be included in the Harms section of published reports of all trials.

2.15 Limitations

As with the analysis, we often advise new investigators to write the limitations section of their report before the study is initiated. A study planner who is aware of the limitations of the approach chosen may elect to modify or enhance the design or at a minimum recognize what he or she will able to conclude from the study. The limitations include issues of reliability of measurement and limitations to internal or external validity.

2.16 Generalizability

2.16.1 External Validity and Applicability

External validity is the appropriateness of applying the conclusions of a clinical trial outside or beyond the context of that study. In other words, applicability is the extent to which the results of the study can be generalized to and across other situations, people, and times. A big issue in drug research is the need to study treatments for children in children and not just adults. The FDA, for example, requires investigators to develop a Pediatric Study Plan providing assurance that children are included in the study population. A historical example is where gingivitis studies were conducted were conducted in male participants only, because investigators felt that effects of menstruation would interfere with the measurement of gingival inflammation. Results of studies not conducted on women may not be valid for women. These validity issues extend to race or to socioeconomic status as well.

2.17 Publishing the Protocol of a Trial

Journal choices
Peer review

Today many investigators publish the peer-reviewed protocols for trials. Journals have evolved that publish the protocols. Examples are Contemporary Clinical Trials, Trials, BMJ Open, and others. These papers go further than the relatively simple listings in the clinical trials registries. If the protocols have been formally peer reviewed, they often are not sent out for review again but instead published as written. This can provide a publication for younger investigators involved in trials who may have to wait several years before being able to have anything in the literature and whose advancement in academic settings might be impacted. Protocols that have not had formal peer review by a funder can still be published. In this case, the journals will follow their normal peer review process.

2.18 Publishing Results of a Trial

CONSORT statement
Journal choices
Conflict of interest

The publication of clinical trials has largely been standardized internationally by the publication of the Consolidated Standards for Reporting Trials (CONSORT) [21]. The comprehensive CONSORT site provides guidance on the elements required for a trial publication, extensions for different designs, and useful templates and checklists. The CONSORT Statement is endorsed by leading scholarly journals in dentistry and medicine. One should not submit a clinical trial report to a journal that does not endorse the CONSORT Statement.

A special concern in clinical trials of devices and drugs is conflict of interest. One has only to turn to the major newspapers to find reports of published research that may have been biased by investigators who have received, but not publicly acknowledged, payments or other rewards for their participation in research. Such investigators may hold patents or other valuable intellectual property. The peer review process is intended to secure the scientific integrity of the trial and report. Public disclosure of potential conflicts of interest are intended to clarify the role of conflicted individuals in the collection, analysis, or interpretation of trial findings. This does not bar individuals from participating in the publication of the research.

2.19 Case Scenario Exercise

2.19.1 Case Scenario

You are the Dental Director a large community health center that serves low-income populations. Over 90% of the adults in your clinic are enrolled in Medicaid. Most of these adults come in for regular check-ups every 6 months. However, many of the adults present with recurrent tooth decay at these check-ups. You and your staff have identified poor diet, particularly too much added sugar intake, as the source of the problem.

Questions

1. What are potential intervention strategies?
2. What is the importance of an advisory group? How would you assemble an advisory group?
3. What is your selected intervention and what is the main outcome?
4. How will you fund your intervention?
5. What are the steps involved in obtaining IRB approval for your intervention?
6. What type of special training will be needed for your study staff?
7. What are the inclusion and exclusion criteria for your intervention?
8. What is your participant recruitment plan?
9. How will you prevent attrition during your study?
10. What are potential harms of your intervention and how will you monitor for these during the intervention?
11. Complete the CONSORT Statement for your study.

Answers

1. What are potential intervention strategies?
   - Chairside motivational interviewing intervention to improve diet
   - Home-based intervention to improve meal quality
   - App-based intervention to monitor and reduce added sugar intake
2. What is the importance of an advisory group? How would you assemble an advisory group?
   - See Sect. 2.1.3
3. What is your selected intervention and what is the main outcome?
   - Respond depends
4. How will you fund your intervention?
   - See Sect. 2.1.6
5. What are the steps involved in obtaining IRB approval for your intervention?
   - See Sect. 2.1.8
6. What type of training will be needed for your study staff?
   - See Sect. 2.1.11
7. What are the inclusion and exclusion criteria for your intervention?
   - See Sect. 2.3

8. What is your participant recruitment plan?
   - Chart review and direct contact
   - Fliers placed in waiting room
   - Recruitment in waiting room
9. How will you prevent attrition during your study?
   - Provide incentives for participation
   - Collect information on alternative ways to contact participant (e.g., phone, e-mail, text, contact for family member or friend)
   - Create social media page with study updates to keep participants engaged
   - Keep study obligations for participants simple
10. What are potential harms of your intervention and how will you monitor for these during the intervention?
   - See Sect. 2.14
11. Complete the CONSORT Statement for your study.
   - See Sect. 2.18

References

1. Gartlehner G, Hansen RA, Nissman D, et al. Criteria for distinguishing effectiveness from efficacy trials in systematic reviews. Rockville, MD: Agency for Healthcare Research and Quality (US); 2006. http://www.ncbi.nlm.nih.gov/books/NBK44024/. Accessed 7 Sept 2020.
2. Singh S, Loke YK. Drug safety assessment in clinical trials: methodological challenges and opportunities. Trials. 2012;13:138. https://doi.org/10.1186/1745-6215-13-138.
3. Schmidt B. Proof of principle studies. Epilepsy Res. 2006;68(1):48–52. https://doi.org/10.1016/j.eplepsyres.2005.09.019.
4. Milgrom P, Tut O, Rothen M, et al. Efficacy evaluation of an anticaries varnish: protocol for a phase II randomized controlled trial. BMJ Open. 2017;7:e017866. https://doi.org/10.1136/bmjopen-2017-017866.
5. Zucker D. Developing your career in an age of team science. J Investig Med. 2012;60(5):779–84. https://doi.org/10.2310/JIM.0b013e3182508317.
6. Tebes JK, Thai ND. Interdisciplinary team science and the public: steps toward a participatory team science. Am Psychol. 2018;73(4):549–62. https://doi.org/10.1037/amp0000281.
7. Orticio LP. Protecting human subjects in research. Insight. 2009;34(3):14–6.
8. Agency for Healthcare Research and Quality (AHRQ). Step 2: form an advisory group. 2011. http://www.ahrq.gov/cahps/surveys-guidance/helpful-resources/planning/Form-an-Advisory-Group.html. Accessed 7 Sept 2020.
9. Chi DL, Hopkins S, O'Brien D, Mancl L, Orr E, Lenaker D. Association between added sugar intake and dental caries in Yup'ik children using a novel hair biomarker. BMC Oral Health. 2015;15(1):121. https://doi.org/10.1186/s12903-015-0101-z.
10. Chi DL, Tut O, Milgrom P. Cluster-randomized xylitol toothpaste trial for early childhood caries prevention. J Dent Child (Chic). 2014;81(1):27–32.
11. Toerioen M, Brookes ST, Metcalfe C, et al. A review of reporting of participant recruitment and retention in RCTS in six major journals. Trials. 2009;10:52. https://doi.org/10.1186/1745-6215-10-52.
12. Roseman M, Milette K, Bero LA, et al. Reporting of conflicts of interest in meta-analyses of trials of pharmacological treatments. JAMA. 2011;305(10):1008–17. https://doi.org/10.1001/jama.2011.257.
13. Food and Drug Administration (FDA). Institutional review boards (IRBs) and protection of human subjects in clinical trials. 2019. http://www.fda.gov/about-fda/center-drug-evaluation-and-research-cder/institutional-review-boards-irbs-and-protection-human-subjects-clinical-trials. Accessed 7 Sept 2020.
14. National Institute of Dental and Craniofacial Research (NIDCR). Data and safety monitoring board (DSMB) guidelines. 2018. http://www.nidcr.nih.gov/research/human-subjects-research/toolkit-and-education-materials/interventional-studies/data-and-safety-monitoring-board-guidelines. Accessed 7 Sept 2020.
15. Huić M, Marušić M, Marušić A. Completeness and changes in registered data and reporting bias of randomized controlled trials in ICMJE journals after trial registration policy. PLoS One. 2011;6(9):e25258. https://doi.org/10.1371/journal.pone.0025258.
16. World Health Organization (WHO). Welcome to WHO ICTRP. International Clinical Trials Registry Platform (ICTRP). http://www.who.int/ictrp/en/. Accessed 7 Sept 2020.
17. World Health Organization (WHO). WHO data set. International Clinical Trials Registry Platform (ICTRP). http://www.who.int/ictrp/network/trds/en/. Accessed 7 Sept 2020.
18. ClinicalTrials.Gov. U.S. National Library of Medicine. http://clinicaltrials.gov. Accessed 7 Sept 2020.
19. National Institute of Dental and Craniofacial Research (NIDCR). Interventional studies—planning & startup. 2020. http://www.nidcr.nih.gov/research/human-subjects-research//toolkit-and-education-

materials/interventional-studies/planning-and-start-up. Accessed 7 Sept 2020.
20. Dorri M, Martinez-Zapata MJ, Walsh T, Marinho VC, Sheiham A (Deceased), Zaror C. Atraumatic restorative treatment versus conventional restorative treatment for managing dental caries. Cochrane Database Syst Rev. 2017;12:CD008072. https://doi.org/10.1002/14651858.CD008072.pub2.
21. Consolidated Standards of Reporting Trials (CONSORT). 2010. http://www.consort-statement.org/. Accessed 7 Sept 2020.
22. Liu J, Ulrich C. Mediation analysis in nursing research: a methodological review. Contemp Nurse. 2016;52(6):643–56. https://doi.org/10.1080/10376178.2015.1041999.
23. Gholami M, Knoll N, Schwarzer R. A brief self-regulatory intervention increases dental flossing in adolescent girls. Int J Behav Med. 2015;22(5):645–51. https://doi.org/10.1007/s12529-014-9459-6.
24. Medical Dictionary for Regulatory Activities (MedDRA). http://www.meddra.org/. Accessed 7 Sept 2020.

Part II

Randomized Controlled Trials in Dental Specialties

3 Randomized Controlled Trials in Dental Public Health

Paulo Nadanovsky, Ana Paula Pires dos Santos, and Richie Kohli

3.1 Introduction

Public health is a broad field that encompasses four dimensions: the health of a whole society; the specific policies, services, programs, and efforts to protect, promote, and restore people's health and its determinants; the institutions—either public or private—that aim to plan, develop, fund, and implement such efforts; and the scientific disciplines and professions [1]. More specifically, dental public health (DPH) may be defined as "the science and art of preventing and controlling dental diseases and promoting dental health through organized community efforts. It is that form of dental practice which serves the community as a patient rather than the individual. It is concerned with the dental health education of the public, with applied dental research, and with the administration of group dental care programs as well as the prevention and control of dental diseases on a community basis" [2]. However, it should be noted that the view that DPH is concerned with the oral health of the community while the clinical dental disciplines and personal dental care are concerned with the oral health of the individual may not be helpful as it implies, wrongly, that the public health approach has little to contribute to the care of the individual patient.

The experimental (or interventional) epidemiological study, preferably the randomized controlled trial (RCT), is the design better suited to answer DPH questions; the experimental study includes clinical trials (with patients), field trials (with healthy people), and community intervention trials (with the intervention assigned to groups of healthy people).

A clinical trial is an experiment designed to test the hypothesis that an intervention (a drug, a procedure, or a technique) favorably alters the natural history of a disease or condition. At least two groups are included: the test (experiment or intervention) group, which is compared to a control group. The control group represents the natural history of the disease in a group similar to the

P. Nadanovsky (✉)
Department of Epidemiology, National School of Public Health, Oswaldo Cruz Foundation (Fiocruz), Rio de Janeiro, Brazil

Department of Epidemiology, Institute of Social Medicine, Rio de Janeiro State University, Rio de Janeiro, Brazil
e-mail: paulo.nadanovsky@fiocruz.br; nadanovsky@ims.uerj.br

A. P. P. dos Santos
Department of Community and Preventive Dentistry, School of Dentistry, Rio de Janeiro State University, Rio de Janeiro, Brazil

R. Kohli
Division of Dental Public Health, School of Dentistry, Oregon Health & Science University, Portland, OR, USA
e-mail: kohli@ohsu.edu

R. Kohli et al. (eds.), *Randomized Controlled Trials in Evidence-Based Dentistry*,
https://doi.org/10.1007/978-3-031-47651-8_3

Table 3.1 Types of experimental (or interventional) epidemiological studies

Types of experimental epidemiological studies	Study population	Recruitment of participants	Intervention
Clinical trials (including cluster randomized trials)	Patients	Patients in health services	A drug; a procedure; a technique (individual intervention)
Field trials (including cluster randomized trials)	Healthy people	People in households, workplaces or schools	Fluoridated toothpaste; dental sealants (individual intervention)
Community intervention trials	Groups of healthy people	Schools in neighborhoods; neighborhoods in regions; cities in countries; countries	Fluoridated water; legislation limiting sugar promotion; a new school curriculum (intervention on a community-wide basis)

test group.[1] Many aspects should be considered in order to ensure the validity of the results from this study design, such as randomization, allocation concealment, baseline comparability, blinding, missing data, and outcome selective reporting.

In the field trials, the recruitment of participants generally takes place at the participant's residence, workplaces, or schools; and not at the health service location. They are typically recruited to evaluate the effectiveness of preventive interventions of either common or serious diseases. Oral diseases are common and, therefore, suitable for field trials. It is difficult to develop an efficient field trial when the incidence of the disease is low. In this case, it is necessary to enroll a large number of participants or high-risk groups to gain efficiency. Field trials in which the treatment is randomly assigned to groups of participants are known as cluster randomized trials. An important aspect to be highlighted is that in studies in which the allocation is at the group (cluster) level, the unit of analysis can be the group or the individual. Analysis at the individual level is more desirable because it reduces the loss of information, but requires that the cluster effect be taken into account. This effect can be quantified by calculating the intra-class correlation coefficient (ICC), defined as the proportion of the total variance (i.e., the variance between individuals plus the variance between the groups) that can be attributed to the variation between groups.

The community intervention trial is an extension of the field trial that applies an intervention on a community-wide basis. For example, fluoride in the toothpaste and dental sealants are administered through individual tubes and professional-patient dyads encounters, respectively; thus, these measures can be applied to one specific individual while refrained from another individual within the same group. On the other hand, fluoride in the water and legislation limiting sugar promotion are administered through the water supplies and promulgation/implementation of laws, respectively; these measures cannot be applied to one individual and not to another in the same community. They can only be applied to the whole community, and so they could not be studied in a conventional field trial, only in a community intervention trial (see Table 3.1).

Some oral health and dentistry themes are central for the practice of DPH and were the focus of major experimental studies. These included clinical, field, and community intervention trials. We selected some of them in order to illustrate the importance of the experimental studies for the practice of DPH as discussed below. Table 3.2 summarizes these important themes that were (or should be) the focus of experimental epidemiological studies in DPH.

[1]Alternatively, the control group may represent not the natural history of the disease, but the history of the disease in a similar group who is receiving another intervention, usually the standard intervention (standard care).

Table 3.2 Important themes that are central for the practice of Dental Public Health and were (or should be) the focus of experimental epidemiological studies

Theme	Effect of intervention or exposure	Study type	Evidence	Comment
Water fluoridation	Reduces caries	Community intervention trials	Strongly in favor of the intervention	In the presence of widespread use of fluoride toothpaste, the additional benefit of water fluoridation has not been clearly established
Fluoride toothpaste	Reduces caries	Mainly field trials, but also community intervention trials of toothpaste distribution	Strongly in favor of the intervention	The use of standard fluoride toothpaste is the default; to recommend any other form of fluoride delivery, in addition to toothpaste, one should demonstrate that this will bring clinically relevant additional benefit that is more cost-effective than fluoride toothpaste alone. To date, this has not been demonstrated
Sugar	Increases caries	Field trials	Strongly against the exposure	Different strategies can be tested in order to assess the effects of sugar restricting measures on caries. One of these strategies is taxing sugar; no RCTs have been performed reporting on dental caries, only model-based studies. Individual level RCTs to test measures to reduce sugar consumption should be generally discouraged. RCTs assessing the effects of nudge on sugar reduction are welcome
Pit and fissure sealants	Reduces caries	Clinical trials	Strongly in favor of the intervention	Cost-effectiveness studies are needed. There seems to be no evidence of the effectiveness of sealants in adults, and insufficient evidence on primary dentition and on the comparison between different materials
The 6-monthly dental check-up	Does not benefit oral health	Clinical trials	Against the intervention	RCTs to assess the benefits and harms of dental check-up are needed; primary outcomes should include tooth loss, dental pain and cavities
Professionally applied fluoride	Reduces caries Arrests cavitated dentin caries	Clinical and field (including cluster) trials	Arguably in favor of the intervention	More RCTs are needed in order to find out whether fluoride gel/foam adds any benefit for people already using fluoride toothpaste. Cost-effectiveness analyses are needed on varnish
Fluoride mouth rinse	Reduces caries	Clinical and field (including cluster) trials	Arguably in favor of the intervention	More RCTs are needed in order to find out whether fluoride rinse adds any benefit for people already using fluoride toothpaste
Supervised toothbrushing	Reduces caries	Field trials	Arguably in favor of the intervention	Whether toothbrushing supervision increases the anticaries effect of fluoride toothpastes is still an open question

(continued)

Table 3.2 (continued)

Theme	Effect of intervention or exposure	Study type	Evidence	Comment
Dental fillings for the treatment of caries in the primary dentition	Does not benefit oral health	Clinical trial	Strongly against the intervention	Despite the existence of a methodologically sound, pragmatic, large trial in the UK, similar RCTs should be replicated in other countries
Screening and interventions to prevent dental caries in children younger than age 5 years	Reduces caries	Clinical and field (including cluster) trials	Varies by the type of intervention	RCTs needed on the accuracy of oral health examination and caries risk assessment by primary care clinicians, primary care referral for dental care, and effective parental and caregiver/ guardian educational and counseling interventions
Dental care delivery systems	Improves access to dental caries treatment	Mainly observational longitudinal studies	Arguably in favor of the intervention	The studies in this area have mostly utilized observational longitudinal study design. RCTs are lacking. One suggestion is to use cluster RCT design and compare patient outcomes via different delivery models

3.2 Water Fluoridation

Water fluoridation is considered, by the USA Centres for Disease Control and Prevention, as one of the 10 great public health achievements of the twentieth century [3]. Epidemiology books [4, 5] cite water fluoridation as a remarkable achievement in public health and an example of an epidemiologic approach that clearly demonstrates a causal relationship, that is, fluoride-reducing dental caries.

Already in the 1940s, observational epidemiological studies had signaled that fluoride in the drinking water was associated with marked lower dental caries levels. The first two controlled experimental studies in the United States to add fluoride to a community water supply in order to bring the fluoride concentration up to 1 ppm began at Grand Rapids-Muskegon, MI [6] and at Newburgh-Kingston, NY in the 1940s [7]. Another important study took place in the decades of 1950 and 1960 at Tiel and Culemborg, The Netherlands [8]. The three studies showed lower caries incidence in the cities in which fluoride was added to the water supply.

These studies are good examples that if only two communities are involved in a study, and only one of them will receive the intervention, it is irrelevant whether the intervention is randomly assigned because differences in baseline characteristics will have the same magnitude irrespective of the method of assignment [5]. In this case, the distribution of the intervention (fluoridation of the water supplies) should be planned in order to ensure maximum comparability between the two communities (the groups). In other words, the investigator should try to choose two communities that are as similar as possible with regard to the known factors that may influence the outcome (caries incidence), such as income (income may be a proxy for sugar consumption and use of effective caries preventive measures such as dental sealants).

A review of water fluoridation collated the evidence from 107 studies that were included in a quantitative synthesis [9]. The three classic community intervention trials mentioned above were among these and were classified as "prospective observational studies" or "controlled before-and-after studies." The main findings were a reduction of 35% and 26% in caries in primary and permanent teeth, respectively, and an increase of 15% and 14% in the percentage of children free of caries in primary and permanent teeth, respectively. The authors emphasized that as most studies dated from before 1975 (71%), prior to the time when the use of fluoridated toothpaste was widespread, the benefit of water fluoridation may not be the same nowadays. Therefore, they concluded that "there is very little contemporary evidence… that has evaluated the effectiveness of water fluoridation for the prevention of caries."

Overall, the review concluded that water fluoridation is effective at reducing dental caries in both primary and permanent teeth of children and that there is a significant association between dental fluorosis—regardless of the level—and fluoride level in the water. However, the authors emphasized that the observational nature of the study designs, the high risk of bias and heterogeneity in the included studies, and the applicability of the evidence to current lifestyles limit their confidence in the estimates. Studies assessing fluorosis are generally more recent than those assessing caries. Nowadays, there are several other sources of fluoride available but this is generally disregarded among the studies, so the risk of different levels of fluorosis attributed to water fluoridation remains unclear.

The main (implicit) conclusion of this review appears sound; that, in the presence of widespread use of fluoride toothpaste, the additional benefit of water fluoridation has not been clearly established. However, this review has been rightly criticized because the authors used inclusion criteria that were exceedingly restrictive, leaving out a large amount of relevant evidence, especially considering the important role of water fluoridation for public health [10]. Another limitation of this review was the absence of an explicit aim to assess the benefit of water fluoridation in communities where there is widespread use of fluoridated toothpaste. Maybe, it was this very exaggerated restrictive inclusion criteria that did not allow the authors to answer this important public health question. Also, authors applied misplaced criteria to judge the adequacy of the study design and the risk of bias; water fluoridation is a community intervention, thus the feasible (and correct) study design to assess its effectiveness is the community intervention trial, not the traditional individual clinical RCT. However, the authors of the review applied the risk of bias tool used for individual clinical RCT to judge the risk of bias in water fluoridation community trials. In addition, as stated by Rugg-Gunn, "In many cases it is simply impossible to make recommendations for public health interventions and policy if reliance is only placed on RCTs" [10].

3.3 Fluoride Toothpastes

Fluoride toothpaste is a highly effective anticaries intervention. Toothbrushing with a toothpaste is a cheap and well-established oral hygiene daily routine. The addition of fluoride to toothpastes makes this form of fluoride application easy to implement, as it does not interfere with habits already established and it does not demand people to seek professional help in order to obtain access to fluoride. Since the 1940s, more than 100 trials have been conducted to test the effects of different fluoride toothpastes on caries control. Some trials have compared fluoride toothpastes to placebo toothpastes, others have compared toothpastes with different fluoride concentrations, and others have compared toothpastes with different fluoride agents. Varied age groups have been involved, from preschoolers to elderly people. Some have assessed the effect of fluoride toothpastes on coronal (enamel, dentine, and enamel plus dentine) caries while others have included root caries. Despite the vast amount of studies on the subject, it was not until the late 1990s and early 2000s that a systematic synthesis of these studies has been published. Today, the amount of evidence available from RCTs enables us to rely on the results of several systematic reviews on the subject [11–17].

Two reviews played important roles in answering whether fluoride toothpastes are effective in the reduction of dental caries incidence. The first one, published in 2003, included 74 trials comparing fluoride toothpaste of any concentration versus placebo, and only five of these trials were not in school settings [11]. In the majority of these trials, toothbrushing was unsupervised at home, so the effect assessed was the distribution and recommendation to use the toothpaste. To be included, trials must have ensured blinded outcome assessment and follow-up of at least 1 year, as the primary outcome was caries at the dentine level and trials with shorter follow-up periods would not allow enough time for caries progression to reach the dentine. Most trials were cautious to ensure that only one type of toothpaste was available in each household; this is important in field trials in order to avoid contamination of the interventions between the groups being compared. The review excluded trials that applied any additional active agent or caries preventive measure, such as chlorhexidine, fluoride varnish, or mouth rinse. Also, as information about the frequency of toothbrushing was not available from many trials, the authors of the review assumed, in those trials, that toothbrushing was performed once per day by the child. This review found that fluoride toothpastes significantly decreased the incidence of caries. This effect was higher with higher baseline caries level, higher concentration of fluoride, higher frequency of toothbrushing, and supervised use. Exposure to water fluoridation did not modify the reduction in the incidence of caries caused by fluoride toothpaste.

Another review updated the evidence on the anticaries effects of toothpastes with different fluoride concentrations [16]. In this review, 96 trials were included, either comparing fluoride toothpastes to placebo or toothpastes with different fluoride concentrations. This review supported the benefits of fluoride toothpaste in preventing caries when compared to non-fluoride toothpaste and showed a dose–response effect for children and adolescents; the higher the concentration of fluoride, the larger the magnitude of the anticaries effect. However, most studies compared 1000–1500 ppm fluoride toothpastes with non-fluoride toothpastes, so there is still uncertainty on the effects of other fluoride concentrations. Also, some toothpastes available in the market use different agents in their formulation, and the extent to which these agents could enhance (or reduce) the anticaries effect of the fluoride in the toothpaste is not established yet.

Regarding the primary dentition, the evidence on the effects of low (<600 ppm) versus standard (1000–1500 ppm) fluoride toothpastes has also been systematically reviewed [13]. The use of low-fluoride toothpastes by preschoolers should not be recommended as they increased the risk of caries (compared to standard fluoride toothpaste) and did not reduce the risk of aesthetically objectionable fluorosis in upper permanent anterior teeth. The largest trial included in this review was carried out in non-fluoridated districts of England, but where most toothpastes in the market contained fluoride [18]. The trial was designed primarily to evaluate the effects on caries of regularly supplying free fluoride toothpaste through the mail to children from the age of 12 months to 5 years. There were three comparison groups: 1450 ppm fluoride toothpaste, 440 ppm fluoride toothpaste, and a control group receiving no toothpaste through the mail. Thus, this trial investigated, rather than the efficacy of the products per se, one public health strategy of delivering an effective product, that is, fluoride toothpaste. For this reason, the design of this trial differed from that of a conventional RCT. It demonstrated that a program distributing free 1450 ppm fluoride toothpaste provided a significant clinical benefit for high caries risk children living in deprived, non-fluoridated districts. When these children were 8–10 years old, dental fluorosis was assessed using standardized digital photographs of the anterior teeth and there was no increased risk of aesthetically objectionable fluorosis [19]. This type of community intervention trial is valuable to test new creative ways of delivering fluoridated toothpaste to populations around the world living in diverse conditions, especially in vulnerable deprived communities.

Finally, we would like to mention the recommendations given by the authors of one systematic review on this theme [16]: "The choice of fluoride toothpaste concentration should also be informed by concurrent fluoride use whether from self-care measures (e.g. fluoride mouthrinse, community water fluoridation) or professionally applied sources (e.g. fluoride varnish), and consideration of the risk of fluorosis in the developing dentition of younger children." The adoption of measures such as fluoride varnish or any other professionally applied fluoride should not take precedence over fluoride toothpaste, especially from a public health perspective. On the contrary, there is no justification to recommend more expensive measures that are not more effective than fluoride toothpaste (or that do not bring clinically relevant additional benefits). As already stated, fluoride in the toothpaste relies on toothbrushing, which is a cheap and well-established routine that does not interfere with daily habits and does not create unnecessary dependency on dental services. The implementation and maintenance of professionally applied fluoride programs, even outside clinical settings, demand extra training and allocation of personnel and resources. The use of standard fluoride toothpaste is the default; to recommend any other form of fluoride delivery, in addition to toothpaste, one should demonstrate that its delivery will bring clinically relevant additional benefit that is more cost-effective[2] than fluoride toothpaste alone. To date, this has not been demonstrated.

3.4 Sugar

Despite being considered a multifactorial disease, dental caries is caused by sugar. The lack of sugar halts all the chain of events that leads to the demineralization of dental tissues [21]. However, during the 1930s, it was still not clear whether dental caries was a deficiency disease or a diet-mediated disease. At that time, oral health was extremely poor in Scandinavia, and a definite study on the relationship between caries and diet was needed [22]. This study took place from 1945 to 1954. It was a controlled field trial with 436 Swedish mentally handicapped people living in the Vipeholm Hospital [23].

This classic study was divided into different phases, one of which aimed to examine how caries activity was influenced by the ingestion of carbohydrates under controlled conditions. There were six experimental groups (sucrose in solution group, sugar-rich bread group, milk chocolate group, 22—caramel group, 8—toffee group, and 24—toffee group). The control group received a low-sugar diet supplied only at meals. Although a similar study would not be conceivable nowadays due to ethical concerns, some considerations of the Vipeholm study should be highlighted: it was performed when the role of sugar in caries (let alone in other diseases) was not clearly established; the daily amount of sugar offered to the participants was similar to that consumed by children in the city where it took place; and the study was planned years before the publication of the Helsinki Declaration. Also, the study had a robust methodology, such as good inter-examiner reliability, well-controlled conditions, concerns regarding contamination among groups and choice of a permanent population in order to avoid losses to follow up. We should also point out that, even nowadays, despite all the evidence of the harm caused by sugar [24], sugar consumption is incentivized by commercial advertisement and culture in general, and authorities hardly ever interfere even where individuals consume very high amounts of sugar, for example, in Latin America [25].

This study is perhaps the most striking evidence establishing frequent consumption of sugar as a direct cause of dental caries. It unequivocally showed that very frequent consumption of sugar in sticky form is a direct cause of caries. The number of caries lesions appearing in the groups of people in the study who were eating sugar several times each day was so great that the research team had to change the research protocol after the first year of the study. The between meal sugar in these groups was stopped and then a dramatic fall in caries increment was observed.

The findings of the Vipeholm study stimulated research on sugar substitutes, which do not lead to acid formation in dental biofilm [26]. One example is a series of relatively small-scale studies that have been conducted in Finland in order to investigate the dental, oral, and general effects of chronic consumption of fructose, sucrose, and xylitol —The Turku studies. One of the studies of

[2]Cost-effectiveness = ratio of the difference in costs between two interventions (incremental costs) and difference in the effects (incremental effects) between them [20]. It expresses how much more it is paid, comparing the intervention with the control group, in order to avoid one event of an undesirable outcome (one episode of dental pain, a loss of a tooth or a new cavitated dentine lesion, e.g.).

this series was a 2-year trial with 125 subjects, with a mean age of 28 years [27]. A massive reduction in caries increment was observed in the xylitol group. Some limitations of this trial were the lack of sample size calculation, of blinding, and of randomization as subjects were assigned to groups partly on individual preference basis. Due to ethical considerations, in the sucrose group, the participants were not requested to consume any specific number of sugar-containing products, but were instructed to maintain their previous usual sugar consumption. Despite the lack of randomization, groups were balanced at baseline regarding age, sex, and caries levels. An important limitation in this trial design was that it created doubts about the interpretation of the very low incidence of caries in the xylitol group: was it due to the absence of sucrose or also due to a direct anticaries effect of xylitol?

Today, there is consistent evidence of moderate quality showing a causal relationship between the amount of sugar intake and dental caries development [21, 28] and, therefore, RCTs testing its effects on health outcomes are no longer ethically acceptable. However, different strategies can be tested in order to assess the effects of sugar-restricting methods on caries. One of these strategies is taxing sugar. No RCTs have been performed reporting on dental caries, only model-based studies, and all showed that the implementation of a 20% tax on sugar-sweetened beverages (SSB) is likely to reduce caries incidence [29–31]. A broad range of different interventions potentially affecting the consumption of SSB and its effects on health have been compiled in a systematic review [32]. Traffic-light labeling, increases in prices, healthier default beverages on children's menus in chain restaurants, and in-store promotion of healthier beverages in supermarkets have been associated with decreasing SSB sales. Other interventions, such as reduced availability of SSBs in schools, government food benefit programs with restrictions on purchasing SSB, and improved availability of low-calorie beverages in the home environment were associated with decreased SSB consumption. It should be noted, however, that the certainty of the evidence was low to moderate for most outcomes. Overall, the evidence is prone to reporting bias as studies were not prospectively registered. Whenever possible, RCTs should be carried out although they may not always be feasible for population-level health interventions and, in this case, alternatives to minimize bias should be implemented. Also, self-report data on diet is problematic. The evidence is not directly generalizable as most studies were carried out in high-income countries.

Reduction in sugar consumption requires action at a community level, not at educating individuals to change their dietary behavior alone [33]. Therefore, experimental studies assessing the effects of community-level interventions on sugar reduction, and consequent oral health improvements, are needed. Despite the anticaries effect of fluoride and its widespread availability in water and toothpaste (and in some communities, through professionally applied fluoride), caries levels increase as people age [34]. Thus, strategies to control caries without tackling sugar intake is deemed to failure. Individual-level RCTs to test measures to reduce sugar consumption should be discouraged. In communities where there is large availability of sugar in the diet, it is unrealistic to expect that individuals would behave differently from most people around them and keep to a low-sugar diet while everybody else does not. Also, even a relative reduction in sugar consumption by some individuals may be insufficient if it does not cross the threshold of the association between sugar and caries [21, 35, 36]. There are large differences in individual susceptibility to caries [37] and it is difficult to obtain reliable information from individuals about their sugar consumption [32]. Finally, it has repeatedly been argued that sugar consumption is not an important cause of caries anymore given the high consumption of sugar by children and their low caries levels in modern societies, especially in rich industrialized countries [38, 39]. In trying to explain the dramatic decline in caries that suddenly occurred in the mid-late 1970s, even if one believes that sugar consumption among children is high and, therefore, fluoride is the reason for the low caries levels, one has to be aware that the strength of a cause depends on the distribution of other component causes in the population. A new factor (widespread use of fluoride in the 1970s) becomes a strong cause if its complementary causes are common (sugar). In other words, it is difficult to depict a cause (sugar) if it does not vary enough between the units of analysis (the individuals). Thus, even believing that fluoride in the toothpaste is the main reason for current low caries levels [40] does not allow one to disregard sugar as the major cause of caries in the rich western countries. Millions of people exposed to fluoridated toothpaste in these countries develop caries, and the number of decayed teeth increases significantly with age [34, 35].

The implication of all these facts is that individual-level RCTs of sugar restriction will likely be unable to detect the strong causal association between sugar consumption and caries in modern societies. The appropriate experimental design to study the effect of measures to reduce sugar and caries is the community intervention trial.

In recent years, interventions based on behavioral economic theory have been increasingly applied in order to change the environment so that it subtly stimulates the individual to make more beneficial choices for themselves, despite exposure to harmful options. Nudge is any aspect of choice architecture capable of changing the behavior of the individual in a predictable way, to improve decisions about health, wealth, and happiness, without prohibiting any option and without any significant change in their economic incentives [41]. This approach is promising for societal attempts to reduce sugar consumption and improve health.

A few examples of how to assess the effects of nudging on dietary choices are RCTs that evaluate whether nudging and social marketing strategies encourage employees to make healthier food choices during their daily worksite cafeteria visits [42], and whether improved positioning and serving of fruit, accompanied by attractive labeling of both fruit and vegetables on offer, encourage children to select and consume more fruit and vegetables in their lunchtime meal in primary school cafeterias [43]. Both trials showed positive results, highlighting that low-cost, simple, and creative strategies may nudge people towards healthier food choices. This type of community intervention trials is a promising way to improve diet and public health in general. Specifically, RCTs assessing the effects of nudge on sugar reduction are welcome.

A comprehensive analysis of sugar industry's internal documents has shown that the sugar industry has heavily influenced public health research priorities, focusing on other aspects of caries, diverting attention from the role of sugar. This strategy included tactics such as funding research into a vaccine against dental caries [44]. Thus, potential conflict of interest is a major concern in studies assessing the effects of sugar on health outcomes.

3.5 Pit and Fissure Sealants

Dental sealant is a professionally applied resin, mainly on the occlusal surface of the teeth, to prevent the appearance or progression of caries on that surface. As this surface is the most susceptible to caries, the preventive potential of sealants is great. By the end of the 1970s, several clinical trials had already been carried out in different populations and the results showed that sealants were very effective [45–48].

The research program on the effectiveness of sealants has a large number of independent RCTs. A systematic review including seven RCTs that randomized 1548 and examined 1322 children found an 88% reduction in the risk of dentine caries in permanent molars followed for at least 2 years in children who received resin-based sealants compared to those who did not receive sealants. The authors estimated that in a scenario where the incidence of caries was 400 molars per 1000, sealant application would reduce this incidence to 63 per 1000 [49].

This review convincingly demonstrated the effectiveness of sealants in preventing caries. However, there are still important questions that have not been answered. It is still necessary to identify factors that increase or decrease sealant effectiveness and to evaluate whether there are enough studies to obtain a conclusive answer as to its cost-effectiveness [50]. For example, sealant effectiveness may vary according to the level of caries in the population, to the material used, to the application technique employed, to the age of the patient, to the type of tooth, and to the stage of tooth eruption. Regarding cost-effectiveness, it may be better to seal only teeth that already show early signs of caries [51]. Also, children at greater risk of developing new cavities benefited more from a school sealant program [52, 53]. Another systematic review concluded that sealant is equally effective when applied to a sound surface or to a non-cavitated carious lesion. In addition, sealant was much more effective than the application of fluoride varnish. In a population with a caries prevalence of 30%, for every 1000 sealed teeth, 207 cavities would be avoided in the next 2–3 years, compared with 1000 unsealed teeth; compared with 1000 unsealed teeth that were treated with fluoride varnish, 196 cavities would be avoided by sealant [54, 55]. So, compared to sealant, the number of cavities avoided by fluoride varnish was negligible.

When comparing sealants to fluoride varnish, there is some evidence favoring sealants. As the quality of evidence as well as the number of studies are low, it is not possible to draw clear conclusions about differences in effectiveness between these two measures for preventing or controlling dental caries on occlusal surfaces of permanent molars. One RCT on the subject found that the proportion of children who developed dentine caries on at least one first permanent molar after 36 months was similar in the sealant (19.6%) and fluoride varnish (17.5%) groups, but slightly lower costs were observed for fluoride varnish application. It should be noted that in this trial the sealant used was resin-based, which requires adequate moisture control and therefore should be applied in a dental setting, while fluoride varnish does not necessarily need to be applied within a clinic or traditional health-care setting. Both fluoride varnish and dental sealant had high acceptability in a school setting [56, 57]. Less than 10% of sealants were lost during the 3-year period of this trial. This implies that sealants could be applied and the individual reassessed only once every 2 or 3 years. Varnish, on the other hand, presumably needs to be reapplied at least once every 6 months. So, sealants can be more cost-effective. This trial was not able to assess this possibility because participants in the sealants arm were reassessed once every 6 months, and the sealants were reapplied when partially or totally lost. Future RCTs should assess the cost-effectiveness of different sealants, such as glass ionomer (GI) sealants, compared to varnish, taking advantage of sealants allowing for only one professional assessment every 2 or 3 years.

One important issue regarding trials assessing the effectiveness of GI sealants is that the use of retention (a surrogate outcome) instead of dentine caries (a true endpoint) as the primary outcome may have misled dentists into rejecting GI sealants in favor of resin-based sealants. Although the retention of GI sealants is lower, they may be as (or even more) effective in avoiding caries cavities, as GI particles remain in the bottom of fissures [58, 59].

It appears that the research program on the effectiveness of sealants has reached a stage where effectiveness has already been demonstrated, but there is still a need for cost-effectiveness studies. In addition, there seems to be no evidence of the effectiveness of sealants in adults, and insufficient evidence on primary dentition and on the comparison between different materials [54].

3.6 Dental Check-Up

The 6-monthly dental check-up is arguably one of the most popular dental public health recommendations and dental programs usually include regular clinical examinations. Paradoxically, this is one of the least evidence-based dental public health recommendations/measures [60]. Until recently, there was only one RCT [61]. This trial was carried out in the early 1990s, included 3, 16, and 18-year-olds and lasted 2 years. The 241 participants were allocated either to 12- or 24-month recall intervals; 12 months were already the norm in the study population, so the test was merely an extension from 12- to 24-month interval, in a 24-month follow-up study. The 24-month interval group showed higher dental caries increments, but it was more economical [62].

There were several limitations in this trial. Participation was restricted to individuals with lower risk of developing caries: 3-year-olds with dmft >0, 16-year-olds with DMFT >10, and 18-year-olds with DMFT >12 were not included. Before entering the trial, all participants were already attending for annual dental checks and the follow-up was only 2 years. There was no information about the randomization process apart from a sentence stating that participants were randomly allocated to two groups. Of the 241 who started the study, only 185 were accounted for at the end of the 2 years, no information was available for this nearly a quarter of participants that were lost and there was no intention to treat or sensitivity analysis. Caries at baseline was unbalanced between the 12- and 24-month interval groups, except among the 3-year-olds. So, already at the baseline, the 24-month interval group had higher caries levels among the 16- and 18-years-old, suggesting that they were more susceptible to caries. All these problems generated a high risk of selection bias. The examiners who assessed caries outcome were not blinded to the intervention group of the participants. In addition, they provided all the dental care and assessed dmfs and DMFS increments. So, there was a high risk of performance (care provided) and detection (caries assessment) bias. Finally, the estimate of higher caries increment in the longer interval group was very imprecise.

The INTERVAL dental recalls trial [63] was registered in 2008 and the results were published in early 2021 [64]. "This is a UK multi-center, parallel-group, randomized controlled trial with blinded outcome assessment. The trial is set in Primary Dental Care, reflecting the setting within which the vast majority of dentistry is delivered in the UK." The authors aimed to recruit 50 general dental practitioners from across the United Kingdom, including dentists in England, Scotland, Wales, and Northern Ireland. The inclusion criteria in this trial were adult patients (≥18 years of age) who were dentate and had visited their dentist in the previous 2 years in the NHS (National Health Service UK). The trial interventions were three recall intervals for dental check-ups, that is: 24-month; 6-month; a variable length interval based on patient risk assessment (varying from 3 to 24 months). The content of the check-up was the usual practice, that is, clinical examination, advice, and monitoring of periodontal status. For participants allocated to the fixed-period recall groups (6 and 24 months), dentists were expected to provide routine care. Not all eligible participants could be allocated to the 24-month interval, only those classified as low risk of dental disease. This trial had two randomization strata, those with a high risk of dental disease could only be randomized to 6-month intervals or to the variable risk-based interval arm. Only those with low risk of dental disease could be part of the randomization strata that included these two arms plus the 24-month interval arm. The selection of participants to be in one of these two randomization strata was based on a clinical exam by their dentist prior to randomization, to determine suitability for randomization to the 24-month recall arm. Follow-up was expected to be 4 years. Primary outcomes were gingival inflammation/bleeding on probing at the gingival margin and a measure of oral health-related quality of life (OHRQoL), specifically the Oral Health Impact Profile 14 instrument (OHIP-14). The main secondary outcomes were dental caries and periodontal pocket depth. There were also some economic outcomes.

This trial had important strengths. The question that it tried to answer, that is, what is the best dental recall interval, is long overdue [60] and is important for dental public health in relation to oral health and in terms of dental services expenditure. It was a "quasi-pragmatic" trial as the patients, health-care settings, and professionals were an extract of the real-life situation of primary dental care within a large country and public health system, that is, the UK NHS ("quasi-pragmatic" because it did not assess true oral health endpoints—see next). It was a multi-center trial, with around 50 dental practices, so that dentists of varied skills and patients of varied socioeconomic status were distributed to all the comparison recall interval groups.

The main limitation of this trial is related to the selection of the primary outcomes. Dental caries (i.e., cavities in teeth) is the most prevalent disease of humanity [65, 66] with indirect costs corresponding to economic losses within the range of the 10 most prevalent global causes of death [67]. It is the most relevant oral health problem for individuals and societies, the main cause of dental pain, infections, and work and school days losses [65, 66]. Surely, dental screening/check-ups must be assessed first and foremost regarding the effect on the incidence of caries and its direct consequences, such as toothache, tooth loss, and need for restorative treatment. Dental check-ups must reduce the risks of these events in order to be considered beneficial. However, dental caries, or its direct consequences, was not selected as a primary outcome in this trial. Contrastingly, gingival bleeding on probing, one of the two primary outcomes, is hardly ever a threat to oral health and seldom tangible for the patient (bleeding on probing is usually a reversible condition that often does not cause any harm to people). The other primary outcome, a measure of OHRQoL (OHIP-14), is a relevant oral health outcome. However, it is not yet established what is the amount of change in this measure that is relevant to the patient (the minimally important difference—MID [68]).

The secondary outcomes, dental caries and periodontal pocket depth, suffer from the same limitations as the primary outcomes. Sample size calculation aimed to detect an effect on white spot lesions. White spot lesions are hardly ever a threat to oral health as they are not tangible for the patient and a large proportion does not progress. Periodontal pocket depth was not considered in the sample size calculation. More importantly, what is a clinically relevant effect? Specifically, how many millimeters would shorter recall intervals have to reduce, in how many teeth sites and in which ages, for the effect to be considered clinically relevant?

Other important limitations were the following: there was no true control group, that is, a group not invited for dental check-up during the 4 years follow-up; patients classified as high-risk were not randomized to the 24-month interval recall group; there was no objective definition of high-risk. The absence of a true control group without check-up and of high-risk patients in the 24-month interval suggests that there was a presumption that these two situations were ethically unacceptable. However, it is ethically questionable to presume the benefit of an intervention that may have no effect or even be harmful. Shorter recall intervals raise dental services costs and may increase the risk of false-positive diagnosis and unnecessary harmful interventions.

The INTERVAL trial found no difference in the risk for dental health between the intervals of 24-month, 6-month, and risk-based for the 30% of adults considered suitable to be recalled at 24 months by their dentist. Thus, the authors concluded that “there is no clinical benefit of a 6-monthly recall compared to a risk-based recall or 24-month recall in those patients considered eligible” [64].

This trial may encourage new large pragmatic trials, as dentists may feel less opposing to randomize their patients to varied and longer recall intervals, regardless of their risk profile. RCTs to assess the benefits and harms of dental check-ups are still needed, as despite the admirable efforts of the INTERVAL trial, there are questions still unanswered. These new RCTs should be Large Simple Trials (LST). These LSTs should be performed with a large and heterogeneous group of patients, preferably multicenter, with several dental practices participating and obeying the same protocol, in which the recruitment of participants occurs with a minimum of restriction. The intervention should be simple, inexpensive, and not sensitive to providers’ skills. Comparison groups should include no recall (i.e., attend only when the participant perceives that there is a problem) versus 12-, 24-, and 36-month intervals. Standard recall visits are kept simple and limited to a minimum standard care including the following: clinical exam plus bite-wing radiograph when needed; oral health and hygiene instructions; professional tooth-cleaning with scale and polishing when needed; professionally applied topical fluoride). The outcomes should be a few health measures that are less prone to measurement error and are clearly relevant to the patient's life, such as tooth loss, dental pain, and cavities.

3.7 Professionally Applied Fluoride

Professionally applied fluoride products include gel/foam, varnish, and silver diamine fluoride (AgF). There are comprehensive systematic reviews of experimental studies showing anticaries effects of all of these products. One main limitation of the evidence collated by the review on fluoride gels is that most of the 28 included trials were carried out in the decades of 1960–1980; only four were carried out in the late 1990s and early 2000s [69]. Old trials make it difficult to perform a thorough risk of bias assessment, as they are usually poorly reported. Also, evidence from a time when participants were not exposed to fluoride toothpaste put into question the extent to which the results can be extrapolated to the present time. In any case, the risk of selection bias was high in the majority of the trials (due to the inclusion of quasi-randomized trials or trials with improper random sequence generation and allocation concealment, and high rates of losses to follow-up), as was the risk of performance bias (due to inclusion of trials lacking a placebo control group that prevented blinding of participants and personnel). Only two trials reported acute toxicity. Although the review found anticaries benefits associated with fluoride gels, the absolute benefit will be small where the expected caries increment is small. The recommendation for dental personnel to apply fluoride gel in children and adolescents every 6-months is based on evidence from RCTs with poor methods, and expected absolute benefits that are negligible for each individual. In order to be able to ethically recommend professionally applied fluoride gel, there is a need for new evidence on the anticaries benefit of gel, additional to fluoride toothpaste, and, if effective, evidence of its cost-effectiveness.

In contrast to trials on fluoride gel, there are many recent trials on fluoride varnish for preschoolers. The American Dental Association (ADA) considers that, for children up to 6 years of age, it is the only fluoridated product for professional use where the risk of adverse effects does not outweigh the potential benefits [70]. One example is a large-scale RCT in 22 general dental practices (GDP) in Northern Ireland [71]. In this trial, dentists screened children according to their own GDP and those eligible were centrally randomized to either the intervention group (varnish, toothbrush, and toothpaste delivered at the child's dental checkup twice a year) or to the control group (no professionally provided fluoride interventions). Both groups received the same standardized dental health advice on optimal use of fluoride toothpaste and restriction of sugar consumption. All children were caries free when recruited at 2–3 years old; this low-risk population comprises the majority of patients seen in dental practices. The trial had high retention and compliance rates, but failed to keep children caries-free. A cost-effectiveness analysis considering a public payer perspective was carried out alongside this trial and showed that the costs of providing this preventive intervention outweighed savings in treatment during the 3–5-year follow-up period [72]. These findings raised concerns about the cost-effectiveness of delivering a combined fluoride intervention designed to prevent caries in preschoolers attending general dental practices.

Another example of a fluoride varnish trial, this time with a high-risk population, was a field cluster randomized trial carried out in 52 classrooms with 3–5-year-old American Indians [73]. The classrooms were randomly assigned to the intervention group (intervention consisting of oral health promotion, fluoride varnish applications, and distribution of toothbrushes and toothpaste for the household, delivered by lay health workers to children/caregivers) or to the control group (only distribution of toothbrushes and toothpaste for the household). At the beginning of the trial, children in the intervention and control groups had high levels of caries (dmfs 20 and 23, respectively) and, after 3 years, no differences in caries increment were observed. In this trial, community tribal health workers trained to deliver the intervention in a preschool setting where children spent substantial time; this resulted in high participation of children. The participation of the community also ensured its cultural relevance. This highlights the need to adopt strategies to reduce losses to follow up in RCTs, such as establishing a relationship between the participant and research personnel by employing well-trained staff with the same social background [74].

A systematic review that aimed to assess the effects of fluoride varnish applications on caries and caries-related hospitalizations in preschoolers included 19 RCTs published between 1979 and 2018 [75]. It compared fluoride varnish alone or associated with an oral health program versus no intervention, usual care, or placebo. Some trials included in this review randomized children (in schools) whereas others were randomized schools or practice settings. No information on caries-related hospitalizations was reported. This review found an arguably modest benefit, that is, a lower increment of caries in the varnish group of one surface per child or less. No significant difference was observed at the tooth level. The risk of developing new dentine caries lesions was reduced by 12% among the children who received fluoride varnish when compared to those who did not (in a population with 50% caries incidence, it would be necessary to apply fluoride varnish in 17 children to avoid one developing new caries lesions in the next 2 years). This was a rather modest benefit considering that many children developed new dentine caries lesions irrespective of fluoride varnish use [75]. This review also showed that older studies had a poorer performance, especially regarding selection bias. They also were poorly reported and, therefore, had more domains assessed as unclear risk of bias in comparison to more recent studies. Non-preregistered subgroup analysis showed no differences in the risk of developing new dentine caries in RCTs comparing fluoride varnish versus placebo. In most trials, children were exposed to fluoride toothpaste, and increasing the fluoride exposure by applying fluoride varnish made hardly any difference in the risk of developing new caries lesions in children. Therefore, cost-effectiveness analyses are needed.

Another vehicle for delivering fluoride is silver diamine fluoride (SDF). Although it has been in use for a long time in some countries, such as Brazil and China, not until recently it only became recently popular in other countries, such as the United States. In the United States, SDF was cleared in 2014 by the US Food and Drug Administration (FDA) to treat dentine hypersensitivity in adults [76] and is commonly used as off-label to arrest dental caries in adults and children. Since then, the number of trials on SDF has greatly increased. Its popularity is due to it being a noninvasive caries management strategy, with easy and quick application, making it attractive to be applied in young children, patients with special needs, and the elderly. There is evidence of the effectiveness of SDF for arresting and preventing coronal carious lesions in children in the primary dentition and root carious lesions in older adults [77–79]. Compared to fluoride varnish, SDF was more effective in arresting cavitated caries in primary teeth [80, 81].

A well-designed 30-month RCT was carried out including 888 3–4-year-old healthy children from 37 kindergartens in Hong Kong [82]. The aim was to compare the effectiveness of two concentrations (12% or 38%) and two periodicity of application (once or twice a year) of SDF on arresting cavitated dentine caries in primary teeth. The sample size calculation took into account the cluster effect. Eligible children were divided into two strata according to the number of carious tooth surfaces they presented (1–3 and >3 surfaces) to achieve baseline balance of caries severity among groups; they were then randomly allocated to one of the following four treatment groups: 12% SDF applied every 6 or 12 months and 38% SDF applied every 6 or 12 months. Authors stated that the lack of a non-intervention group was due to ethical reasons. The bottles of SDF were wrapped in aluminum foil to ensure blinding. It should be noted that all children received the intervention every 6 months, but in the groups where SDF should be applied every 12 months, a placebo ("saline solution") was applied in order to ensure blinding. The 38% SDF solution was more effective in arresting dentine caries compared to 12% SDF, but the application of SDF was not sufficient to prevent the development of new caries. Apart from the black staining on the arrested caries lesions, SDF did not cause other adverse effects. Parental acceptance of the staining of caries lesions after SDF application can significantly differ among communities. Thus, future SDF trials in different settings must ensure parents are fully informed about this negative aesthetic effect.

3.8 Fluoride Mouth Rinse

Fluoride mouth rinses have been extensively used in the last decades as a caries preventive method in children and adolescents. They were widely adopted in school-based programs in the 1970s and 1980s in the form of weekly supervised application of solutions of 0.2% sodium fluoride. Nowadays, they are a popular self-applied oral health-care product (daily home use of solutions of 0.05% sodium fluoride). The most updated evidence on the anticaries effects of fluoride mouth rinses is a systematic review that included 37 trials; only one of these trials was carried out in the 2000s whereas the vast majority was carried out before the 1990s [83]. As with fluoride gels, the body of evidence on fluoride mouth rinses consists of old trials mainly with participants who were probably not exposed to fluoride toothpaste. The extent to which this evidence is applicable today is questionable.

The most recent trial, published in 2005, was carried out in a non-fluoridated Swedish city [84]. It was a 3-year RCT of a school-based fluoride mouth rinsing that aimed to assess its effects on approximal caries development in 13-year-olds with low-to-moderate caries risk. Five schools were included and each had five classes within the age group—each class was randomized to one of the five groups: in four groups, the intervention was mouth-rinse supervised by a dental nurse at different intervals and the control group did not rinse. Randomization was not clearly described in this trial. Authors performed no sample size calculation. All participants brushed their teeth twice a day with fluoride toothpaste and received fluoride varnish applications at their yearly check-ups at the public dental clinics. Caries was assessed in bite-wing radiographs with no clinical visual examination. No information was given whether the lesions were cavitated, at the dentine level; thus, there was no information about how tangible/clinically relevant these lesions were. Although the authors concluded that "supervised school-based fluoride mouth rinsing is an excellent method to prevent caries incidence in 13–16-year-olds in low to medium caries risk areas," at the end of the study, most caries lesions that developed were enamel lesions, while new dentine lesions were negligible. Also, in all five groups, few enamel caries lesions progressed into the dentine or to fillings. The only "significant" effect was related to enamel demineralization, arguably an irrelevant outcome: the authors reported "a large" effect (prevented fraction 59%—see Sect. 3.13.2) on approximal caries at enamel level detected by radiographs when fluoride mouth rinses were used on the first and the last three schooldays every semester (it is difficult to understand the plausibility that few days of rinsing could reduce 3 years caries incidence). There was a drop-out rate of 21%, including changing classes, schools or moving out of town, bad quality of bite-wing radiographs, and non-compliance. Also, losses were not balanced among the groups. The lack of an intention-to-treat analysis, as only participants present at initial and final examinations were included in the data analysis, introduced a high risk of selection bias.

The above-mentioned review [83] claimed that the anticaries benefits of fluoride mouth rinses were so clear that additional randomized comparisons of fluoride mouth rinses with placebo alone would be difficult to justify. However, as already mentioned, there is no evidence on the effects of unsupervised home use, trials are old, with high or unclear risk of bias and the most recent trial, where participants were exposed to fluoride toothpaste, has failed to add relevant information. Moreover, as in this more recent trial, participants were exposed to other forms of fluoride, including toothpaste, it was expected that the rinsing effect would be smaller than the effect from older trials where the only fluoride exposure was rinsing; however, this trial presented the largest preventive fraction among the 35 studies included in the DMFS meta-analysis. This unexpected larger effect increases the uncertainty regarding the risk of bias.

It is unfortunate that such a common practice (fluoride mouth rinse) lacks robust evidence and continues to be recommended by dentists and adopted in public health programs. Clearly, more RCTs are needed (including placebo comparison groups) in order to find out whether fluoride rinse adds any benefit for people already using fluoride toothpaste. Provided that it does, RCTs should include head-to-head comparisons of different frequencies of use and types of mouth rinses, as well as economic evaluations alongside the trials.

Orthodontic patients with fixed appliances are often prescribed daily fluoride mouth rinses as it is assumed that they are at a higher risk of developing white-spot lesions [85]. However, there is no evidence that topical fluorides reduce the risk of white-spot lesions in these patients [86]. Only one trial comparing fluoride mouth rinses to placebo was included in the latest update of a review that compared the effects of different types of fluoride on the incidence of white spot lesions during orthodontic treatment [86]. This trial assessed the effect of a 250 ppm F mouth rinse compared to a placebo mouth rinse on the number of participants with new white spot lesions measured by quantitative light-induced fluorescence. There was no evidence for a difference in the outcome between the groups. This study had a high risk of attrition bias as 33% of the randomized patients were lost to follow-up. Thus, the widespread recommendation to use fluoride mouth rinses during orthodontic treatment is not evidence-based. The authors of this review called for adequately powered and better-designed RCTs, including the use of factorial designs, which allows two or more interventions to be simultaneously assessed and enables the evaluation of possible interactions between them. Also, the outcome should be assessed by more than one evaluator using standard photographs. Future trials should compare fluoride to placebo mouth rinses in orthodontic patients using fluoride toothpaste, and assess patient-reported outcomes, such as aesthetic concerns.

3.9 Supervised Toothbrushing

Supervised toothbrushing may increase the anticaries effect of fluoride toothpastes. However, the evidence in favor of supervised toothbrushing accrued from secondary analyses that investigated its role as a potential source of heterogeneity in trials that compared fluoride versus placebo toothpastes [11]. Authors of RCTs of school-based programs of supervised toothbrushing have claimed that it reduces caries incidence, but the trials supporting their claims lacked a proper control group. In order to know whether toothbrushing supervision increases the anticaries effect of fluoride toothpastes, the ideal head-to-head comparison would be test and control groups using or receiving the same fluoride toothpaste, but in addition, the test group being supervised during toothbrushing whereas the control group not. This would isolate the anticaries effect of the fluoride toothpaste from the potential effect of toothbrushing supervision. However, in some trials, there was a control group with no intervention at all, and the type of toothpaste used by the children in the control group was unknown [87, 88], or the control group knowingly used a fluoride toothpaste with a different concentration and formulation from that of the test group [89]; these are not fair comparisons.

A systematic review that aimed specifically to assess the effects of supervised toothbrushing per se on caries incidence in children and adolescents found no conclusive evidence that supervised toothbrushing increases the anticaries benefit already provided by fluoride toothpaste [90]. Only four RCTs with proper control groups were identified, but these were heterogeneous, had a high risk of bias, and showed conflicting results. Whether toothbrushing supervision increases the anticaries effect of fluoride toothpastes is still an open question. That is not to say that toothbrushing supervision should be dismissed, as it is important to control the amount of toothpaste used by children, especially preschoolers.

3.10 Management of Dental Caries in Primary Teeth

Much time and resources are spent by dental services to treat caries in primary teeth. However, there was no evidence from RCT about the benefits of this intervention until recently. For that reason, attitudes towards the treatment of dental caries in primary teeth vary widely; from complete disregard due to the belief that the restoration of a primary tooth is unnecessary as the tooth will exfoliate; to valuing it due to the belief that the placement of a filling is necessary to avoid pain and infection.

The FICTION trial was an RCT that assessed "(1) the clinical effectiveness and cost-effectiveness of three strategies for managing caries in primary teeth and (2) quality of life, dental anxiety, the acceptability and experiences of children, parents and dental professionals, and caries development and/or progression." FICTION was a multicenter trial set in primary dental care in Scotland, England, and Wales, including NHS patients aged 3–7 years who were at a high risk of caries and had at least one primary molar with dentine caries, but no pain/sepsis. The three interventions compared were the following: (1) local anesthetic, carious tissue removal, filling placement; (2) sealing-in with crowns, selective carious tissue removal and fissure sealants; (3) dietary and toothbrushing advice, topical fluoride, and fissure sealing of permanent teeth. Groups 1 and 2 received their specific interventions plus the group 3 intervention. Primary outcomes were dental pain or dental sepsis whereas secondary outcomes were dental caries in primary and permanent teeth, and the cost-effectiveness of managing dental caries in primary teeth [91, 92].

A total of 72 dental practices were recruited and 1144 participants were randomized (of these, 1058 were included in an intention-to-treat analysis). The median follow-up time was 33.8 months and the median number of dental visits in each group was 7. The incidence of dental pain and/or infection during the 2–3 years of follow-up was high in all groups: around 40% in each of the three groups. So, despite having access to comprehensive dental health services in a developed country, the incidence of dental pain and/or infection was high among high-risk 3–7-year-old children who presented at least one decayed primary tooth at the start of the study. The risk of pain and/or infection did not differ much between the three groups. The less expensive treatment was prevention only (group 3), but it was a little less beneficial than sealant + prevention (group 2). Society would need to decide how much it is willing to pay in order to avoid dental pain and/or infection due to decayed primary teeth. Based on the estimates from this trial, the most cost-effective alternative for children with dentine caries in primary teeth is sealant + prevention (group 2) if society is willing to pay a minimum of £130 to avoid one episode of dental pain and/or infection.

This RCT's findings are generalizable to the UK population of children who regularly attend primary care and are at high risk of developing caries in the primary or mixed dentition. However, the placing of fillings and sealants are sensitive to dental practitioner's techniques and skills [93] and these may vary across countries. Thus, despite being a methodologically sound, pragmatic, large, and simple trial, similar RCTs should be replicated in other countries.

The US Preventive Services Task Force recently published a report on systematic review on screening and interventions to prevent dental caries in children younger than age 5 years [94]. They concluded that dietary fluoride supplementation and fluoride varnish appear to be effective at preventing caries outcomes in higher risk children younger than 5 years of age. Dietary fluoride supplementation in early childhood is associated with risk of enamel fluorosis, which is usually mild. In terms of gaps, they found that no randomized trial or observational study compared clinical outcomes between children younger than 5 years of age screened and not screened by primary care clinicians for dental caries. Almost all trials of topical fluoride were conducted in higher risk populations or settings. Evidence on other preventive interventions was limited (xylitol) or unavailable (silver diamine fluoride). Evidence on educational or counseling interventions was very sparse and no studies directly evaluated the effectiveness of primary care referral to a dentist versus no referral. This taskforce recommended more research on the accuracy of oral health examination and caries risk assessment by primary care clinicians, primary care referral for dental care, and effective parental and caregiver/guardian educational and counseling interventions.

3.11 Dental Care Delivery Systems

Emerging dental care delivery systems, e.g., virtual dental home or hub and spokes model, have shown promising results to improve dental access [95, 96]. This model generally comprises of a dental team connected through teledentistry where trained and licensed allied dental professionals provide the most basic screening and primary and secondary prevention services in the community settings, medical clinics, etc. (spokes) under the supervision of off-site dentists (central hub). Patients needing more extensive services are referred to the dentist at the central hub clinic. The studies in this area have mostly utilized longitudinal study design. For example, Kohli et al. (2021) (senior author) demonstrated that Oregon's virtual dental home project was successful in training Expanded Practice Dental Hygienists to perform Interim Therapeutic Restorations safely in school settings after caries diagnosis by the supervising dentist via teledentistry and in integrating this component into a regular school-based preventive dental program. Parents reported a decrease in dental access barriers and very high levels of satisfaction with this dental care program. Since it is difficult to standardize various components of health-care delivery systems and measure the true effect of the program in terms of clinical outcomes, the RCTs in this area are lacking. One suggestion is to use cluster RCT design and compare patient outcomes via different delivery models.

Table 3.2 summarizes these important themes that were (or should be) the focus of experimental epidemiological studies in Dental Public Health.

3.12 Practical Considerations of RCTs in Dental Public Health (Table 3.3)

3.12.1 Investigator Bias

In some instances, the investigator's preconceived belief in that the intervention is certainly effective can lead to investigator bias. Thus, it is critical to carefully examine the risk of bias of the study and interpret the results, especially if the effectiveness of an intervention is only reported by the same authors and in the same population.

Table 3.3 Practical considerations of RCTs in Dental Public Health

Funding	Government; industry; academic; foundation
Budgeting	Personnel; study intervention and per-patient costs; travel and meetings; technology; statistical analysis and data management support; the institutional review board
Drug regulation	Food and Drug Administration and Environmental Protection Agency (USA); Food Inspection Agency and the Department of Health (Canada); European Medicines Agency; The Medicines and Healthcare Products Regulatory Agency (UK)
Administration and quality control	Protocol review; recruitment; negotiation of agreements; development and negotiation of budgets; protocol compliance; billing; risk management and analysis; review the data collected during the trial; quality control of agents (toothpaste for example) used in the trial

3.12.2 Funding

Clinical trials related to Dental Public Health are mostly sponsored by government, industry, academic, or foundation. The researchers generally first generate pilot data via small foundation and academic grants to apply the funding for large-scale government grants.

Some examples of previously funded studies on the effect of water fluoridation on caries include the US Environmental Protection Agency, the Indian Council of Medical Research, the National Institute of Dental Research (NIDR), now called, the National Institute of Dental and Craniofacial Research (NIDCR), the Mexican National Council of Science and Technology ConacytSivilla, the Norwegian State Educational Loan fund, etc. Fluoride toothpastes, dental sealants, professionally applied fluoride, and fluoride mouth rinses trials have also been previously supported by the industry. The degree of funding and the type of involvement of industry funders vary. Mostly the industry would support a trial by providing free study medication. In rare cases, a company fully funds and controls a trial. The risk of bias due to industry-sponsored studies in dental public health trials has generally been low. Because of different priorities of health-care organizations and government bodies in different countries, the investigators in those countries seem to have a laser focus on many key issues. E.g. the National Institute for Health and Care Excellence (NICE) in the United Kingdom, an agency of the National Health Service (NHS) is charged with promoting clinical excellence in NHS service providers in England and Wales. Their role is to develop clinical guidelines and recommendations on the effectiveness of treatments and medical procedures, including technology. It is observed that countries that have national health-care delivery systems or financing have an increased motivation to assess the value of public health interventions.

3.12.3 Budgeting

The major costs of a dental public health clinical trial in a budget are: personnel who do trial work including those in the field; study-related care, including study intervention and per-patient costs; travel and meetings; technology; statistical analysis and data management support; and the Institutional Review Board (IRB) charges fees for the review of clinical trials from for-profit sponsors. Budget development also allows for a reflection on the processes involved and the feasibility of the study. Clinical trials are assumed to be expensive and generally have a budget of millions depending on the type of the study. Most academic institutions have research clinical centers that provide support in preparing a budget for trial costs, but ultimately, it is the PI's responsibility to take all the factors into account based on the activities laid out in the protocol.

3.12.4 Drug Regulation

In the United States, the Food and Drug Administration (FDA) is responsible for protecting the public health by ensuring the safety, efficacy, and security of human and veterinary drugs, biological products, and medical devices; and by ensuring the safety of food supply, cosmetics, and products that emit radiation. Similar examples of agencies from other countries are: the Canadian Food Inspection Agency (CFIA) and the Department of Health Canada (Health Canada), the European Medicines Agency, The Medicines and Healthcare products Regulatory Agency, UK, etc. In regards to the products used in Dental Public Health trials, the US Environmental Protection Agency (EPA) is responsible for the safety and quality of drinking water in the United States and sets a maximum allowable limit for fluoride in community drinking water. The FDA is responsible for approving prescription-related products (e.g. 5000 ppm fluoride toothpaste) and over-the-counter fluoride products, e.g., fluoride toothpaste and mouth rinse, e.g., the new researchers, if intending to bring a new product to the market should familiarize themselves with the drug regulation and approval process and seek guidance from the experts who have gone through the process. Due to globalization, collaborations across the world and the evolution of industries, there have been efforts to homogenize drug regulation across the world. This initiative will especially be helpful for particular countries where drug regulations appear to be ignored.

3.12.5 Administration and Quality Control

All members of the study are responsible for quality control and assurance. It is very critical to have experienced clinical trial administrators as they are responsible for protocol review, recruitment, negotiation of agreements, development and negotiation of budgets, protocol compliance, billing, international studies, and risk management and analysis. The study team should meet regularly to review the data collected to date, address any issues, and for continual study quality improvement. It is also critical to have quality control of agents used in the RCTs including the independent verification of contents of agents such as toothpaste or varnishes. This is especially important when studies are conducted in the areas of the world where the drug regulation process is not as stringent.

3.13 Key Considerations in RCTs

3.13.1 Outcomes

Caries and periodontitis are the most prevalent oral diseases. RCTs assessing interventions to prevent and treat them should focus on tangible outcomes (true endpoints). These are clinically relevant to patients [97], and include the following: tooth loss, dental pain, dentine cavity, tooth mobility, excessive loss of periodontal attachment according to age [98–100], and patient-reported outcomes [101] (aesthetics, function, comfort, psychological and social well-being). Researchers should avoid designing RCTs to prevent or treat outcomes that are intangible to patients.

Surrogate outcomes are valid only when they predict true endpoints [97, 102]. Unfortunately, effects on surrogate outcomes often fail to predict the true clinical effects of interventions [97]. For example, most white-spot lesions will not lead to tooth loss, dental pain, or even dentine cavity, therefore, they are not valid surrogates in caries RCTs. Similarly, gingivitis most often does not lead to tooth mobility, tooth loss or pain, so it is not a valid surrogate outcome in periodontal disease RCTs. The same reasoning applies to mild/moderate malocclusion in orthodontics trials [103].

RCTs are hard to conduct, take time, resources, and effort, and, therefore, it is not ethical to randomize participants when assessing surrogate outcomes that will bring no reliable or useful answers to clinical decision-making or public health policies. The aim of any treatment is to provide tangible patient benefits [104].

3.13.2 Risk Communication

The uncertainty surrounding the process of clinical decision-making gives rise to several cognitive biases that may affect dentists' reasoning. Some forms of risk communication reinforce cognitive bias, while others mitigate them. Good risk communication allows people to have a clear thinking when population and individual risks are evaluated in order to implement preventive health programs. Numerical formats are key to understanding health risk communication [105] and, therefore, when communicating the results of RCTs, authors should report absolute numbers and the base rate [106].

One effect measure widely used in caries trials and systematic reviews is the prevented fraction (PF). Its popularity derives from the fact that it allows the combination of different methods of measuring caries, such as DMFT (S), DFT (S), dmft (s), and dft (s). It is calculated by subtracting the increment of caries in the test group from the increment of caries in the control group and dividing this difference by the increment of caries in the control group, generating the percentage of the increment of caries in the control group that can be reduced by the intervention/treatment. However, as it is a relative measure, the PF fails to show the true differences in the caries increment observed between the groups being compared, and substantial PFs may, in fact, mean a clinically irrelevant caries reduction. Thus, PF is a misleading way of communicating risk reduction in RCTs and should be avoided [106].

3.14 Concluding Remarks

All types of RCTs play an important role in DPH. However, community intervention trials are better suited for addressing questions related to population health. The Nobel Prize in Economics in 2019 was won by three economists who used RCTs to determine how best to lift people out of poverty and improve their health [107, 108]. This is an excellent illustration of the power of the RCTs to investigate the effectiveness of public policies. The example of these Nobel prize-winning economists should serve as an inspiration for Dental Public Health researchers. They applied large simple trials to compare policies at a population level (clusters), focused on tangible outcomes, easy-to-implement interventions, and no restriction regarding eligible participants. Researchers carrying out such trials are urged not only to pre-register them in appropriate platforms but also to report them according to the Consolidated Standards of Reporting Trials (CONSORT) [109] and its extension for cluster trials [110]. This allows a comprehensive and careful analysis by readers of the trials' results, and especially, by reviewers when trials are included in evidence syntheses.

3.15 Case Scenario Exercise

3.15.1 Case Scenario

You are interested in conducting a study on children to test whether specially trained community lay health workers who administer fluoride varnish and oral health promotion education reduce caries as compared to nonintervention children.

Questions

1. What settings would you use to conduct this trial?
2. What is the most practical way to randomize children in the school setting in this case?
3. How would you get schools to participate in your study?
4. How would you obtain consents from the children who are minors in this case?

Answers

1. One of the factors determining the settings would be the age of children you are interested in, e.g., Head Start centers can be targeted for 4–5 years age groups, and elementary schools can be targeted for 5–11 years age groups.
2. Cluster randomized controlled trial (RCT) design is generally used in such situations. Eligible schools are randomly allocated either to an intervention or a control group.
3. Common strategies include meetings with the school district and school administrators, principals, teachers, and staff as well as parents to establish trust and explain the study, different steps involved, and overall benefits to the community. It is also important to plan the study so the children and staff have minimal disruption during the school time. Be appreciative of the work everyone is doing to make your study a success. Even small but meaningful tokens of appreciation, e.g., buying staff lunch on a specific day, certificates, holiday cards, etc., provide encouragement to everyone involved.

4. Parental consent is needed ahead of time. Teachers generally put these consents in the child's daily folder and send it electronically if needed. Always use clear and lay language in consent forms for better understanding. It is also wise not to burden the parents with too much paperwork and multiple consents. In addition, the child's assent is needed at the time of treatment. Unlike informed consent, assent is not always required by law, though IRBs may require it.

References

1. Porta M. A dictionary of epidemiology. 6th ed. New York: Oxford University Press; 2014.
2. American Dental Association. Specialty definitions. https://www.ada.org/en/ncrdscb/dental-specialties/specialty-definitions. Adopted Mar 2018.
3. Centers for Disease Control and Prevention. Ten great public health achievements. United States, 1900–1999. https://www.cdc.gov/mmwr/preview/mmwrhtml/00056796.htm.
4. Gordis L. Epidemiology. 5th ed. Philadelphia, PA: Elsevier Saunders; 2014.
5. Rothman KJ, Greenland S. Types of epidemiological studies. In: Rothman KJ, Greenland S, editors. Modern epidemiology. 2nd ed. Philadelphia, PA: Lippincott-Raven; 1998.
6. Arnold FA Jr, Dean HT, Jay P, Knutson JW. Effect of fluoridated public water supplies on dental caries prevalence. Public Health Rep. 1956;71(7):652–8.
7. Ast DB, Finn SB, Mc CI. The Newburgh-Kingston caries fluorine study; dental findings after three years of water fluoridation. Am J Public Health Nations Health. 1950;40(6):716–24. https://doi.org/10.2105/ajph.40.6.716.
8. Backer Dirks O, Houwink B, Kwant GW. The results of 6 1/2 years of artificial fluoridation of drinking water in The Netherlands. The Tiel-Culemborg experiment. Arch Oral Biol. 1961;5:284–300. https://doi.org/10.1016/0003-9969(61)90065-6.
9. Iheozor-Ejiofor Z, Worthington HV, Walsh T, O'Malley L, Clarkson JE, Macey R, et al. Water fluoridation for the prevention of dental caries. Cochrane Database Syst Rev. 2015;2015(6):CD010856. https://doi.org/10.1002/14651858.CD010856.pub2.
10. Rugg-Gunn AJ, Spencer AJ, Whelton HP, Jones C, Beal JF, Castle P, et al. Critique of the review of 'Water fluoridation for the prevention of dental caries' published by the Cochrane Collaboration in 2015. Br Dent J. 2016;220(7):335–40. https://doi.org/10.1038/sj.bdj.2016.257.
11. Marinho VC, Higgins JP, Sheiham A, Logan S. Fluoride toothpastes for preventing dental caries in children and adolescents. Cochrane Database Syst Rev. 2003;2016(1):CD002278. https://doi.org/10.1002/14651858.CD002278.
12. Santos AP, Nadanovsky P, Oliveira BH. A systematic review and meta-analysis of the effects of fluoride toothpastes on the prevention of dental caries in the primary dentition of preschool children. Community Dent Oral Epidemiol. 2013;41(1):1–12. https://doi.org/10.1111/j.1600-0528.2012.00708.x.
13. Santos AP, Oliveira BH, Nadanovsky P. Effects of low and standard fluoride toothpastes on caries and fluorosis: systematic review and meta-analysis. Caries Res. 2013;47(5):382–90. https://doi.org/10.1159/000348492.
14. Twetman S. Caries prevention with fluoride toothpaste in children: an update. Eur Arch Paediatr Dent. 2009;10(3):162–7. https://doi.org/10.1007/BF03262678.
15. Twetman S, Axelsson S, Dahlgren H, Holm AK, Kallestal C, Lagerlof F, et al. Caries-preventive effect of fluoride toothpaste: a systematic review. Acta Odontol Scand. 2003;61(6):347–55. https://doi.org/10.1080/00016350310007590.
16. Walsh T, Worthington HV, Glenny AM, Marinho VC, Jeroncic A. Fluoride toothpastes of different concentrations for preventing dental caries. Cochrane Database Syst Rev. 2019;3:CD007868. https://doi.org/10.1002/14651858.CD007868.pub3.
17. Wright JT, Hanson N, Ristic H, Whall CW, Estrich CG, Zentz RR. Fluoride toothpaste efficacy and safety in children younger than 6 years: a systematic review. J Am Dent Assoc. 2014;145(2):182–9. https://doi.org/10.14219/jada.2013.37.
18. Davies GM, Worthington HV, Ellwood RP, Bentley EM, Blinkhorn AS, Taylor GO, et al. A randomised controlled trial of the effectiveness of providing free fluoride toothpaste from the age of 12 months on reducing caries in 5-6 year old children. Community Dent Health. 2002;19(3):131–6.
19. Tavener JA, Davies GM, Davies RM, Ellwood RP. The prevalence and severity of fluorosis in children who received toothpaste containing either 440 or 1,450 ppm F from the age of 12 months in deprived and less deprived communities. Caries Res. 2006;40(1):66–72. https://doi.org/10.1159/000088909.
20. Listl S, Grytten JI, Birch S. What is health economics? Community Dent Health. 2019;36(4):262–74. https://doi.org/10.1922/CDH_4581Listl13.
21. Sheiham A, James WP. Diet and dental caries: the pivotal role of free sugars reemphasized. J Dent Res. 2015;94(10):1341–7. https://doi.org/10.1177/0022034515590377.
22. Krasse B. Why was the Vipeholm study done and why have this symposium? Scand J Dent Res. 1989;97(2):99–102. https://doi.org/10.1111/j.1600-0722.1989.tb01436.x.
23. Gustafsson BE, Quensel CE, Lanke LS, Lundqvist C, Grahnen H, Bonow BE, et al. The Vipeholm dental caries study; the effect of different lev-

els of carbohydrate intake on caries activity in 436 individuals observed for five years. Acta Odontol Scand. 1954;11(3–4):232–64. https://doi.org/10.3109/00016355308993925.
24. Guideline: sugars intake for adults and children. Geneva: World Health Organization; 2015.
25. OECD/FAO. OECD-FAO agricultural outlook 2019-2028. Rome: OECD Publishing, Paris/Food and Agriculture Organization of the United Nations; 2019. https://doi.org/10.1787/agr_outlook-2019-en.
26. Birkhed D. Sugar substitutes—one consequence of the Vipeholm study? Scand J Dent Res. 1989;97(2):126–9. https://doi.org/10.1111/j.1600-0722.1989.tb01441.x.
27. Scheinin A, Makinen KK, Ylitalo K. Turku sugar studies. V. Final report on the effect of sucrose, fructose and xylitol diets on the caries incidence in man. Acta Odontol Scand. 1976;34(4):179–216. https://doi.org/10.3109/00016357608997711.
28. Moynihan PJ, Kelly SA. Effect on caries of restricting sugars intake: systematic review to inform WHO guidelines. J Dent Res. 2014;93(1):8–18. https://doi.org/10.1177/0022034513508954.
29. Jevdjevic M, Trescher AL, Rovers M, Listl S. The caries-related cost and effects of a tax on sugar-sweetened beverages. Public Health. 2019;169:125–32. https://doi.org/10.1016/j.puhe.2019.02.010.
30. Schwendicke F, Thomson WM, Broadbent JM, Stolpe M. Effects of taxing sugar-sweetened beverages on caries and treatment costs. J Dent Res. 2016;95(12):1327–32. https://doi.org/10.1177/0022034516660278.
31. Sowa PM, Keller E, Stormon N, Lalloo R, Ford PJ. The impact of a sugar-sweetened beverages tax on oral health and costs of dental care in Australia. Eur J Pub Health. 2019;29(1):173–7. https://doi.org/10.1093/eurpub/cky087.
32. von Philipsborn P, Stratil JM, Burns J, Busert LK, Pfadenhauer LM, Polus S, et al. Environmental interventions to reduce the consumption of sugar-sweetened beverages and their effects on health. Cochrane Database Syst Rev. 2019;6:CD012292. https://doi.org/10.1002/14651858.CD012292.pub2.
33. Moynihan P, Miller C. Beyond the chair: public health and governmental measures to tackle sugar. J Dent Res. 2020;99(8):871–6. https://doi.org/10.1177/0022034520919333.
34. Broadbent JM, Thomson WM, Poulton R. Trajectory patterns of dental caries experience in the permanent dentition to the fourth decade of life. J Dent Res. 2008;87(1):69–72. https://doi.org/10.1177/154405910808700112.
35. Nadanovsky P. Sugar consumption and dental caries. Br Dent J. 1994;177(8):280–1. https://doi.org/10.1038/sj.bdj.4808586.
36. Sheiham A. Why free sugars consumption should be below 15 kg per person per year in industrialised countries: the dental evidence. Br Dent J. 1991;171(2):63–5. https://doi.org/10.1038/sj.bdj.4807606.
37. Haworth S, Esberg A, Lif Holgerson P, Kuja-Halkola R, Timpson NJ, Magnusson PKE, et al. Heritability of caries scores, trajectories, and disease subtypes. J Dent Res. 2020;99(3):264–70. https://doi.org/10.1177/0022034519897910.
38. van Loveren C. Sugar restriction for caries prevention: amount and frequency. Which is more important? Caries Res. 2019;53(2):168–75. https://doi.org/10.1159/000489571.
39. Woodward M, Walker AR. Sugar consumption and dental caries: evidence from 90 countries. Br Dent J. 1994;176(8):297–302. https://doi.org/10.1038/sj.bdj.4808437.
40. Nadanovsky P, Sheiham A. Relative contribution of dental services to the changes in caries levels of 12-year-old children in 18 industrialized countries in the 1970s and early 1980s. Community Dent Oral Epidemiol. 1995;23(6):331–9. https://doi.org/10.1111/j.1600-0528.1995.tb00258.x.
41. Thaler RH, Sunstein CR. Improving decisions about health, wealth, and happiness. New York: Penguin Books; 2008.
42. Velema E, Vyth EL, Hoekstra T, Steenhuis IHM. Nudging and social marketing techniques encourage employees to make healthier food choices: a randomized controlled trial in 30 worksite cafeterias in The Netherlands. Am J Clin Nutr. 2018;107(2):236–46. https://doi.org/10.1093/ajcn/nqx045.
43. Marcano-Olivier M, Pearson R, Ruparell A, Horne PJ, Viktor S, Erjavec M. A low-cost Behavioural Nudge and choice architecture intervention targeting school lunches increases children's consumption of fruit: a cluster randomised trial. Int J Behav Nutr Phys Act. 2019;16(1):20. https://doi.org/10.1186/s12966-019-0773-x.
44. Kearns CE, Glantz SA, Schmidt LA. Sugar industry influence on the scientific agenda of the National Institute of Dental Research's 1971 National Caries Program: a historical analysis of internal documents. PLoS Med. 2015;12(3):e1001798. https://doi.org/10.1371/journal.pmed.1001798.
45. Alvesalo L, Brummer R, Le Bell Y. On the use of fissure sealants in caries prevention. A clinical study. Acta Odontol Scand. 1977;35(3):155–9. https://doi.org/10.3109/00016357709056004.
46. Llodra JC, Bravo M, Delgado-Rodriguez M, Baca P, Galvez R. Factors influencing the effectiveness of sealants—a meta-analysis. Community Dent Oral Epidemiol. 1993;21(5):261–8. https://doi.org/10.1111/j.1600-0528.1993.tb00771.x.
47. Mitchell L, Murray JJ. Fissure sealants: a critique of their cost-effectiveness. Community Dent Oral Epidemiol. 1989;17(1):19–23. https://doi.org/10.1111/j.1600-0528.1989.tb01819.x.
48. Ripa LW. Sealants revisted: an update of the effectiveness of pit-and-fissure sealants. Caries Res. 1993;27(Suppl 1):77–82. https://doi.org/10.1159/000261608.

49. Ahovuo-Saloranta A, Forss H, Walsh T, Nordblad A, Makela M, Worthington HV. Pit and fissure sealants for preventing dental decay in permanent teeth. Cochrane Database Syst Rev. 2017;7:CD001830. https://doi.org/10.1002/14651858.CD001830.pub5.
50. Weintraub JA, Stearns SC, Rozier RG, Huang CC. Treatment outcomes and costs of dental sealants among children enrolled in Medicaid. Am J Public Health. 2001;91(11):1877–81. https://doi.org/10.2105/ajph.91.11.1877.
51. Heller KE, Reed SG, Bruner FW, Eklund SA, Burt BA. Longitudinal evaluation of sealing molars with and without incipient dental caries in a public health program. J Public Health Dent. 1995;55(3):148–53. https://doi.org/10.1111/j.1752-7325.1995.tb02358.x.
52. Himida T, Promise U. School-based dental sealant programmes may be effective in caries prevention. Evid Based Dent. 2017;18(1):13–4. https://doi.org/10.1038/sj.ebd.6401218.
53. Muller-Bolla M, Lupi-Pegurier L, Bardakjian H, Velly AM. Effectiveness of school-based dental sealant programs among children from low-income backgrounds in France: a pragmatic randomized clinical trial. Community Dent Oral Epidemiol. 2013;41(3):232–41. https://doi.org/10.1111/cdoe.12011.
54. Deery C. Clinical practice guidelines proposed the use of pit and fissure sealants to prevent and arrest noncavitated carious lesions. J Evid Based Dent Pract. 2017;17(1):48–50. https://doi.org/10.1016/j.jebdp.2017.01.008.
55. Wright JT, Crall JJ, Fontana M, Gillette EJ, Novy BB, Dhar V, et al. Evidence-based clinical practice guideline for the use of pit-and-fissure sealants: a report of the American Dental Association and the American Academy of Pediatric Dentistry. J Am Dent Assoc. 2016;147(8):672–82.e12. https://doi.org/10.1016/j.adaj.2016.06.001.
56. Chestnutt IG, Hutchings S, Playle R, Morgan-Trimmer S, Fitzsimmons D, Aawar N, et al. Seal or varnish? A randomised controlled trial to determine the relative cost and effectiveness of pit and fissure sealant and fluoride varnish in preventing dental decay. Health Technol Assess. 2017;21(21):1–256. https://doi.org/10.3310/hta21210.
57. Chestnutt IG, Playle R, Hutchings S, Morgan-Trimmer S, Fitzsimmons D, Aawar N, et al. Fissure seal or fluoride varnish? A randomized trial of relative effectiveness. J Dent Res. 2017;96(7):754–61. https://doi.org/10.1177/0022034517702094.
58. Frencken JE, Wolke J. Clinical and SEM assessment of ART high-viscosity glass-ionomer sealants after 8-13 years in 4 teeth. J Dent. 2010;38(1):59–64. https://doi.org/10.1016/j.jdent.2009.09.004.
59. Alsabek L, Al-Nerabieah Z, Bshara N, Comisi JC. Retention and remineralization effect of moisture tolerant resin-based sealant and glass ionomer sealant on non-cavitated pit and fissure caries: randomized controlled clinical trial. J Dent. 2019;86:69–74. https://doi.org/10.1016/j.jdent.2019.05.027.
60. Sheiham A. Is there a scientific basis for six-monthly dental examinations? Lancet. 1977;2(8035):442–4. https://doi.org/10.1016/s0140-6736(77)90620-1.
61. Riley P, Worthington HV, Clarkson JE, Beirne PV. Recall intervals for oral health in primary care patients. Cochrane Database Syst Rev. 2013;(12):CD004346. https://doi.org/10.1002/14651858.CD004346.pub4.
62. Wang N, Marstrander P, Holst D, Ovrum L, Dahle T. Extending recall intervals-effect on resource consumption and dental health. Community Dent Oral Epidemiol. 1992;20(3):122–4. https://doi.org/10.1111/j.1600-0528.1992.tb01544.x.
63. INTERVAL Dental Recalls Trial. ISRCTN95933794. https://doi.org/10.1186/ISRCTN95933794.
64. Clarkson JE, Pitts NB, Fee PA, Goulao B, Boyers D, Ramsay CR, et al. Examining the effectiveness of different dental recall strategies on maintenance of optimum oral health: the INTERVAL dental recalls randomised controlled trial. Br Dent J. 2021;230(4):236–43. https://doi.org/10.1038/s41415-021-2612-0.
65. Disease GBD, Injury I, Prevalence C. Global, regional, and national incidence, prevalence, and years lived with disability for 354 diseases and injuries for 195 countries and territories, 1990-2017: a systematic analysis for the Global Burden of Disease Study 2017. Lancet. 2018;392(10159):1789–858. https://doi.org/10.1016/S0140-6736(18)32279-7.
66. Kassebaum NJ, Smith AGC, Bernabe E, Fleming TD, Reynolds AE, Vos T, et al. Global, regional, and national prevalence, incidence, and disability-adjusted life years for oral conditions for 195 countries, 1990-2015: a systematic analysis for the global burden of diseases, injuries, and risk factors. J Dent Res. 2017;96(4):380–7. https://doi.org/10.1177/0022034517693566.
67. Listl S, Galloway J, Mossey PA, Marcenes W. Global economic impact of dental diseases. J Dent Res. 2015;94(10):1355–61. https://doi.org/10.1177/0022034515602879.
68. Guyatt GH, Osoba D, Wu AW, Wyrwich KW, Norman GR. Clinical Significance Consensus Meeting Group. Methods to explain the clinical significance of health status measures. Mayo Clin Proc. 2002;77(4):371–83. https://doi.org/10.4065/77.4.371.
69. Marinho VC, Worthington HV, Walsh T, Chong LY. Fluoride gels for preventing dental caries in children and adolescents. Cochrane Database Syst Rev. 2015;2021(6):CD002280. https://doi.org/10.1002/14651858.CD002280.pub2.
70. Weyant RJ, Tracy SL, Anselmo TT, Beltran-Aguilar ED, Donly KJ, Frese WA, et al. Topical fluoride for caries prevention: executive summary of the updated clinical recommendations and supporting systematic review. J Am Dent Assoc. 2013;144(11):1279–91. https://doi.org/10.14219/jada.archive.2013.0057.
71. Tickle M, O'Neill C, Donaldson M, Birch S, Noble S, Killough S, et al. A randomized con-

trolled trial of caries prevention in dental practice. J Dent Res. 2017;96(7):741–6. https://doi.org/10.1177/0022034517702330.
72. O'Neill C, Worthington HV, Donaldson M, Birch S, Noble S, Killough S, et al. Cost-effectiveness of caries prevention in practice: a randomized controlled trial. J Dent Res. 2017;96(8):875–80. https://doi.org/10.1177/0022034517708968.
73. Braun PA, Quissell DO, Henderson WG, Bryant LL, Gregorich SE, George C, et al. A cluster-randomized, community-based, tribally delivered oral health promotion trial in Navajo head start children. J Dent Res. 2016;95(11):1237–44. https://doi.org/10.1177/0022034516658612.
74. Kaur M, Sprague S, Ignacy T, Thoma A, Bhandari M, Farrokhyar F. How to optimize participant retention and complete follow-up in surgical research. Can J Surg. 2014;57(6):420–7. https://doi.org/10.1503/cjs.006314.
75. Sousa FSO, Santos APP, Nadanovsky P, Hujoel P, Cunha-Cruz J, Oliveira BH. Fluoride varnish and dental caries in preschoolers: a systematic review and meta-analysis. Caries Res. 2019;53(5):502–13. https://doi.org/10.1159/000499639.
76. U.S. Department of Health and Human Services, Public Health Service, Food and Drug Administration. Memo regarding K102973—silver dental arrest. Available at: https://www.accessdata.fda.gov/cdrh_docs/pdf10/K102973.pdf. Accessed 2 Aug 2021.
77. Oliveira BH, Cunha-Cruz J, Rajendra A, Niederman R. Controlling caries in exposed root surfaces with silver diamine fluoride: a systematic review with meta-analysis. J Am Dent Assoc. 2018;149(8):671–9 e1. https://doi.org/10.1016/j.adaj.2018.03.028.
78. Oliveira BH, Rajendra A, Veitz-Keenan A, Niederman R. The effect of silver diamine fluoride in preventing caries in the primary dentition: a systematic review and meta-analysis. Caries Res. 2019;53(1):24–32. https://doi.org/10.1159/000488686.
79. Seifo N, Cassie H, Radford JR, Innes NPT. Silver diamine fluoride for managing carious lesions: an umbrella review. BMC Oral Health. 2019;19(1):145. https://doi.org/10.1186/s12903-019-0830-5.
80. Duangthip D, Wong MCM, Chu CH, Lo ECM. Caries arrest by topical fluorides in preschool children: 30-month results. J Dent. 2018;70:74–9. https://doi.org/10.1016/j.jdent.2017.12.013.
81. Mabangkhru S, Duangthip D, Chu CH, Phonghanyudh A, Jirarattanasopha V. A randomized clinical trial to arrest dentine caries in young children using silver diamine fluoride. J Dent. 2020;99:103375. https://doi.org/10.1016/j.jdent.2020.103375.
82. Fung MHT, Duangthip D, Wong MCM, Lo ECM, Chu CH. Randomized clinical trial of 12% and 38% silver diamine fluoride treatment. J Dent Res. 2018;97(2):171–8. https://doi.org/10.1177/0022034517728496.
83. Marinho VC, Chong LY, Worthington HV, Walsh T. Fluoride mouthrinses for preventing dental caries in children and adolescents. Cochrane Database Syst Rev. 2016;7:CD002284. https://doi.org/10.1002/14651858.CD002284.pub2.
84. Moberg Skold U, Birkhed D, Borg E, Petersson LG. Approximal caries development in adolescents with low to moderate caries risk after different 3-year school-based supervised fluoride mouth rinsing programmes. Caries Res. 2005;39(6):529–35. https://doi.org/10.1159/000088191.
85. Kerbusch AE, Kuijpers-Jagtman AM, Mulder J, Sanden WJ. Methods used for prevention of white spot lesion development during orthodontic treatment with fixed appliances. Acta Odontol Scand. 2012;70(6):564–8. https://doi.org/10.3109/00016357.2011.640282.
86. Benson PE, Parkin N, Dyer F, Millett DT, Germain P. Fluorides for preventing early tooth decay (demineralised lesions) during fixed brace treatment. Cochrane Database Syst Rev. 2019;2019(11) https://doi.org/10.1002/14651858.CD003809.pub4.
87. Curnow MM, Pine CM, Burnside G, Nicholson JA, Chesters RK, Huntington E. A randomised controlled trial of the efficacy of supervised toothbrushing in high-caries-risk children. Caries Res. 2002;36(4):294–300. https://doi.org/10.1159/000063925.
88. Jackson RJ, Newman HN, Smart GJ, Stokes E, Hogan JI, Brown C, et al. The effects of a supervised toothbrushing programme on the caries increment of primary school children, initially aged 5-6 years. Caries Res. 2005;39(2):108–15. https://doi.org/10.1159/000083155.
89. Petersen PE, Hunsrisakhun J, Thearmontree A, Pithpornchaiyakul S, Hintao J, Jurgensen N, et al. School-based intervention for improving the oral health of children in southern Thailand. Community Dent Health. 2015;32(1):44–50.
90. Santos APP, Oliveira BH, Nadanovsky P. A systematic review of the effects of supervised toothbrushing on caries incidence in children and adolescents. Int J Paediatr Dent. 2018;28(1):3–11. https://doi.org/10.1111/ipd.12334.
91. Innes NP, Clarkson JE, Douglas GVA, Ryan V, Wilson N, Homer T, et al. Child caries management: a randomized controlled trial in dental practice. J Dent Res. 2020;99(1):36–43. https://doi.org/10.1177/0022034519888882.
92. Maguire A, Clarkson JE, Douglas GV, Ryan V, Homer T, Marshman Z, et al. Best-practice prevention alone or with conventional or biological caries management for 3- to 7-year-olds: the FiCTION three-arm RCT. Health Technol Assess. 2020;24(1):1–174. https://doi.org/10.3310/hta24010.
93. Griffin SO, Jones K, Gray SK, Malvitz DM, Gooch BF. Exploring four-handed delivery and retention of resin-based sealants. J Am Dent Assoc. 2008;139(3):281–9; quiz 358. https://doi.org/10.14219/jada.archive.2008.0157.

94. Screening and interventions to prevent dental caries in children younger than age 5 years: a systematic review for the U.S. Preventive Services Task Force. 11 May 2021. https://www.uspreventiveservicestaskforce.org/uspstf/document/draft-evidence-review/prevention-of-dental-caries-in-children-younger-than-age-5-years-screening-and-interventions1. Accessed 22 Sept 2021.
95. Glassman P, Subar P, Budenz AW. Managing caries in virtual dental homes using interim therapeutic restorations. J Calif Dent Assoc. 2013;41(10):744–7, 50–2.
96. Kohli R, Clemens J, Mann L, Newton M, Glassman P, Schwarz E. Training dental hygienists to place interim therapeutic restorations in a school-based teledentistry program: Oregon's virtual dental home. J Public Health Dent. 2021;82:229. https://doi.org/10.1111/jphd.12465.
97. Fleming TR, DeMets DL. Surrogate end points in clinical trials: are we being misled? Ann Intern Med. 1996;125(7):605–13. https://doi.org/10.7326/0003-4819-125-7-199610010-00011.
98. Pilot T. Periodontal diseases. In: Pine CM, editor. Community oral health. Oxford: Wright; 1997. p. 82–8.
99. Wennstrom JL, Papapanou PN, Grondahl K. A model for decision making regarding periodontal treatment needs. J Clin Periodontol. 1990;17(4):217–22. https://doi.org/10.1111/j.1600-051x.1990.tb00016.x.
100. Papapanou PN, Sanz M, Buduneli N, Dietrich T, Feres M, Fine DH, et al. Periodontitis: consensus report of workgroup 2 of the 2017 world workshop on the classification of periodontal and peri-implant diseases and conditions. J Clin Periodontol. 2018;45(Suppl 20):S162–70. https://doi.org/10.1111/jcpe.12946.
101. John MT. Health outcomes reported by dental patients. J Evid Based Dent Pract. 2018;18(4):332–5. https://doi.org/10.1016/j.jebdp.2018.09.001.
102. Prentice RL. Surrogate endpoints in clinical trials: definition and operational criteria. Stat Med. 1989;8(4):431–40. https://doi.org/10.1002/sim.4780080407.
103. Shaw WC. Dentofacial irregularities. In: Pine CM, editor. Community oral health. Oxford: Wright; 1997. p. 104–11.
104. Hujoel PP. Endpoints in periodontal trials: the need for an evidence-based research approach. Periodontol. 2000;2004(36):196–204. https://doi.org/10.1111/j.1600-0757.2004.03681.x.
105. Nadanovsky P, Santos A, Lira-Junior R, Oliveira BH. Clinical accuracy data presented as natural frequencies improve dentists' caries diagnostic inference: evidence from a randomized controlled trial. J Am Dent Assoc. 2018;149(1):18–24. https://doi.org/10.1016/j.adaj.2017.08.006.
106. Nadanovsky P, Costa LR, Santos APP. Risk communication in the context of clinical research. Braz Oral Res. 2020;34(Suppl 2):e078.
107. Tollefson J. Revolt of the randomistas. Nature. 2015;524:150–3.
108. Callaway E. 'Randomistas' who used controlled trials to fight poverty win economics Nobel. Nature. 2019; https://doi.org/10.1038/d41586-019-03125-y.
109. Moher D, Hopewell S, Schulz KF, Montori V, Gotzsche PC, Devereaux PJ, et al. CONSORT 2010 explanation and elaboration: updated guidelines for reporting parallel group randomised trials. BMJ. 2010;340:c869. https://doi.org/10.1136/bmj.c869.
110. Campbell MK, Piaggio G, Elbourne DR, Altman DG, CONSORT Group. Consort 2010 statement: extension to cluster randomised trials. BMJ. 2012;345:e5661. https://doi.org/10.1136/bmj.e5661.

4 Randomized Controlled Trials in Endodontics

Richie Kohli, Harjit Singh Sehgal, and Danielle Wingrove

4.1 Introduction

Well-designed and executed randomized controlled trials (RCTs) provide the reliable evidence on the effectiveness of healthcare interventions and thus decision-making in healthcare. Poorly done studies waste resources and raise ethical issues regarding the rights of participants. The Consolidated Standards of Reporting Trials (CONSORT) statement, originally developed in 1996 [1] and updated in 2010 [2] provides guidance to investigators in conducting and reporting clinical trials. The quality of RCTs in dental research and other fields of medicine is typically assessed using the CONSORT checklist as a reference to the standards, and trials following the CONSORT standards are more readily published. Top-flight journals will not publish studies that do not follow this guidance.

There have been two studies that have reviewed the quality of clinical studies in endodontics. First, Lucena et al. (2016) [3] assessed the quality of 89 RCTs in endodontics published from 1997 to 2012 using a checklist based on Jadad criteria [4], CONSORT statement, and SPIRIT [5] (Standard Protocol Items: Recommendations for Interventional Trials), the overall quality was poor. Many had serious methodological flaws. This is a devastating finding and suggests that both novice and more experienced researchers need to adopt a higher standard in future studies. Only 45% of the published work had a low risk of bias for random sequence generation, 75% did not provide information on allocation concealment, and in 19% of the investigators were not blinded. Only 55% of the RCT reports reviewed provided adequate sample size estimation, and only 16% included confidence intervals in reporting results. Almost all (87%) of the reports failed to provide sufficient information to determine whether the statistical methodology was appropriate. Higher quality was found in reports of multi-center studies, RCTs authored by more than five authors, reports published in journals ranked above the Journal of Citation Reports (JCR) median, and papers fully complying with the CONSORT guidelines.

Second, in a scoping review [6] of 354 randomized controlled trials, cohort, case–control

R. Kohli (✉)
Division of Dental Public Health, School of Dentistry, Oregon Health & Science University, Portland, OR, USA
e-mail: kohli@ohsu.edu

H. S. Sehgal
Division of Periodontology, Department of Regenerative and Reconstructive Sciences, School of Dentistry, Oregon Health & Science University, Portland, OR, USA
e-mail: sehgal@ohsu.edu

D. Wingrove
Endodontics, School of Dentistry, University of Utah, Salt Lake City, UT, USA
e-mail: danielle.wingrove@hsc.utah.edu

R. Kohli et al. (eds.), *Randomized Controlled Trials in Evidence-Based Dentistry*,
https://doi.org/10.1007/978-3-031-47651-8_4

studies, and case series of endodontic articles published after 1980 through 2020, two overarching limitations were identified: missing information and misreporting. Often missing were details on the prospective, retrospective, or ambispective nature of the study (especially for cohort and case series), the blinding of patient or outcome assessor/treatment provider, and reasons for the loss of participants at follow-up assessments. Misreporting of data was reported for units of sample size (count and percentage of patients, teeth, roots); overestimated outcome measure in multi-rooted teeth; exclusion of dropouts from the analyses (e.g., per protocol and not intention to treat analyses); and lack of standardized terminology for pulpal and periapical diagnosis.

The objective of this chapter is to critically review the existing key endodontics RCTs in terms of (1) research focus and outcomes and (2) research design, methods, and reporting issues, and to identify the strengths and limitations of these studies and give examples. We also discuss the unique challenges of conducting RCTs in endodontics, (3) gaps in the existing studies and future recommendations for novice and experienced researchers, and (4) newly introduced Preferred Reporting Items for RAndomized Trials in Endodontics (PRIRATE) guidelines.

4.2 Research Focus and Outcomes

A fundamental skill in designing RCTs is the ability to ask well-built clinical questions directly relevant to patients' problems and designed to precisely answer a question that addresses a gap in knowledge. To answer such a question requires clearly defined, reliable, and valid outcomes. The existing literature reports highly variable, and often idiosyncratic methods for measuring and reporting outcomes. Endodontic treatment outcomes assessment has evolved from landmark Strindberg's disease-based criteria [7] to patient-centered outcomes [8].

Strindberg's disease-based criteria defined treatment success as the absence of symptoms and normal radiographic appearance of the periapical tissues, which implies clinical, radiologic, and histologic resolution of inflammation whereas the presence of symptoms or radiographic changes is considered a treatment failure. This criterion was rigid and it also often led to erroneous conclusions because many studies were too short to really assess the physical or radiographic outcomes. This is particularly true with healing after root-end surgery. Hence, with more advancement in the endodontics field, patient-centered outcomes gained importance to determine success. Examples are oral health-related quality of life, total treatment time for the patient, number of visits, functional teeth not needing extraction, and treatment cost.

Lucena et al. (2016) [3] reported that the majority of RCTs in endodontics published between 1997 and 2012 posed questions regarding the efficacy of drugs or anesthesia or analgesia techniques (38.2%), the effectiveness of different materials or techniques in application to pulpotomy, pulpectomy or direct pulp capping (30.3%). The minority focused on the retreatment of periapical lesions [9], outcomes of a single visit and multiple visit RCTs [10], interventions for avulsed and replanted permanent front teeth [11], and regenerative endodontic procedures and outcomes [12]. The main findings from the top cited key RCTs, systematic reviews, Cochrane reviews, and meta-analyses are summarized in Box 4.1.

Box 4.1 Summary of the Main Findings from the Top Cited Key RCTs, Systematic Reviews, Cochrane Reviews, and Meta-analyses in Endodontics

- For the success of anesthesia, 4% articaine, 1:100,000 epinephrine is superior to 2% lidocaine, 1:100,000 epinephrine when root canal treatment is performed in teeth with irreversible pulpitis. For surgical procedures and surgical procedures/periodontal treatment of teeth with irreversible pulpitis, 2% lidocaine,

1:100,000 epinephrine is superior to 3% prilocaine, 0.03 IU felypressin, and 4% prilocaine plain, respectively [14].
– MTA seems to be the gold standard material in the pulpotomy of primary teeth. Promising results were also found with calcium silicate-based cement [27].
– There is no evidence to suggest differences in clinical outcomes or short- and long-term complications of root canal treatment in a single visit or in multiple visits [10].
– There is no evidence that a surgical approach leads to better results compared with non-surgical retreatment of teeth with apical periodontitis at 1 year or at 4 or 10 years after intervention [9].
– Due to a lack of robust evidence, the benefits and risks of different materials used for retrograde filling in root canal therapy are unclear [71].
– There is insufficient evidence to assess the difference in the effects of restoration of root canal-treated teeth with or without post and core by indirect restorations (e.g., crowns, inlays, or onlays) compared to conventional restorative materials placed directly into the teeth [65].
– There is also no evidence that antibiotics attenuate endodontic pain, thus antibiotics prescription in the absence of systemic involvement must be avoided to prevent antimicrobial resistance in patients [90, 91].
– There is a great need for further research on diagnostic procedures, risk factors, the management of root resorption, and the prognosis of affected teeth to help clinicians and patients to make informed choices about treatment options for root resorption [80, 103].
– There are significantly improved outcomes in laser-assisted endodontic therapy, suggesting the use of lasers as useful adjunctive treatment modalities, but the existing studies are heterogeneous and have design limitations [97]. Better quality studies are needed to confirm these findings.
– There is insufficient evidence to draw conclusions regarding the superiority of different interventions for avulsed (knocked out) and replanted teeth (e.g., hyperbaric oxygen, root canal pastes like Ledermix versus Ultracal, pulp extirpation, and soaking the knocked out tooth in thymosin alpha) with clinical outcomes of periodontal healing, tooth survival, pulpal healing, pain, and aesthetics (discoloration) [11].
– For immature and mature teeth with pulpal necrosis and apical periodontitis, the comparison of tooth survival and periapical health with revitalization versus RCT treatment options has shown mostly inconclusive findings due to a lack of well-designed robust studies as well as relatively newer treatment options for revitalization [105].

4.2.1 Efficacy of Drugs or Anesthesia or Analgesia Techniques

Local anesthetics (LA) are widely used in endodontics to control pain during dental treatment. There are different local anesthetic formulations and techniques available to dentists, but the success of local anesthesia has been reported to vary as a result of underlying pathology, materials, and procedural factors like dosage, presence of inflammation, tooth type, operative procedure (e.g., dental extraction vs. root canal treatment), and type of technique used, and patient factors like presence or absence of anxiety. Patients with high levels of anxiety usually exhibit lower pain thresholds [13] and, therefore, there is a decreased anesthesia success rate among these patients. However, patients with anxiety or who are on antianxiety medications are generally excluded from the clinical trials determining the success of local anesthesia and resulting in reduced generalizability and validity, especially since most of the investigators did not measure dental anxiety systematically, resulting in confounding. There are also challenges comparing RCTs to assess the success of one type of LA with another because of the difference in LA formulations available in different countries and that formulations with higher vasoconstrictor concentration may be contraindicated in patients with certain medical conditions.

A recent Cochrane Review by George et al. (2018) [14] concluded that low-quality evidence plagues these study reports decreasing confidence that the results are valid. Examples are: success (absence of pain), 4% articaine, 1:100,000 epinephrine was superior to 2% lidocaine, 1:100,000 epinephrine when root canal treatment was performed in posterior teeth with irreversible pulpitis, and 2% lidocaine, 1:100,000 epinephrine was superior to 4% prilocaine when surgical procedures/periodontal treatment was provided. Moderate-quality evidence gives greater confidence: the studies showed that 2% lidocaine, 1:100,000 epinephrine was superior to 3% prilocaine, 0.03 IU felypressin when surgical procedures were performed. An additional problem is that to assess any subgroup differences between injection types, a priori power analysis, and appropriate subgroup sample sizes are needed, which was found lacking.

The major considerations for RCTs studying analgesia and techniques are to use validated criteria of success and clinical outcomes and clearly report them. Validity of a measure refers to results being measured accurately and that the measure actually measures what it is supposed to measure. Examples of measures that are commonly used and reported, but likely, not valid are the presence/absence of pain measured by Visual Analogue Scale (VAS), pulpal anesthesia check by an electric pulp tester (EPT) or cold stimulus, and speed of onset and duration of anesthesia measured with a clock. Since EPT and thermal pulp tests are not 100% accurate, the accurate diagnosis should not be based on one test result. Similarly, for self-reported pain measurement with the VAS measure, proper patient instructions are very important. It is suggested to have a training exercise with the investigator and the participant so the participant really understands what the investigator is looking for. Additional such measures are the area of soft tissue anesthesia measured by probing, patient self-reported experiences, volume and type of injection, type of procedure, tissues involved, real treatments versus simulated scenarios, local adverse events, and systemic effects [15].

In their review, George et al. (2018) [14] found a substantial number of simulated scenario trials testing healthy pulps with an electric pulp tester. Although studies (or testing) using simulation are convenient to carry out, they may not be valid and clinical anesthesia may be present at values less than a maximum pulp tester reading, which is a common criterion for success. For many clinical procedures, only a clinical intervention can be used to test the oral tissues or soft tissues anesthetized. Therefore, these study design elements and the results of the studies cited should be interpreted with caution.

4.2.2 Effectiveness of Different Materials or Techniques in Application to Pulp Capping, Pulpotomy, and Pulpectomy

4.2.2.1 Vital Pulp Therapy (VPT) Procedures

VPT procedures are ways of preserving the vitality and function of the dental pulp after an injury resulting from trauma, caries, or restorative procedures [16]. There have been a myriad of different materials and techniques tried over the years in an effort to find clinical methods to improve the success of pulp therapy. VPT includes indirect or direct pulp capping and partial or complete pulpotomy. According to the American Association of Endodontics (AAE) current diagnostic terminology, a vital pulp can be diagnosed in one of three categories: normal, reversible pulpitis, or irreversible pulpitis, which could be symptomatic or asymptomatic [17, 18].

Pulpotomy Techniques and Materials

Although both partial and full pulpotomy can be recommended in symptomatic irreversible pulpitis, there is a lack of consensus on which treatment is better. Partial pulpotomy maintains physiologic dentine deposition in the coronal area, which aids in the protection of the radicular pulp against dystrophic calcification caused by various pulpotomy agents [19]. However, it is difficult to assure the full removal of diseased tissue. Coronal pulpotomy eliminates all inflammatory pulp tissue and creates a solid layer of the pulp chamber's bottom for correct placement and condensation of the pulp-capping agent.

A meta-analysis by Elmsmari et al. (2019) [20] evaluated the effect of partial pulpotomy (PP) in caries-exposed permanent teeth and found 96% overall success, with 75% success in symptomatic irreversible pulpitis (SIP) at 1-year follow-up. Cushley et al. (2019) [21] conducted a systematic review to determine whether coronal pulpotomy is clinically effective in treating carious teeth with signs and symptoms indicative of irreversible pulpitis. The authors reported 97.4% clinical and 95.4% radiographic success of complete pulpotomy (CP) at 1-year follow-up in caries-exposed permanent teeth with signs indicative of symptomatic irreversible pulpitis (SIP). The success rates reduced with longer follow-up at 36 months with 93.97% clinical and 88.39% radiographic success. A comparative clinical trial included in this study [22] showed pulpotomy to have comparable success to pulpectomy (also called as root canal treatment) at 12-month follow-up (92.2% vs. 89% radiographic success) 24-month follow-up (86.7% vs. 79.5% radiographic success) and 60-month follow-up (71.3% vs. 65.8%), respectively. The clinical success at 12 and 24 months follow-up remained high for both treatments (97.6–98.1%).

However, the authors pointed out that the included studies showed evidence of high and unclear risk of bias, both detection and performance bias. And because of inadequate reporting by these studies, it was not possible for them to perform analyses for the secondary outcomes such as quality of life or cost-effectiveness. The authors also found additional limitations that the included studies varied in design, number of participants, and materials used for pulp capping. There was heterogeneity in reporting outcomes, with some studies reporting clinical and radiographic success, while others reported overall combined success or clinical success alone. Both outcomes are essential to determine periapical health. Most studies were conducted in hospital and university settings, and thus are difficult to apply to general dental practices. Further, the follow-up periods in existing studies have ranged from 6 months and 5 years. Future studies need to determine what is the most appropriate follow-up period when the healing process is unlikely to reverse its course, and when treatment can be concluded as success or failure, without a further need for follow-up. In situations when RCTs are done by endodontics graduate students, the follow-up periods are short due to the limited time they have during their specialty program. In these cases, we recommend faculty members design the studies and then different residents overtime work on these studies so the follow-up is adequate.

There are different medications used for pulpotomy procedures. These include formocresol, glutaraldehyde, ferric sulfate, and calcium hydroxide. As noted earlier also, the success rate for pulpotomy decreases over time, i.e., 90% or more in 6–12 months follow-up to 70% or less after 3 years or more [23, 24]. More recently mineral trioxide aggregate (MTA) has been used for pulpotomies for primary molars and has shown a 97% success rate [25]. Indirect pulp capping has shown higher long-term success rates than any pulpotomy procedures other than MTA [26]. Bossù et al. (2020) [27] concluded that mineral MTA is the gold standard material in the pulpotomy of primary teeth with a clinical and radiographical success rate ranging from 88% to 100% in studies with at least 12 months of follow-up. Even these seemingly adequate follow-up periods likely upwardly bias the results and need to be repeated with more realistic follow-up periods. This is often because regulatory agencies treat MTA as a medical device rather than a drug and lower standards exist for studies of devices. Promising results were similarly found with calcium silicate-based cement (Biotene). Nevertheless, there is considerable heterogeneity in the methods used in these RCTs making study comparisons difficult and likely biasing the clinical outcomes. Examples of unaccounted-for variations in methods are the use of rubber dams, pulpotomy using electrosurgery versus bur or sharp instrument, hemostasis with different agents, different compositions of restorative materials and their management, and clinician expertise. Thus, these factors should be carefully controlled while study planning, implementation, and reporting.

Pulp Capping

In direct pulp capping, at the site of pulpal exposure, the pulp is covered with a protective dressing or base, which aims to protect the pulp from additional injuries and permits healing and repair [18]. In indirect pulp capping, a protective cement or dressing is placed over a thin layer of remaining sound or slightly softened dentine which if removed, might expose the pulp [18].

The success rate of direct pulp capping varies between 70% and 98% in reported RCTs. The variation is unexplained: confounders (mediators, moderators) affecting the interpretation of the results, e.g., age, type of pulp exposure, size of the exposure and degree of pulp bleeding, type of dentition, and provider expertise are not accounted for. Future studies are needed that address these limitations. A 2016 systematic review and meta-analysis by Schwendicke et al. (2016) [28] evaluated studies of materials for direct capping that were evaluated clinically and/or radiographically after a minimum of 3 months. Studies are clearly needed where follow-up is more clinically realistic. Most studies used calcium hydroxide as a control and compared it to MTA, bonding without prior etching/conditioning, or bonding with prior etching/conditioning, enamel matrix proteins, resin-modified glass ionomer cement, calcium sulfate, zinc oxide eugenol, corticosteroids, antibiotics, or formocresol. One study compared MTA and calcium-enriched cement. The authors found that in permanent teeth, the risk of failure was significantly decreased if MTA instead of calcium hydroxide was used (risk ratio (RR) [95% confidence intervals (CI)] 0.59 [0.39/0.90]); no difference was found for primary teeth. The other comparisons did not find significant differences or were supported by only one study.

The authors found that there was insufficient data to provide definite recommendations for the use of a specific pulp capping material, and noted that dentists might consider using MTA instead of calcium hydroxide for direct capping to reduce the risk of failure. There are other several gaps in these studies. For example, the findings from studies that used pulp capping models using artificially exposed pulps in sound teeth are mostly applicable to situations with traumatic pulp exposure and studies are needed including teeth with carious exposures. Studies evaluating short-term histological reactions, which may be easy for graduate students to carry out, have little clinical significance. Typically, failures occur 2 years or longer after direct capping. Further other factors like special technique required for MTA, its high cost, long setting time, and difficult storage can result in the provider choosing one material over another for direct pulp capping.

Recently, indirect pulp treatment has been suggested to be more successful than direct pulp cap and pulpotomy in long-term studies, according to a review by the American Association of Pediatric Dentistry (AAPD) [29, 30]. In addition, indirect pulp treatment allows for normal exfoliation. It can be chosen instead of direct pulp capping or pulpotomy when the pulp is normal or has a diagnosis of reversible pulpitis and there is no pulp exposure [30]. There has also been a question about the effectiveness of vital pulp therapies as compared to pulpectomy. Wells et al. (2019) [31] evaluated the clinical evidence regarding the clinical effectiveness and safety of vital pulp therapies compared with pulpectomy. They reported that evidence from one very low-quality systematic review, and four very low to moderate-quality primary studies suggested that clinical success rates for teeth treated with vital pulp therapy or pulpotomy may not significantly differ from teeth treated with root canal therapy or pulpectomy. They also pointed out that findings were comparable between vital pulp therapy and a root canal or in favor of vital pulp therapy for short-term (1 week) postoperative pain reduction. Thus, future high-quality studies with longer follow-ups are needed to confirm these findings.

4.2.2.2 Pulpectomy Procedures and Materials

The goal of pulpectomy is the prevention and elimination of periapical disease [32]. The key steps involved in endodontic therapy aim to maintain asepsis in vital teeth and to provide decontamination of non-vital teeth [32]. These include the placement of a rubber dam, the use of a pre-sterilized armamentarium, and the use of antimicrobial irrigation solutions. Multiple studies have shown that even with advancements in chemomechanical preparation techniques, it is difficult to achieve complete cleaning and disinfection of the root canal system [33, 34]. A well-sealed canal system can also reduce leakage into the tooth and prevent coronal contamination as well as out of the tooth by remaining bacteria and their byproducts from the apex which has a significant impact on the success of treatment [35]. The filling of root canals, commonly known as obturation, is an important step in successful pulpectomy. The comparison of the effectiveness of different pulpectomy steps, procedures, and materials is described below.

Irrigation Techniques, Materials, and Activation Methods

Irrigation is critical in endodontic treatment and for apical periodontitis as it helps to reduce the bacterial load to ensure long-term healing. Different irrigation techniques and materials have been studied. Examples are conventional needle irrigation with only sodium hypochlorite (NaOCl), the combination of NaOCl with 1-hydroxyethane-1,1-diphosphonate, or etidronate (HEDP) and MTAD, the combination of NaOCl and chlorhexidine (CHX), and different irrigation activation methods (passive ultrasonic irrigation-PUI, XP-endo finisher, F-file activator, and EndoVac activator).

NaOCl is a commonly used irrigant due to its antimicrobial activity, ability to dissolve organic matter [36], and low cost [37]. Studies have reported that MTAD and HEDP in combination with either 2.5% or 1.3% NaOCl has been shown to reduce the bacterial load to a level below that is required as compared to NaOCl alone [36, 38–41]. Although both HEDP and MTDA are highly effective in completely removing the smear layer, MTDA's action is enhanced when a lower concentration of NaOCl (1.3%) [36–38]. Chlorhexidine (CHX) is used as an alternative to NaOCl because of its antimicrobial activity, effectiveness lasting for days to weeks, and prevention of root canal reinfection [36, 42]. Studies have shown that an increased CHX concentration of 2% reduces the bacterial load as effectively as 1% NaOCl [43, 44].

More recent research has suggested that 3.8% SDF (silver diamine fluoride) exerts antibacterial characteristics against an *Enterococcus faecalis* biofilm and should be further tested as a root canal irrigant to reduce treatment failure in both primary and permanent teeth [45]. Future clinical studies also need to have an adequate sample size and consider other variables such as present microbial species and their spatial location in the root canal system, their access to nutrients, and their ability to adapt and survive [46].

When comparing irrigation systems, activation methods, i.e., ultrasonic irrigation, have shown statistically significant action in reducing bacterial load when compared to conventional needle irrigation systems [41, 46, 47]. In their systematic review, Tonini et al. (2022) [37] found that activation methods provide significantly higher biofilm reduction than conventional needle irrigation methods. Based on their literature review, Prada et al. (2019) [48] concluded that the most adequate irrigation protocol consists of using 2.5% NaOCl activated with ultrasound followed by a final wash with 7% maleic acid (MA) or 0.2% cetrimide (CTR) combined with 2% CHX. Crozeta et al. (2020) [49] evaluated the efficacy of passive ultrasonic irrigation (PUI) and the GentleWave system as supplementary techniques to remove remaining filling materials from oval-shaped root canals. They found that the use of PUI and GentleWave as supplementary techniques significantly reduced the volume of remaining filling material after initial instrumentation. PUI removed 18% of the remaining filling material, whereas the GentleWave system removed approximately 10% ($P < 0.05$). The strength of this study was the use of micro-CT to allow equitable tooth selection of single and oval-shaped distal canals. This minimized the effects of variable root canal anatomy, improved sample standardization, and facilitated an equal sample distribution between the experimental groups based on the remaining volume of filling material. This study had a major limitation that there was difficulty in the standardization of irrigant volumes because the GentleWave system delivers approximately 50 mL of irrigation solution per minute. The authors suggested the development of new techniques and protocols to enhance root canal cleanliness during nonsurgical endodontic retreatment to improve treatment outcomes.

In their systematic reviews, Goncalves et al. [50] and Tonini et al. [37] found that the details on the irrigating protocols, especially regarding irrigants' application time or total volumes, have not been adequately reported in the literature. Tonini et al. [37] noted that for the included studies, describing their protocols was very complex, application time and volume of irrigants were not always reported, and comparing the results was impossible due to the heterogeneity of the methodologies. They concluded that the existing literature lacks high-quality studies, and the level of evidence is moderate. Based on the available evidence, the authors reported that activation methods provide significantly higher biofilm reduction than conventional needle irrigation methods. Combinations of NaOCl with different chelating agents were ineffective in terms of antimicrobial, but it could potentially increase the risk of irrigant extrusion. The irrigating protocols, especially those regarding the irrigant's application time or total volume, were not carefully detailed in the included studies.

They also pointed out that the lack of double-blind procedures and concerns regarding the selectivity of the reported results reduced the quality of the studies. And that the lack of a universal standard for assessing the antibacterial efficacy of endodontic treatment prevents determining standard protocols for optimal irrigation methods. Considering the limitations of the included studies and the review itself, the authors acknowledged that activated irrigation procedures are fundamental for reducing the bacterial load in the whole root canal system and that NaOCl continues to be a key element in all protocols. They recommended that improving the quality of studies requires identifying more efficient protocols and more suitable approaches that facilitate the work of clinicians, reduce chairside time, and have more reliable outcomes.

Obturation Techniques and Materials

The ideal root canal filling material should be easy to introduce into the root canal, seal the canal laterally and apically, not shrink after being inserted, and be impervious to moisture, bacteriostatic, radiopaque, not stain tooth structure or irritate periradicular tissues [51, 52]. It should also be sterile or easily and quickly sterilized immediately before insertion. Further, it should be easily removable from the root canal if retreatment is required. Gutta-percha is the most popular and commonly used root canal filling material, generally placed with a sealer [53, 54]. The main difference in how dental practitioners fill a root canal system depends on the technique to place the gutta-percha and the sealer system used.

In combination with gutta-percha, endodontic sealers play a critical role in obturation techniques. They fill the gaps not obturated with gutta-percha. Epoxy resin-based sealers are frequently used as a reference material for comparisons with newly developed sealers [55] as they provide a stable apical seal [56]. These materials used with gutta-percha in vertical (warm) or lateral (cold) compaction techniques are considered the gold standard for sealer cements [57, 58]. Many alternatives to the traditional gutta-percha-based systems have been proposed to enhance the seal at sealer–core obturation material and sealer-radicular dentine interfaces [59].

The warm vertical technique is one of the most utilized obturation techniques [57], with cold lateral condensation used frequently for comparison with other filling techniques. Tooth survival has been reported as similar in teeth treated using cold lateral condensation and warm gutta-percha obturation technique, Thermafil [58, 60, 61]. The overall success rate was 96% with Thermafil and 98% in the cold lateral condensation group, with slightly lower success rates over a 2-year recall period in the Thermafil group [57]. But this difference was not statistically significant ($P > 0.05$). With regard to radiographic evidence of the reduction in apical lesion size and normal periodontal ligament space, cold lateral condensation resulted in the resolution of periapical lesions from 44% to 15% while in the thermoplasticized experimental gutta-percha group, it decreased from 59% to 5% [61, 62], In this study, the absence of calcium hydroxide-based sealer did not make any difference to the outcome.

A carrier-based system (Softcore) used with Diaket sealer has also shown similar outcomes to laterally condensed gutta-percha for the healing of apical periodontitis (AP) [63]. Comparison of hand filing/lateral condensation to NiTi/single matched cone showed that both protocols lead to a similar healing rate of AP. The success rate ranged from 73% to 78% after 12 months [64]. When assessing a single-file Reciproc system and a single-cone technique with hand filing as compared to the crowndown technique and obturation with gutta-percha and AH Plus sealer using lateral condensation technique for the management of anterior teeth with AP, no difference in incidence, the intensity of postoperative pain, and the incidence of flare-up were observed [64].

In their comprehensive review, Komabayashi et al. (2020) [54] reported that as compared to AH Plus, tricalcium silicate sealers show the lowest relative microleakage among the sealers assessed, followed by silicone sealers and other non-AH Plus epoxy resin sealers. Tricalcium silicate sealers are the most favorable antimicrobial effect and excellent biocompatibility. The authors recommended that future sealers developed should combine a hermetic seal with therapeutic effects.

In their systematic review, Pirani et al. (2022) [61] compared alternatives (non-lateral compaction techniques) to the standard cold laterally condensed gutta-percha and also assessed the efficacy of different sealers compared with epoxy resin, AH Plus sealer in the management of apical periodontitis in permanent teeth. The authors did not find any difference between different procedures and materials in relation to tooth survival, pain, tenderness, swelling, and need for medication. Only a few studies included information on radiographic evidence of a reduction in apical lesion size or improvement in oral health-related quality of life. The risk of bias was high, thus the findings need to be replicated in better-designed studies. The authors suggested that well-designed RCTs should be carried on with follow-up of at least 4 years and supported by an adequate sample size calculation to identify clinically significant differences in the long term between the efficacy of the various alternative filling techniques and sealers.

Single Visit Versus Multiple Visits to Perform Root Canal Therapy

Another frequent area of research in endodontics is the number of treatment visits needed to perform root canal therapy (RCT), also called pulpectomy. Historically, the filling of infected canals was delayed until bacterial cultures were negative but today most clinicians do not follow this practice. A 2018 Cochrane review found that there is no evidence to suggest differences in clinical outcomes or short and long-term complications of root canal treatment in a single visit or in multiple visits [10]. Single-visit treatment, however, has a higher frequency of late postoperative pain. Most of these studies were done before engine-driven techniques were introduced and might be repeated with a higher standard. The existing studies mostly do not describe the gender and race/ethnicity of the participants. Many of the study populations do not include older adults or patients with special health care needs. Thus, the populations are likely not representative of the population in need of care and results cannot be generalized. Studies are needed in which the study participants mirror those seeking care. In addition, studies done in public hospitals or university clinics, where the expertise of clinicians and postgraduate students performing root canal treatments, may be less than those in private clinics raise validity issues that need to be addressed in designing future work. Rarely do studies describe the training and calibration or certification of the clinicians or provide any measure of fidelity of the treatment to the protocol.

Restoration of Endodontically Treated Teeth With or Without Posts

There are limited studies assessing the outcomes of restoration of endodontically treated teeth by indirect compared to direct conventional restorations. It is argued that indirect restorations help to protect root-filled teeth by reducing fractures while direct restorations are less time and cost-demanding and require less tooth structure removal. A 2015 Cochrane review [65] concluded that there is insufficient evidence to assess the difference in the effects of restoration of endodontically treated teeth with or without post and core by indirect restorations (e.g., crowns, inlays, or on-lays) compared to conventional restorative materials placed directly into the teeth. This review included only a single study [66] with a high risk of performance, detection, and attrition bias. Higher quality RCTs are needed to reach clinically meaningful conclusions. These studies must include random assignment as selection bias is a common problem in this type of study.

In their clinical study, Prakash et al. (2022) [67] compared the clinical survival rates of custom-fabricated cast metal post-and-cores in cases of anterior and posterior teeth while controlling for the population's age and gender, type of post material, length of the post, amount of alveolar bone tissue supporting the roots, tooth location in the dental arch, and type of cement used, as well as the effect of opposing dentition and the type of definitive prosthetic treatment received. They reported that no significant changes were observed between the stability of the post structures in the anterior and posterior teeth that were examined, and the survival rates were found to be similar in both instances. Thus they concluded that anterior and posterior teeth with cast metal posts performed at a similar success rate for the 1-year period, but suggested longer follow-up periods to further assess the findings for future studies.

The studies would also have been improved had the researchers used standardized evaluation methods such as modified United States Public Health Service Commissioned Corps (USPHS) guidelines for clinical evaluation of dental restorative materials [68]. These criteria focus on (a) choices of clinically relevant criteria; (b) assessment using simple nominal scales; (c) calibration of evaluators; (d) two independent evaluations; (e) nonparametric statistical analysis that recognizes the patient (and not the restoration) as the independent variable; and (f) additional parameters such as postoperative sensitivity, fracture, interproximal contact, and occlusal contact [68].

4.2.3 Endodontic Procedures for Retreatment of Periapical Lesions

4.2.3.1 Surgical Versus Non-surgical Therapy

When there is a failure of primary root canal therapy, periapical lesions can be retreated with or without surgery. Non-surgical root canal retreatment involves the removal of root canal filling materials from the tooth followed by cleaning, reshaping, and re-obturation of the canals. Surgical root-end resection involves exposure of the periapical lesion through osteotomy, surgical curettage of the soft tissue infected tissue, removal of part of the root-end tip to enable access, disinfection, and, retrograde sealing or filling of the apical portion of the remaining root canal.

In their systematic review, Torabinejad et al. (2009) [69] compared the clinical and radiographic outcomes of nonsurgical retreatment with those of root end resection to determine which modality offers more favorable outcomes. The authors found a significantly higher success rate for endodontic surgery at 2–4 years (77.8%) compared with nonsurgical retreatment (70.9%; $P < 0.05$). At 4–6 years, however, this relationship was reversed, with nonsurgical retreatment having a higher success rate of 83.0% compared with 71.8% for endodontic surgery ($P < 0.05$). They concluded that endodontic surgery has more favorable initial success, but nonsurgical retreatment offers a more favorable long-term outcome. Kang et al. (2015) [70] reported that endodontic microsurgery and nonsurgical retreatment have 92% and 80% of overall pooled data success rates, respectively. However, when the data were organized and analyzed according to their follow-up periods, a significantly higher success rate was found for the microsurgery group in the short-term follow-up (<4 years), whereas no significant difference was observed in the long-term follow-up (>4 years), consistent with what was found in the other studies comparing conventional and surgical treatment [70].

More recently, Del Fabbro et al. (2016) [9] assessed (1) the effects of surgical and non-surgical therapy for retreatment of teeth with apical periodontitis; and (2) the effects of surgical root-end resection under various conditions, like different materials, devices, or techniques. Outcomes were assessed by the healing of the periapical lesion assessed after a 1-year follow-up or longer; postoperative pain and discomfort; and adverse effects evaluated through radiographs. The authors found that there is no evidence that a surgical approach leads to better results compared with non-surgical retreatment at 1 year or at 4 or 10 years after intervention. But people who were treated surgically reported more pain and swelling during the first week after treatment. With regard to different surgical techniques, healing at 1-year follow-up was improved by the use of ultrasonic devices, instead of the traditional bur, for root-end preparation. There was some evidence of better healing at a 1-year follow-up when root ends were filled with MTA as compared to smoothing of orthograde gutta-percha root filling. The application of a graft composed of a gel enriched with the patient's own platelets to the defect during the surgical procedure significantly reduced postoperative pain. The use of a low-energy level laser did not reduce pain at the surgical site. There was no evidence for the use of antibiotics to reduce postoperative infection occurrence. The enhancement of the surgeon's view through different ways (surgical microscope, loupes, and endoscope) did not lead to different results at least 1 year after the operation, and results of retreatment were independent of the radiographic technique used to make the diagnosis.

In all, the authors judged the quality of the evidence to be poor [9]; therefore, we cannot rely on the findings. Out of 20 studies assessed, only one study had a low risk of bias and the majority of them had a high risk of bias. Most bias was due to a lack of allocation concealment and blinding of operators, participants, and evaluators, and omission of most information regarding the source of funding, the characteristics of participants, the teeth, and the lesions. In many studies, some participants had more than one tooth treated and data were provided with only the tooth and not the participant considered as the analysis unit. The authors concluded that future high-quality studies are needed to understand whether a surgical or a non-surgical approach should be used, and which surgical procedures may provide the best and most predictable results for the healing of periapical lesions and patient's quality of life. They also recommended that future studies should use standardized techniques and success criteria, precisely defined outcomes, specific features of the periapical lesion and use the participant, not the tooth, as the analysis unit, and follow the CONSORT recommendations for reporting.

4.2.3.2 Retrograde Filling Materials

In a recent Cochrane Review, Li et al. (2021) [71] compared studies of different retrograde filling materials with the reported success rate assessed by clinical or radiological methods and a follow-up period of at least 12 months. The authors included eight RCTs published between 1995 and 2019 and they were assessed as being at a high overall risk of bias. The authors concluded that due to a lack of robust evidence, the benefits and risks of different materials used for retrograde filling in root canal therapy are unclear. Future studies are needed with a large number of participants from different ethnicities and increased follow-up periods to observe the long-term effects and safety. More research is also needed on the use of a chelating agent or accelerator to overcome the main drawback of MTA and its long setting time. Most studies only have the participants and the statistical assessor blinded and not the surgeon or the radiograph observer. Christiansen (2009) [72] used a practical method to blind the radiograph observers in which they exported radiographs from the Digora system in TIFF format to Adobe Photoshop format, masking the apical root filling with grey patches. Future studies could use this methodology for blinding.

4.2.4 Antibiotic Use

Symptomatic apical periodontitis and acute apical abscess are common causes of dental pain due to inflamed or necrotic dental pulp, or infection of the pulpless root canal system. The treatment requires the removal of the source of inflammation or infection by local operative measures. Systemic antibiotics are currently only recommended for situations where there is evidence/signs of spreading infection or systemic involvement or in medically/immunocompromised patients [73–75]. Endodontic conditions like symptomatic reversible and irreversible pulpitis, pulpal necrosis, acute apical periodontitis, acute apical abscess with no systemic involvement, and chronic apical abscess do not need antibiotic coverage and have no added therapeutic benefit [73–75].

In a Cochrane review, Cope et al. (2018) [76] evaluated the effects of systemic antibiotics provided with or without surgical intervention (such as extraction, incision and drainage of swelling, or endodontic treatment), with or without analgesics, for symptomatic apical periodontitis and acute apical abscess in adults. Based on the two trials included in this review, the authors found no clear differences in the pain or swelling reported by participants who received oral antibiotics compared with a placebo when provided alongside the first stage of root canal treatment and analgesics. However, the authors pointed out that the studies were small and of poor quality with a high and unclear risk of attrition bias. Neither study assessed the effect of antibiotics on their own, without surgical dental treatment, so future studies in this area will be helpful.

In an update of the 2016 Cochrane Review [77], Agnihotry et al. (2019) [78] assessed the randomized controlled trials which compared pain relief with systemic antibiotics and analgesics, against placebo and analgesics in the acute preoperative phase of irreversible pulpitis. Only one study [79] of 103 studies screened met the inclusion criteria and was included in the review. Although this study had a low risk of bias, it was underpowered with only 20 participants in each study arm and thus the results were not valid. The authors still stated that penicillin administration did not significantly reduce either the pain perception or the quantity of analgesic medication required by patients with irreversible pulpitis, not recognizing the limitations of their work. The evidence certainty was rated low in the Cochrane Review for different outcomes. Future studies are needed with robust methodology including a priori power analyses and appropriate sample sizes that can provide additional evidence as to whether antibiotics, prescribed in the preoperative phase, can affect treatment outcomes for irreversible pulpitis.

4.2.5 Root Resorption

Root resorption is a progressive process that leads to the loss of dentin and cementum. This process is essential for primary dentition as it leads to the exfoliation of deciduous teeth. But root resorption in permanent teeth is pathological and can be classified according to its location, i.e., internal/external and cervical/apical.

External and internal root resorption can occur due to mechanical or chemical stimuli such as infection, pressure, trauma, or rapid orthodontic tooth movement. Resorption is detected primarily by radiography, but in some cases, it will manifest clinical symptoms such as pain, swelling, and tooth mobility; and for internal root resorption, color changes in tooth crown. The treatment of root resorption is focused on addressing the cause of the resorption and aiding the restoration or regeneration of the resorptive lesion.

4.2.5.1 External Root Resorption

Ahangari et al. (2015) [80] conducted a systematic review to assess studies of the effectiveness of different interventions (root canal medications and canal filling, splinting or extraction of teeth, or the surgical removal of any relevant pathology) for the management of external root resorption in permanent teeth. No randomized controlled trials were found. Most of the studies in this area are either retrospective with unclear inclusion criteria or observational studies, especially since the latter is a better choice for studying prognostic factors. Moreover, the commonly used two-dimensional (2D) images are not enough for the accuracy required for the diagnosis in these cases. Because of the low quality of the available evidence, Sondeijker et al. (2020) [81] could only provide weak recommendations regarding the prevention of external apical root resorption and its treatment.

4.2.5.2 Internal Root Resorption

Treatment of internal root resorption ranges from conventional root canal treatment to endodontic surgery and emerging treatment using revascularization. Based on three clinical reports, Ashraf et al. (2020) [82] reported promising results with revascularization of teeth with internal root resorption, i.e., previous symptoms disappeared, existing root resorption was arrested, and the root canal walls increased in thickness after treatment. Since these treatments were only carried out in the last 5 years with 12–24 months follow-up, no information is available on the revascularization procedure's long-term results and durability.

In conclusion, there is a great need for further research on the management of root resorption to help clinicians and patients make informed choices about treatment options for root resorption.

4.2.6 Managing Endodontic Emergencies

Endodontic emergencies (toothaches) account for 60–82% of the incidence of all dental emergencies [83]. The goal of the treatment of endodontic emergencies is to quickly and effectively manage pain and infections. Procedural interventions, i.e., pulpotomy and pulpectomy have been the first line and gold standard for endodontic emergency treatment with pulpectomy being the preferred choice of treatment [84].

Overall, studies related to the management of endodontic emergencies are of low to moderate quality with short-term follow-ups and limited generalizability.

There are several adjuncts available for use with emergency pulpotomy and pulpectomy procedures: incision and drainage, as adjunctive therapy is indicated for localized, firm or fluctuant intraoral soft tissue swelling to release fluid pressure, reduction in microbial and inflammatory mediators, and prevention of spread of infection to deeper fascial tissues. In their systematic review and meta-analysis, Zanjir et al. (2020) [85] found that very low- to moderate-quality evidence suggests that NSAIDs or NSAIDs plus acetaminophen administered after nonsurgical endodontic treatment lead to a clinically relevant decrease in postoperative pain for patients with irreversible pulpitis or pulpal necrosis and are the most effective treatments available. Postoperative corticosteroids or opioids did not significantly decrease postoperative pain [85].

A recent systematic review and meta-analysis by Smith et al. (2017) [86] demonstrated that a combination of ibuprofen 600 mg and acetaminophen 1000 mg is more effective than a placebo but not significantly different than ibuprofen 600 mg at 6 h postoperatively. Ibuprofen 600 mg is more effective than placebo at 6 h postoperatively; however, there are insufficient data to recommend the most effective NSAID, dosage, and dose interval for postoperative endodontic pain relief of longer duration in patients with preoperative pain. Taggar et al. (2017) [87] compared a newer ibuprofen formulation with 512 mg dose, ibuprofen sodium dihydrate with conventional ibuprofen acid in endodontic pain patients. They found that in endodontic pain patients, a single dose of ibuprofen sodium dihydrate provides a faster onset of pain relief and a greater reduction in spontaneous and evoked pain compared with ibuprofen acid. Although no endodontic treatment was provided in this study, a quicker onset of action of ibuprofen sodium dehydrate is likely to benefit patients with post-endodontic pain. These treatments need to be evaluated over days or weeks after drug administration but before completion of endodontic therapy. Future research is needed to assess the long-term effectiveness of these drugs.

In addition, intramuscular or infiltration injection of ketorolac trimethamine has been shown to significantly decrease moderate to severe pulpal pain over a 3-h tested time or oral administration of ibuprofen sodium dihydrate over a 1-h time period [88]. Future studies are needed to evaluate pain relief over days or weeks after drug administration but before the completion of endodontic therapy.

In their systematic review, Alves et al. (2021) [89] analyzed the influence of occlusal reduction on the postoperative pain levels after instrumentation and obturation of the root canal. The results did not reveal a significant difference in the reduction of postoperative pain levels for endodontic instrumentation at 6, 12, 24, 48 h and for endodontic obturation at 6 or 12 h after occlusal reduction. There is also no evidence that antibiotics attenuate endodontic pain [90], thus antibiotics prescription in the absence of systemic involvement must be avoided to prevent antimicrobial resistance in patients [91].

Another issue that requires attention in endodontics research is inter-appointment flare-ups during endodontic treatment or post-endodontic treatment flare-ups, which are the most common and major problems faced by endodontists [92]. Flare-ups are multifactorial in origin and can occur due to mechanical, chemical, and microbial factors [93]. During endodontic flare-ups, patients have pain and/or swelling leading to emergency visits for relief of the associated symptoms [94]. The incidence of endodontic flare-ups ranges from 1.4% to 16% and even up to 50% [95, 96]. Most of these studies are retrospective in nature. The ones which are prospective have smaller sample sizes. In addition, such variability in frequency may be attributed to the different populations, cultures, and attitudes to pain, different pathologies, and different treatment and obturation materials and techniques [95].

Treatment of flare-ups includes cortical trephination, reinstrumentation, intracanal medicaments, incision and drainage, occlusal relief, and the use of systemic medication [93]. Because of the multifactorial nature of flare-ups, there is no guarantee for a particular treatment strategy to prevent flare-ups, thus requiring further studies to develop a procedure to prevent flare-ups [93].

4.2.7 Lasers as Adjunctive Endodontic Treatment Modalities

In endodontic treatment, lasers are used therapeutically inside the root canal for additional disinfection, as an adjunct to irrigants placed into the canals in combination with a photosensitizer (antimicrobial photodynamic therapy, aPDT), and in pain management (photobiomodulation, PBMT). Studies are needed to confirm the current evidence of success as there are major gaps in the studies. These include lack of: (a) laser parameter and calculations reporting, e.g., power, tip or spot size, fluence incorrectly calculated, pulse duration, energy per pulse, frequency, wet, or dry canal; and (b) standardized irradiation protocols reporting regarding the thermal increase in the root canal system and surrounding tissues.

The majority of studies show improved outcomes [97]. These studies have used pain, bacterial counts, and radiographic healing as outcome measures with little consistency between studies and thus conclusions are hard to draw. Studies evaluating pain intensity are found to be very heterogeneous [98]. Some studies have used a quantification of calcitonin gene-related peptide (CRGP) in gingival crevicular fluid (GCF) and its correlation with pain or self-reported visual analog scale (VAS)-pain evaluation [99].

4.2.8 Endodontic Management of Trauma Dental Injuries

The International Association of Dental Traumatology [100, 101] and the American Association of Endodontists [102] developed guidelines to aid the practitioner in the management and treatment of dental injuries. They emphasized that although it is impossible to guarantee permanent retention of a traumatized tooth, timely treatment of the tooth using recommended procedures can maximize the chances for success. Further, they pointed out that these guidelines are not fixed protocols and the variations in an individual patient's health, teeth, physical condition, and personal preferences are important factors in an endodontist's treatment recommendation. Refer to the original guidelines [100, 101] for details on the management of different types of traumatic injuries. Interventions for avulsed teeth and reimplanted teeth will be covered later in this section.

Krastl et al. (2021) [103] reviewed the present status and future directions of endodontic management of traumatic injuries to permanent teeth. They found that there is a lack of high-quality well-designed studies in this area and suggested relevant research areas that could contribute to an improvement in the diagnosis and treatment of traumatized permanent teeth. The authors noted that future research should pay greater attention to: (1) diagnostic methods to assess the perfusion of the pulp and enhance detection of tooth cracks and initial signs of root resorption; (2) improved materials for vital pulp treatment; (3) studies focusing on type and duration of splinting after root fractures; (4) antiresorptive intracanal medication in case of posttraumatic pulp necrosis and infection-related resorption; and (5) long-term data on the apical barrier technique compared to revitalization.

4.2.8.1 Interventions for Avulsed (Knocked Out) and Replanted Teeth

One of the most severe tooth injuries is when the tooth is knocked totally out of the mouth. Often, it is suggested that the best treatment in this situation for a permanent tooth is to replant the tooth as soon as possible. Beyond this logical recommendation, there is inadequate research. The International Association of Dental Traumatology [100] recommends handling the avulsed tooth by the crown only to minimize contamination, washing in cold running water to remove loose debris, and immediate reimplantation, if possible. If immediate reimplantation is not possible, the guidelines recommend placement of an avulsed tooth in milk, Hanks Balanced Salt Solution, patient's saliva in a clean container), or saline in the order of decreasing preference. The expectation is that the replanted tooth would heal by periodontal healing if managed correctly. If the periodontal ligaments are damaged, healing occurs by bony replacement where the root is replaced with bone and the tooth is eventually lost.

A 2019 Cochrane review by Day et al. [11] investigated the treatments that encourage the replanted tooth to repair by periodontal healing. Different treatment modalities included hyperbaric oxygen, root canal pastes (Ledermix versus Ultracal), removal of the nerve of the tooth (pulp extirpation), and soaking the knocked-out tooth in thymosin alpha 1. The review concluded that the majority of the studies did not follow CONSORT guidance and thus there was insufficient evidence to draw conclusions regarding the superiority of different interventions for avulsed (knocked out) and replanted teeth (e.g., hyperbaric oxygen, root canal pastes like Ledermix versus Ultracal, pulp extirpation, and soaking the knocked out tooth in thymosin alpha) with clinical outcomes of periodontal healing, tooth survival, pulpal healing, pain, and aesthetics (discoloration).

Kenny et al. (2018) [104] developed an internationally agreed core outcome set (COS) for Traumatic Dental Injuries for both children and adults using the Delphi research methodology. These outcomes provide guidance on when, how, and by whom these outcomes should be measured; and are drawn from six domains: injury activity, physical consequences of the disease, functional status, social outcomes and quality of life, side effects of therapy, and health resource utilization. The authors emphasized that COS is dynamic, needs to be validated, and requires implementation research to ensure the COS is "fit for purpose."

4.2.9 Endodontic Tissue Engineering

Endodontic tissue engineering consists of various approaches based on the orthograde introduction of scaffolds or biomaterials (with or without cells) into the root canal to achieve pulp tissue regeneration [105]. This term is also used synonymously with regenerative endodontic procedures or pulp revitalization [106]. These therapeutic procedures are mostly used for immature teeth with pulp necrosis and apical periodontitis. Recently, these procedures have been tested in mature teeth as well. Revitalization is a regenerative endodontic treatment option for immature teeth where bleeding is induced into the root canal resulting in a blood coagulum that is covered with collagen and sealed with a hydraulic calcium silicate cement. The coagulum transforms into a repair tissue enabling the regaining of vitality and cold sensitivity. The additional advantage is an increased chance of increasing root length and dentine wall thickness can improve the tooth's mechanical strength.

For mature teeth with fully developed roots and pulp necrosis, the comparison of tooth survival and periapical health with revitalization versus RCT treatment options has shown mostly inconclusive findings due to a lack of robust studies as well relatively newer treatment options for revitalization. In their systematic review, Widbiller et al. [105] reported finding a high survival with endodontic tissue engineering in mature and immature teeth, but there was a moderate risk of bias due to methodological limitations in the included studies. There was a lack of a robust control group and outcomes besides dental survival. Future clinical trials are needed to address methodological as well as assessment concerns and report long-term results.

4.2.10 Use of Cone Beam Computed Tomography (CBCT) in Endodontics

Intraoral and panoramic radiography provides a 2D representation of three-dimensional anatomic structures. However, in some cases, complex anatomy and surrounding structures can make the interpretation of planar images difficult. With CBCT, one can visualize the dentition, the maxillofacial skeleton, and the relationship of anatomic structures in three dimensions. However, CBCT has limitations, including a possible higher radiation dose to the patient, potential for artifact generation, high levels of scatter and noise, and variations in dose distribution within a volume of interest [107]. In 2015, the AAE and the American Academy of Oral and Maxillofacial Radiology issued a joint position statement on the use of CBCT in endodontics and provided 14 specific recommendations and supporting evidence for when CBCT should be considered [107] (Box 4.2). They recommended that CBCT should be used only when the patient's history and a clinical examination demonstrate that the benefits to the patient outweigh the potential risks, and it should be used only when the need for imaging cannot be met by lower dose 2D radiography [107]. CBCT should not be used routinely for endodontic diagnosis or for screening purposes in the absence of clinical signs and symptoms.

Box 4.2 Recommendations from the AAE and the American Academy of Oral and Maxillofacial Radiology [107] on the Use of CBCT in Endodontics

Diagnosis

Recommendation 1: Intraoral radiographs should be considered the imaging modality of choice in the evaluation of the endodontic patient.

Recommendation 2: Limited FOV (field of view) CBCT should be considered the imaging modality of choice for diagnosis in patients who present with contradictory or nonspecific clinical signs and symptoms associated with untreated or previously endodontically treated teeth.

Initial treatment

Preoperative

Recommendation 3: Limited FOV CBCT should be considered the imaging modality of choice for initial treatment of teeth with the potential for extra canals and suspected complex morphology, such as mandibular anterior teeth, and maxillary and mandibular premolars and molars, and dental anomalies.

Intraoperative

Recommendation 4: If a preoperative CBCT has not been taken, limited FOV CBCT should be considered as the imaging modality of choice for intra-appointment identification and localization of calcified canals.

Postoperative

Recommendation 5: Intraoral radiographs should be considered the imaging modality of choice for immediate postoperative imaging.

Nonsurgical retreatment

Recommendation 6: Limited FOV CBCT should be considered the imaging modality of choice if clinical examination and 2D intraoral radiography are inconclusive in the detection of vertical root fracture.

Recommendation 7: Limited FOV CBCT should be the imaging modality of choice when evaluating the nonhealing of previous endodontic treatment to help determine the need for further treatment, such as nonsurgical, surgical, or extraction.

Recommendation 8: Limited FOV CBCT should be the imaging modality of choice for nonsurgical retreatment to assess endodontic treatment complications, such as overextended root canal obturation material, separated endodontic instruments, and localization of perforations.

Surgical retreatment

Recommendation 9: Limited FOV CBCT should be considered as the imaging modality of choice for presurgical treatment planning to localize root apex/apices and to evaluate the proximity to adjacent anatomical structures.

Special conditions

Implant placement

Recommendation 10: Limited FOV CBCT should be considered as the imaging modality of choice for surgical placement of implants.

Traumatic injuries

Recommendation 11: Limited FOV CBCT should be considered the imaging modality of choice for diagnosis and management of limited dento-alveolar trauma, root fractures, luxation, and/or displacement of teeth and localized alveolar fractures, in the absence of other maxillofacial or soft tissue injury that may require other advanced imaging modalities.

Resorptive defects

Recommendation 12: Limited FOV CBCT is the imaging modality of choice in the localization and differentiation of external and internal resorptive defects and the determination of appropriate treatment and prognosis.

Outcome assessment

Recommendation 13: In the absence of clinical signs or symptoms, intraoral radiographs should be considered the imaging modality of choice for the evaluation of healing following nonsurgical and surgical endodontic treatment.

Recommendation 14: In the absence of signs and symptoms, if limited FOV CBCT was the imaging modality of choice at the time of evaluation and treatment, it may be the modality of choice for follow-up evaluation. In the presence of signs and symptoms, refer to Recommendation #7.

A recent narrative literature review by Patel et al. (2019) [108] concluded that it is clear that the additional information provided by CBCT may improve diagnostic accuracy and confidence in decision-making as well as have an impact on treatment planning. And that more clinical studies are required to assess the long-term impact of CBCT on the outcomes of endodontic treatment. The authors also noted that each scan must be optimized to reduce patient exposure by adjusting the CBCT settings to allow each examination to be personalized to the individual patient and the diagnostic needs, rather than just using the manufacturer's default settings. Finally, if CBCT is used in research, then the study protocols need to include training and certification of the radiologist or technician to assure fidelity.

4.2.11 Clinical Versus Histological Endodontic Diagnosis

One of the critical steps in randomized clinical trials is choosing valid classification measures, criteria, and diagnostic tests. Histological examination is the most accurate method for assessment of pulpal status by which the extent of inflammation or presence of necrosis is observed [109, 110]. However, it is difficult to determine that clinically.

Naseri et al. (2017) [111] assessed the accuracy of sensibility tests by correlating them with histologic pulp condition. They found that there was a significant difference in the normal and a sharp lingered response to heat and cold tests. There was also a significant difference in the negative response to electric pulp testing (EPT) between histological groups. The kappa agreement coefficient between clinical and histological diagnosis of pulp condition was 0.843 ($P < 0.001$), and the accuracy of cold and heat tests and EPT to detect treatable pulp or untreatable pulp states were 78%, 74%, and 62%, respectively. In addition, the sensibility tests diagnosed untreatable pulpitis with a higher probability (negative predictive value, NPV = 63%, 67%, 54%, positive predictive value, PPV = 83%, 91%, 95% for heat, cold, and EPT, respectively). The authors noted that to increase the diagnostic accuracy patient history, clinical signs and symptoms, and also radiographic findings in conjunction with sensibility tests must be used.

Walid et al. (2019) [110] proposed a classification of the different in situ observations to refine the initial pulp diagnosis. The rationale is that histologically when the pulp is irritated, the vascular reaction is observed. This also influences the color and flow of pulp blood which can be seen with the naked eye. The authors conducted a 22-month prospective conducted cross-sectional epidemiological study of 133 cases where for each case, the initial pulpal diagnosis was confronted with the in situ direct observation of the pulp state, i.e., color change and the flow of pulp blood. The initial pulpal diagnosis was either retained or corrected according to the in situ observation. They found no correlation between the initial pulpal diagnosis and the final diagnosis after the in situ observation. The authors reported that their study results confirm the clinical ambiguity of diagnosis. They noted that out of 73 cases of asymptomatic irreversible pulpitis, only 35 cases were diagnosed correctly. Of 25 cases of reversible pulpitis, 7 cases were diagnosed as total necrosis and of 34 cases of symptomatic irreversible pulpitis, 6 cases were diagnosed with partial necrosis. Further studies are needed to test the validity of this proposed classification system based on the color and flow of pulp blood.

4.3 Research Design and Methodology

The quality of RCT reporting plays a key role in assessing the value of the trial. The CONSORT Statement is an evidence-based, minimum set of recommendations for reporting randomized trials. It offers a standardized approach for authors to report trial findings in a transparent way which helps in their critical appraisal and interpretation [112]. The CONSORT Statement includes a 25-item checklist focusing on reporting how the trial was designed, analyzed, and interpreted; and a flow diagram displaying the progress of all participants through the trial. We will discuss selected items from this checklist assessing the reporting quality of RCTs in endodontics. The point here and made in other sections of this book is that the CONSORT checklist is a good guide to use in being sure that study protocols are complete.

4.3.1 Trial Design

The researchers should clearly describe the type of design and other aspects (e.g. participants individually randomized to one of two "parallel" groups, multi-arm parallel, crossover, cluster, and factorial designs, trials identifying the superiority of a new intervention, non-inferiority, or equivalence). The design should also include the unit of randomization (such as patient, type of dental practice, lesion, and tooth), allocation ratio, and phase of the trial for drugs (I-IV).

For example,

> "This prospective study was conducted at the Department of Oral and Maxillofacial Surgery of the Academic Medical Centre of Amsterdam. Patients who were referred for endodontic surgical procedures were recruited to participate in this

double-blind placebo-controlled clinical trial. Patients received either a single dose of 600 mg clindamycin or placebo orally 1 h before incision. Envelopes contained a study-identification number with two capsules of either placebo or clindamycin. Blind administration of study drugs was ensured through the use of labelled sets of identical-looking tablets. The assisting nurse supervised drug administration procedure. Patients, oral and maxillo-facial surgeons (JL, JF) and investigators (PV, HA) were blinded to random allocation throughout the study" [113] (well-explained study design and allocation).

4.3.2 Study Setting

Reporting information on the settings and locations is critical to assess the applicability and generalizability of a trial. Description of types of settings used in the endodontics RCTs includes clinics, community centers, academic institutions, single settings versus multicenter, country, etc. The majority of the RCTs in endodontics have been conducted in academic settings.

For example,

"A total of 80 patients were selected for the study who reported to the OPD of Conservative Dentistry and Endodontics, KGMU, Lucknow, India, out of which only 69 patients fulfilled the criteria of inclusion and exclusion and were randomly divided into three treatment groups ($n = 23$)." [114] (well-explained study setting).

"Study subjects were recruited from the pool of patients referred to the Endodontic Clinic for non-surgical root canal treatment for anterior teeth" [115] (incomplete description of study setting).

In this example, the study participants are poorly described but moreover, they are unlikely to be representative. It is essential for investigators to design recruitment procedures such that the study population better represents a typical population. The US Food and Drug Administration (FDA) and many other country drug regulators require this in order for medical devices to be cleared or drugs to be approved. Since the majority of people receive their dental care in community dental settings and these settings are representative of the contemporary clinical workforce and patient populations, RCTs in dental practice-based research networks (DPBRNs) are encouraged. One example is the practice-based, randomized clinical trial which evaluated and compared the success of direct pulp capping in permanent teeth with MTA or CaOH (calcium hydroxide) [116].

4.3.3 Randomization

Participants should be assigned to a treatment group or comparison group randomly. The non-random process leads to bias and possibly invalid clinical interpretations. Selection bias, where clinicians try to match what they think is the best treatment for a particular participant in clinical studies, leads to uninterpretable results. Authors should report the method of sequence generation, for example, a random-number table or a computerized random number generator. The type of randomization and any details on randomization restriction (e.g., blocking, blocking size, etc.) should be clearly described.

For example,

"The randomization was performed at the patient level. Eight patients were included with two teeth, and for these patients the lot was drawn for the first tooth whilst the second tooth was assigned to the opposite treatment method. Both teeth were operated on the same day. The randomization procedure was as follows: a pool contained 52 marbles (26 red = Gutta Percha/26 white = MTA); each drawn marble was given a successive number (1–52) and then removed from the pool. The procedure was performed and documented in a diary by a clinical chair-side assistant. The surgeon did not participate in drawing the lots" [72] (well-explained randomization).

"The incision technique applied to the mesial or distal interproximal space was randomly selected" [117] (incomplete explanation of randomization).

4.3.4 Blinding

Blinding refers to withholding information about the assigned interventions from participants and personnel involved (e.g. participants, healthcare providers, researchers, those assessing outcomes) in the clinical trial who may be influenced by this knowledge. The blinding of participants and treatment providers in endodontics trials is sometimes difficult to achieve because the involved treatments are visually distinguishable. Blinding can be achieved by using assessors that have no knowledge of treatment assignment. It remains critical to blind outcome assessors; if not blinded, they bias the outcomes or may fail to record possible side effects. The lack of blinding in randomized trials can result in under- or overestimation of the treatment effect size [118].

For example,

> "Two endodontists with 16 and 20 years of clinical experience extraneous to involved patients and study design were calibrated. All radiographs were blindly examined twice at an interval of at least 30 days… After the 1st radiographical recall, only one patient of the platelet-rich fibrin (PRF) test group was classified as healed by the blinded examiners and no significant differences were found between the two groups [119]" (adequate blinding of outcome assessors).

It seems that it was not possible in this study to blind the operator using PRF and participants from whom blood was drawn for PRF preparation.

4.3.5 Incomplete Outcome Data

It is important to take into consideration if the missing data is managed and reported in a satisfactory way. For example, there may be situations when participants did not receive the intended intervention, inadvertently receives an intervention meant for the other trial arm, or where participants dropped out or did not come back for evaluation. The best practice is to assess all outcomes on all participants and include them in all analyses, also known as an intention to treat analysis (INT) [120]. INT analysis is typically required for research published in high-quality journals. It ensures the maintenance of comparability between groups as obtained through randomization, maintains sample size, and eliminates bias. In addition, results obtained in such analysis more closely represent clinical practice, dealing with the "effectiveness" of the intervention rather than "efficacy." This is in contrast to per-protocol analysis which refers to the inclusion in the analysis of only those participants who strictly adhered to the protocol or completed the follow-up. Although per-protocol analysis provides an estimate of the true efficacy of an intervention, i.e., among those who completed the treatment as planned, its results do not represent the real-life situation and likely show an exaggerated treatment effect.

Incomplete outcome data can lead to attrition bias if the characteristics of participants with missing data are different between the randomized groups. In studies where there is a loss to follow-up, the authors typically provide a table comparing the baseline characteristics of participants/teeth of the groups that complete the study and those lost to follow-up. Most high-quality journals require a flow chart that documents the number of participants by stage of the study and the reasons for any loss to follow-up.

For example,

> "In a period of 14 months, 399 patients could be included. Adequate follow-up was obtained from 290 patients (141 bur and 149 ultrasonic). The relatively large number of patients who were lost to follow-up was categorized as "missing at random" with no relation to the outcome of treatment. In the group treated with the ultrasonic device, 24.4% were lost to follow-up and in the group treated with a bur, 30.2% of cases had no adequate follow-up. This difference was not significant ($P = 0.191$). Moreover, there was no difference in the distribution of the type of teeth that were treated between groups (i.e., lost to follow-up, adequate follow-up, bur, and ultrasonic) and the number of dropouts was due to factors unrelated to the intervention of the treatment" [121]. Only the remaining participants ($n = 290$ patients), were included in the analysis. Thus this study has a high risk of bias due to incomplete outcome data inclusion and analysis.

> "Eighteen patients with periapical lesions were treated with a modern endodontic surgical procedure (control group). In another 18 patients, as an adjunct to the surgical procedure, platelet concentrate was applied on the root end in liquid form, within the bone defect in clot form, and over the suture in liquid form (test group). All patients completed a questionnaire for evaluation of main symptoms and daily activities during the first week after surgery. The outcomes of the questionnaires of the 2 groups were statistically compared" [122]. All the data was included and reported in the analysis in a satisfactory manner.

4.3.6 Duration of Follow-Up

Most RCTs in endodontics are quite short, i.e., outcome assessment in either less than 1 year or 2–5 years. Long-term follow-up studies are needed to assess the persistence of periapical and periodontal tissue healing, endodontic treatment success outcomes, and factors affecting tooth survival. A 10-year follow-up study of teeth treated with apical surgery and root-end filling with MTA found that although the outcomes declared as healed after 1 year remained so in 86.8% of the cases after 10 years and there was a 10% decrease in healed cases as compared to success rate seen within 5 years [123]. The major limitation for the long-term follow-up RCTs is the rapid technological advancement (e.g., use of operating microscopes or loupes, rotary endodontic instruments for nonsurgical retreatment, and microsurgery with ultrasonic preparation and MTA, retrograde fillings for surgical retreatment) because of which the treatment method under question may become obsolete before long-term results are available [124].

4.3.7 Sample Size Calculations

The sample size determination for a trial should be planned considering medical, statistical, ethical, and economic considerations. The clinical trials should be designed to have enough power to detect statistically significant and clinically meaningful treatment effects. The primary and secondary hypotheses should be clearly defined when calculating sample size and reported with the results of the trials. The sample size calculation requires different components, i.e., type I and type II errors, effect size, or clinical importance difference. Shahravan et al. (2013) [125] found that sample size calculations in endodontic clinical trials have significantly improved in 2009–2010 compared to 2000–2001. The mean sample size for each intervention and control group in clinical trials published in 2009–2010 was 37.88 compared to 21.69 in 2000–2001 with increasing sample size possibly related to improved sample size calculation in endodontic clinical trials in recent years. On the other hand, type I and type II errors were not reported in 10% and 60% of reviewed clinic trials, respectively, thus further improvements are needed.

For example,

> The criterion for significance (alpha) was set at 0.050. The test was two-tailed, which means that an effect in either direction was interpreted. The proposed sample size was 140 for each of the 2 groups. The study had a power of 80.1% to yield a statistically significant result. This computation assumed that the difference in proportions was −0.15 (specifically, 0.65 versus 0.80). This effect was selected as the smallest effect that would be important to detect, in the sense that any smaller effect would not be of clinical or substantial significance. It is also assumed that this effect in size is reasonable, in the sense that an effect of this magnitude could be anticipated in this field of research [121] (appropriately defined sample size).

4.4 Current Knowledge Gaps and Future Directions

As discussed in this chapter, higher quality scientific studies are needed within the field of endodontics. There are many knowledge gaps and important topics worth of future investigation [126]. For example,

- Factors affecting long-term survival and loss of root canal-treated tooth
- Frequency of pain and swelling in root canal-treated tooth with persistent but asymptomatic periapical inflammation
- Prognostic factors to predict an exacerbation of asymptomatic periapical inflammation in a root-filled tooth
- Comparative effectiveness and cost-effectiveness of root canal treatment and restoration versus extraction and replacement with fixed prosthesis or an implant
- Comparative effectiveness of surgical versus non-surgical root canal treatment
- Comparative effectiveness and safety of different surgical procedures for periapical lesion healing and postoperative quality of life
- Risks to general health when teeth with a periodical inflammatory process remain untreated
- Assessment of new methods of endodontic diagnosis, treatment modalities, and technology, such as devices and materials
- Regeneration of a functional pulp-dentin and periradicular complex
- Standardized clinical and patient-centered outcomes for determining the endodontic success
- Evidence-based effective patient recruitment techniques for endodontic trials

- Qualitative research on socioeconomic determinants in endodontics
- Improving provider and patient participation in practice-based research networks

Future studies should use standardized techniques and success criteria, precisely defined outcomes and specific features of the periapical lesion. Investigators should use the participant—not the tooth—as the analysis unit, if possible. While studying endodontic success, the relative effects of some important but easily neglected factors should be taken into account. E.g., differing loss of tooth structure when restoring endodontically treated teeth, the enrollment of participants with high and low caries risk, and the provision of care in different settings. The survival rate in the posterior endodontically treated tooth (ETT) should be separately investigated by tooth type, i.e., premolars versus molars and the remaining tooth structure or tooth surface loss. In addition, the benefit of post-placement in posterior ETT restored with resin composite restoration should be also be verified.

4.5 Preferred Reporting Items for RAndomized Trials in Endodontics (PRIRATE Guidelines)

To improve the quality of RCT reporting in endodontics, the PRIRATE 2020 guidelines [127] were developed by modifying and integrating the CONSORT guidelines [1, 2] and Clinical and Laboratory Images in Publications (CLIP) principle [128] specifically for endodontics. The PRIRATE guidelines consist of a checklist of 11 sections with 58 individual items and a flow chart (see Appendix). Some of the major inclusions in PRIRATE 2020 guidelines are a list of keywords, the strength of the trial, the conclusion, the implications of the work on future research, and clinical practice as well as the quality of images. Since these guidelines are new, future studies are needed to assess the advantages, limitations, and effects of the inclusion of these guidelines while reporting.

4.6 Case Scenario Exercise (Adapted from Diniz de-Figueiredo et al., 2020 [64])

4.6.1 Case Scenario

This trial aims to assess post-operative pain and healing of apical periodontitis following endodontic therapy with a reciprocating system compared to a crown-down technique with hand files and lateral compaction filling.

Questions

1. Provide examples for assessing the outcomes.
2. Discuss an example of study design for this study.
3. How would you do randomization and allocation concealment?

Answers

1. Postoperative pain will be assessed during the 7 days after the treatment, using a visual analog scale and a verbal rating scale. Apical healing will be assessed using the periapical index score after a 12-month follow-up.
2. This study will be performed from years 1 to 3 in four public endodontic dentistry services in four different cities in Brazil. This randomized pragmatic clinical trial will utilize a two-arm, parallel design (1:1 allocation ratio equivalency). The endodontic treatments will be performed either by combining a single-file and single-cone technique using the Reciproc system (experimental group) or by associating the crown-down hand files with the lateral compaction obturation technique (control group).
3. A random list for each study setting will be created using the website www.sealedenvelope.com. The treatment to be performed on each patient will be placed into opaque and sealed envelopes by a third party not involved in the study intervention. The dentists who will perform the clinical procedures will only

open the envelope at the moment of the intervention. Because this is an intervention study, clinicians cannot be blinded by the procedures they are performing. The patients will not be informed of which group they will be allocated to.

Appendix

PRIRATE 2020: Checklist of items to be included when reporting Randomized Trials in Endodontics[a]

Section/topic	Item number	Checklist items	Reported on page number
Title	1a	The phrase "randomized clinical trial" or "randomized controlled trial" must be included in the title.	
	1b	Details of the specific area(s) of interest using words and phrases that identify the clinical problem and the intervention(s) must be provided	
Keywords	2a	Keywords indicating the specific area(s) of interest using MeSH terms must be included	
Abstract	3a	The introduction of the abstract must explain briefly the rationale for the trial	
	3b	The aim/objective(s) of the trial must be provided at the end of the introduction section within the abstract	
	3c	The methodology section within the abstract must provide essential information on the nature of the trial (e.g., superiority, non-inferiority, equivalence), its design (e.g., parallel, split-mouth, crossover), the inclusion/exclusion criteria, randomization process, blinding process, and statistical analysis	
	3d	The results section within the abstract must describe the number of participants that were randomized and analyzed, the size and direction (group favored) of the difference(s) between the intervention(s) and control groups with statistical analysis (p values and 95% CI). Adverse events or side-effects (if any) must also be reported or if none occurred, that must be mentioned explicitly	
	3e	The conclusion section within the abstract must summarize the findings and emphasize the clinical implication(s) of the results	
	3f	The prospective registration (number and name of the registry) and source(s) of funding must be provided	
Introduction	4a	The scientific background and rationale for the trial must be provided, including the gap(s) or inconsistencies in knowledge	
	4b	The specific aim/objective (s) of the trial must be provided and the main clinical research question formulated clearly, preferably using the PICO framework (Problem/Population, Intervention, Control, and Outcome)	
Methods *Trial design*	5a	Details of the nature of the trial (superiority, non-inferiority, equivalence of experimental intervention(s)), its design (parallel, split mouth, crossover, single/double blinded) and test: control allocation ratio must be provided. If applicable, important information about the study design must also be provided, e.g., pragmatic or preference trial, phase (drug trials), patient or public involvement in planning, etc.	
	5b	Changes to the methodology after the trial commenced (such as eligibility criteria) must be provided along with detailed explanations	
A priori *protocol*	5c	Details of the ethical approval of the protocol and the process for obtaining informed consent must be provided	
	5d	Details of the trial protocol including registration number and name of registry/clinical database and where it can be accessed (open access webpage, if applicable) must be provided	

(continued)

Section/topic	Item number	Checklist items	Reported on page number
Participants (patients, operators, evaluators)	5e	A list of inclusion and exclusion criteria at the individual/tooth/root level must be provided	
	5f	Details of the setting/environment of the trial must be provided. Details on how many operators were involved in performing the intervention and control and their relevant experience/qualifications are essential. The setting where the data were collected must be described. If several operators are included and/or if it is a multi-center set-up, details of how standardization/calibration between individuals or centres was achieved must be provided	
	5g	The treatments in the intervention (experimental) group(s) must be described with sufficient detail to allow replication, including how and when they were actually administered	
	5h	The intervention(s) or absence of intervention(s) in the control group must be described with sufficient details to allow replication, including how and when the intervention(s) was actually administered	
Outcomes measures	5i	The primary and secondary (if any) outcome measures must be described, including how and when they were assessed and by whom	
	5j	Details of any changes made to the study outcomes after the commencement of the trial must be described	
	5k	If primary or secondary outcomes are to be regarded as surrogate outcomes, the rationale and empirical support for the connection between surrogate(s) and the outcome(s) of clinical relevance must be provided	
Sample size	5l	How the sample size was determined must be described with reference to the published literature, or a pilot study. The sample size may be modified after an internal feasibility study. Sample size calculations should generally refer to the primary outcome measure. If secondary outcome measures constitute the base for sample size calculation, an explanation must be provided	
	5m	Any interim analyses and stopping guidelines must be described, when applicable	
Randomization and allocation concealment	5n	The method used to generate the random allocation sequence along with any details of the type of restriction (e.g., blocking) if applicable must be described. The persons responsible for randomization and recruitment must be provided. For multi-centre trials, a central randomization procedure is preferred and must be described. The unit of randomization should be specified and justified. Any stratification variables must be detailed	
	5o	Methods for allocation concealment up to the assignment of the participants into the intervention groups must be described	
Blinding	5p	Information on who was/were blinded after assignment to the interventions (e.g., participants, care-givers, evaluators) must be described in detail. Blinding through masking of interventions (e.g., similar looking drugs/instruments) should be described. Detailed reasons for lack of blinding (if applicable) must be described	
Statistical analysis	5q	The statistical methods used for analysis of the primary and secondary (if any) outcomes, additional subgroup analyses and adjusted analyses (if applicable) must be described in detail. Consideration of drop-outs should be included in the calculations	
	5r	How any cluster effects were managed during the analysis must be described	

Section/topic	Item number	Checklist items	Reported on page number
Results	6a	The number of participants who were randomly assigned, received the intended treatment, and were analysed for the primary and secondary (if any) outcome(s) for each group must be described. A flowchart must be provided	
	6b	Reasons for losses/drop-outs and exclusions after randomization must be described for each group and included in the flow chart. If intention to treat analyses are used, details of the process must be provided	
	6c	The dates of recruitment, follow-up, and study duration must be described	
	6d	Reason(s) for any early termination of the trial must be described	
	6e	The baseline demographic and clinical characteristics of each group must be provided	
	6f	The results for each group for each primary and secondary (if any) outcome(s), along with the estimated effect size and its precision, must be provided	
	6g	Both absolute and relative effect sizes for binary outcomes must be provided	
	6h	The results from any other analyses performed must be described, including subgroup analyses and adjusted analyses, distinguishing pre-specified from exploratory	
	6i	The incidence and management of any adverse effects or unintended effects in each group must be described	
Discussion	7a	An estimate of the overall internal validity must be provided as well as the generalizability (external validity, applicability, real-world relevance) of the trial findings	
	7b	The rationale for inclusion, exclusion criteria, and study duration must be provided	
	7c	An explanation of the clinical relevance of the primary and secondary outcomes must be provided	
	7d	A detailed interpretation consistent with results, balancing benefits and harms, and considering other relevant evidence must be provided	
	7e	The strength(s) of the trial must be provided	
	7f	The limitations of the study must be provided, addressing the sources of potential bias, imprecision and, if applicable, multiplicity of analyses	
	7g	Implication for future research and clinical practice must be described	
Conclusion	8a	A rationale for the conclusion(s) must be provided, and the clinical significance highlighted	
	8b	Explicit conclusion(s) from the trial must be provided	
Funding details	9a	Sources of funding and other support (such as supply of drugs, equipment) as well as the role of funders must be acknowledged and described	
Conflict of interest	10a	An explicit statement on conflicts of interest must be provided	

(continued)

Section/topic	Item number	Checklist items	Reported on page number
Quality of images (if applicable)	11a	Details of the equipment, software, and settings used to acquire the image(s) must be described in the text or legend	
	11b	The reason why the image(s) was acquired and the rationale for its inclusion in the manuscript must be provided in the text. A justification for all images which involve radiation must be included	
	11c	The circumstances (conditions) under which the image(s) were viewed and evaluated by the authors must be provided in the text	
	11d	The resolution and any magnification of the image(s) or any modifications/enhancements (e.g., adjustments for brightness, color balance, or magnification, image smoothing, staining, etc.) that were carried out must be described in the text or legend	
	11e	Patient(s) identifiers (names, patient numbers) must be removed to ensure they are anonymized	
	11f	An interpretation of the findings (meaning and implications) from the image (s) must be provided in the text	
	11g	The legend associated with each image must describe clearly what the subject is and what specific feature(s) it illustrates. Images of patients must describe the age, gender, and ethnicity of the person, if relevant	
	11h	Markers/labels must be used to identify the key information in the image(s) and defined in the legend	
	11i	The legend of each image must include an explanation whether it is pre-treatment, intra-treatment, or post-treatment and, if relevant, how images were standardized over time	

[a] From Nagendrababu V, Duncan HF, Bjørndal L, Kvist T, Priya E, Jayaraman J, Pulikkotil SJ, Pigg M, Rechenberg DK, Vaeth M, Dummer P. (2020) PRIRATE 2020 guidelines for reporting randomized trials in Endodontics: a consensus-based development. *International Endodontic Journal*, Mar 20. https://doi.org/10.1111/iej.13294. For further details visit: http://pride-endodonticguidelines.org/prirate/

PRIRATE 2020 Flowchart

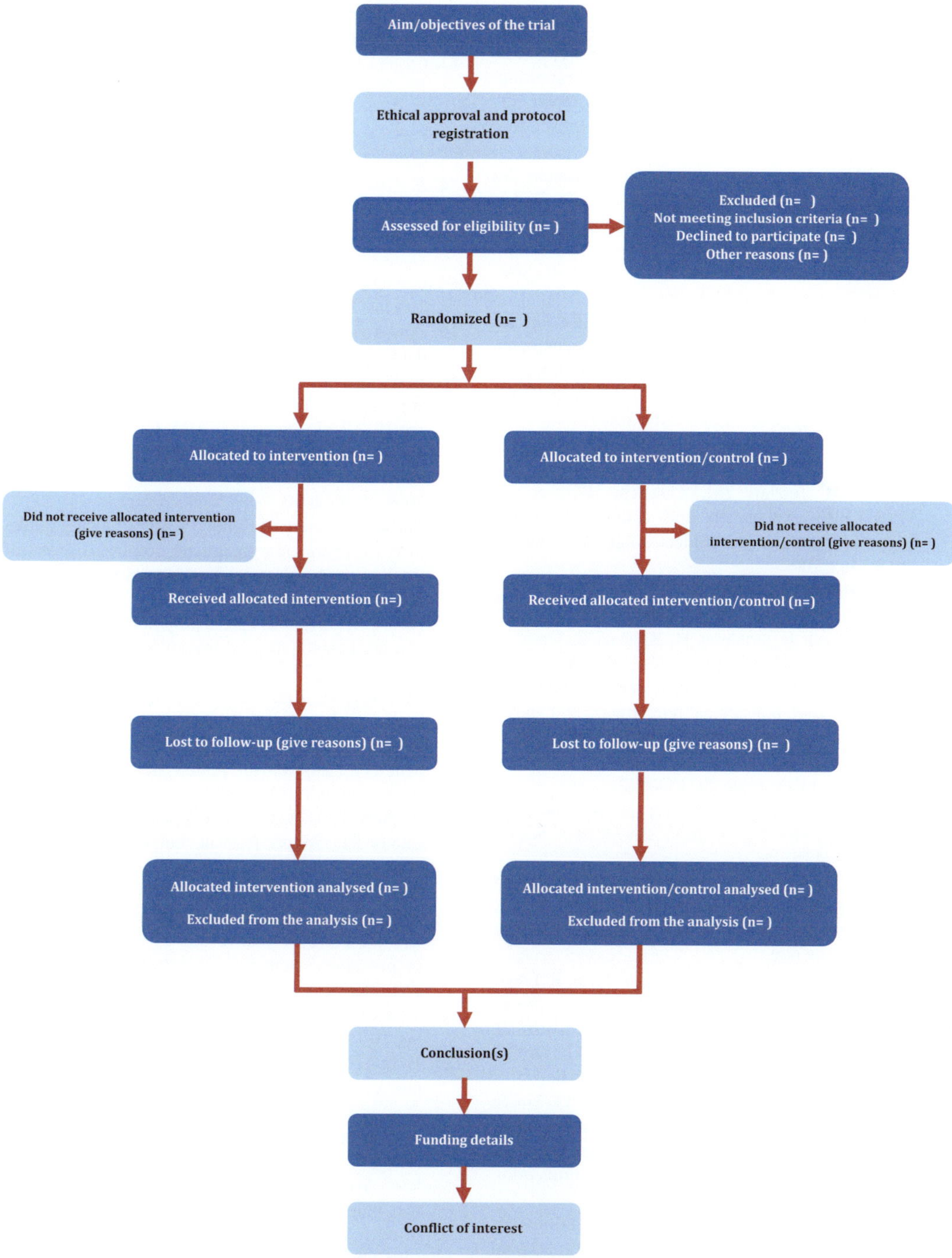

PRIRATE 2020: Flowchart. (From Nagendrababu V, Duncan HF, Bjørndal L, Kvist T, Priya E, Jayaraman J, Pulikkotil SJ, Pigg M, Rechenberg DK, Vaeth M, Dummer P. (2020) PRIRATE 2020 guidelines for reporting randomized trials in Endodontics: a consensus-based development. International Endodontic Journal, Mar 20. https://doi.org/10.1111/iej.13294. For further details, visit: http://pride-endodonticguidelines.org/pirate/)

References

1. Begg C, Cho M, Eastwood S, Horton R, Moher D, Olkin I, Pitkin R, Rennie D, Schulz KF, Simel D, Stroup DF. Improving the quality of reporting of randomized controlled trials. The CONSORT statement. JAMA. 1996;276(8):637–9. https://doi.org/10.1001/jama.276.8.637.
2. Moher D, Hopewell S, Schulz KF, Montori V, Gøtzsche PC, Devereaux PJ, Elbourne D, Egger M, Altman DG. CONSORT 2010 explanation and elaboration: updated guidelines for reporting parallel group randomized trials. BMJ. 2010;340:c869. https://doi.org/10.1136/bmj.c869.
3. Lucena C, Souza EM, Voinea GC, Pulgar R, Valderrama MJ, De-Deus G. A quality assessment of randomized controlled trial reports in endodontics. Int Endod J. 2017;50(3):237–50. https://doi.org/10.1111/iej.12626. Epub 2016 Mar 15.
4. Jadad AR. Randomised controlled trials. London: BMJ Books; 1998.
5. Chan AW, Tetzlaff JM, Gøtzsche PC, et al. SPIRIT2013 explanation and elaboration: guidance for protocols of clinical trials. Br Med J. 2013;346:e7586.
6. Azarpazhooh A, Cardoso E, Sgro A, Elbarbary M, Laghapour Lighvan N, Badewy R, Malkhassian G, Jafarzadeh H, Bakhtiar H, Khazaei S, Oren A, Gerbig M, He H, Kishen A, Shah PS. A scoping review of 4 decades of outcomes in nonsurgical root canal treatment, nonsurgical retreatment, and apexification studies-part 1: process and general results. J Endod. 2022;48(1):15–28. https://doi.org/10.1016/j.joen.2021.09.018. Epub 2021 Oct 22.
7. Strindberg LZ. The dependence of the results of pulp therapy on certain factors. Acta Odontol Scand. 1956;14:1–175.
8. Chugal N, Mallya SM, Kahler B, Lin LM. Endodontic treatment outcomes. Dent Clin N Am. 2017;61(1):59–80. https://doi.org/10.1016/j.cden.2016.08.009.
9. Del Fabbro M, Corbella S, Sequeira-Byron P, Tsesis I, Rosen E, Lolato A, Taschieri S. Endodontic procedures for retreatment of periapical lesions. Cochrane Database Syst Rev. 2016;(10):CD005511. https://doi.org/10.1002/14651858.CD005511.pub3.
10. Manfredi M, Figini L, Gagliani M, Lodi G. Single versus multiple visits for endodontic treatment of permanent teeth. Cochrane Database Syst Rev. 2016;(12):CD005296. https://doi.org/10.1002/14651858.CD005296.pub3.
11. Day PF, Duggal M, Nazzal H. Interventions for treating traumatised permanent front teeth: avulsed (knocked out) and replanted. Cochrane Database Syst Rev. 2019;2(2):CD006542. https://doi.org/10.1002/14651858.CD006542.pub3.
12. Glynis A, Foschi F, Kefalou I, Koletsi D, Tzanetakis GN. Regenerative endodontic procedures for the treatment of necrotic mature teeth with apical periodontitis: a systematic review and meta-analysis of randomized controlled trials. J Endod. 2021;47(6):873–82. https://doi.org/10.1016/j.joen.2021.03.015. Epub 2021 Mar 31.
13. Carter LE, McNeil DW, Vowles KE, Sorrell JT, Turk CL, Ries BJ, et al. Effects of emotion on pain reports, tolerance and physiology. Pain Res Manag. 2002;7(1):21–30. https://doi.org/10.1155/2002/426193.
14. St George G, Morgan A, Meechan J, Moles DR, Needleman I, Ng YL, Petrie A. Injectable local anaesthetic agents for dental anaesthesia. Cochrane Database Syst Rev. 2018;(7):CD006487. https://doi.org/10.1002/14651858.CD006487.pub2. Accessed 19 May 2022.
15. Spivakovsky S. Injectable local anaesthetic agents for dental anaesthesia. Evid Based Dent. 2019;20:42–3.
16. AAE position statement on vital pulp therapy. J Endod. 2021;47(9):1340–44. https://doi.org/10.1016/j.joen.2021.07.015. Epub 2021 Aug 3.
17. Glickman G. AAE consensus conference recommended diagnostic terminology. J Endod. 2009;35:1634–20.
18. European Society of Endodontology. Quality guidelines for endodontic treatment: consensus report of the European Society of Endodontology. Int Endod J. 2006;39(12):921–30.
19. Fong CD, Davis MJ. Partial pulpotomy for immature permanent teeth, its present and future. Pediatr Dent. 2002;24:29–32.
20. Elmsmari F, Ruiz XF, Miró Q, Feijoo-Pato N, Durán-Sindreu F, Olivieri JG. Outcome of partial pulpotomy in cariously exposed posterior permanent teeth: a systematic review and meta-analysis. J Endod. 2019;45:1296–306.
21. Cushley S, Duncan HF, Lappin MJ, Tomson PL, Lundy FT, Cooper P, et al. Pulpotomy for mature carious teeth with symptoms of irreversible pulpitis: a systematic review. J Dent. 2019;88:103158.
22. Asgary S, Eghbal MJ, Fazlyab M, Baghban AA, Ghoddusi J. Five-year results of vital pulp therapy in permanent molars with irreversible pulpitis: a non-inferiority multicenter randomized clinical trial. Clin Oral Investig. 2015;19(2):335–41. https://doi.org/10.1007/s00784-014-1244-z. Epub 2014 Apr 27.
23. Farooq NS, Coll JA, Kuwabara A, Shelton P. Success rate of formocresol pulpotomy and indirect pulp therapy in the treatment of deep dentinal caries in primary teeth. Pediatr Dent. 2000;22:278–86.
24. Vidya K, Patil S, Anegundi R. Is pulpotomy obsolete? A clinical study on the success rates of indirect pulp capping and pulpotomy in the treatment of deep dentinal caries in primary second molars. J Int Clin Dent Res Organ. 2015;7(1):24. https://doi.org/10.4103/2231-0754.153491.
25. American Academy of Pediatric Dentistry. Clinical guidelines on pulp therapy for primary and young permanent teeth: reference manual 2006-07. Pediatr Dent. 2006;28:144–8.

26. Coll JA. Indirect pulp capping and primary teeth: is the primary tooth pulpotomy out of date? Pediatr Dent. 2008;30:230–6.
27. Bossù M, Iaculli F, Di Giorgio G, Salucci A, Polimeni A, Di Carlo S. Different pulp dressing materials for the pulpotomy of primary teeth: a systematic review of the literature. J Clin Med. 2020;9(3):838. https://doi.org/10.3390/jcm9030838.
28. Schwendicke F, Brouwer F, Schwendicke A, Paris S. Different materials for direct pulp capping: systematic review and meta-analysis and trial sequential analysis. Clin Oral Investig. 2016;20(6):1121–32. https://doi.org/10.1007/s00784-016-1802-7. Epub 2016 Apr 2.
29. American Academy of Pediatric Dentistry. Pulp therapy for primary and immature permanent teeth. The reference manual of pediatric dentistry. Chicago, IL: American Academy of Pediatric Dentistry; 2022. p. 415–23.
30. Marchi JJ, de Araújo FB, Froner AM, Straffon LH, Nör JE. Indirect pulp capping in the primary dentition: a 4 year follow-up study. J Clin Pediatr Dent. 2006;31(2):68–71.
31. Wells C, Dulong C, McCormack S. Vital pulp therapy for endodontic treatment of mature teeth: a review of clinical effectiveness, cost-effectiveness, and guidelines. Ottawa, ON: Canadian Agency for Drugs and Technologies in Health; 2019.
32. Malmberg L, Björkner AE, Bergenholtz G. Establishment and maintenance of asepsis in endodontics—a review of the literature. Acta Odontol Scand. 2016;74(6):431–5. https://doi.org/10.1080/00016357.2016.1195508.
33. Heard F, Walton RE. Scanning electron microscope study comparing four root canal preparation techniques in small curved canals. Int Endod J. 2003;30(5):323–31. https://doi.org/10.1046/j.1365-2591.1997.00090.x.
34. Hulsmann M, Peters OA, Dummer PMH. Mechanical preparation of root canals: shaping goals, techniques and means. Endod Top. 2005;10(1):30–76. https://doi.org/10.1111/j.1601-1546.2005.00152.x.
35. Li G-H, Niu L-N, Zhang W, et al. Ability of new obturation materials to improve the seal of the root canal system: a review. Acta Biomater. 2014;10(3):1050–63. https://doi.org/10.1016/j.actbio.2013.11.015.
36. Zehnder M. Root canal irrigants. J Endod. 2006;32:389–98. https://doi.org/10.1016/j.joen.2005.09.014.
37. Tonini R, Salvadori M, Audino E, Sauro S, Garo ML, Salgarello S. Irrigating solutions and activation methods used in clinical endodontics: a systematic review. Front Oral Health. 2022;3:838043. https://doi.org/10.3389/froh.2022.838043.
38. Verma N, Sangwan P, Tewari S, Duhan J. Effect of different concentrations of sodium hypochlorite on outcome of primary root canal treatment: a randomized controlled trial. J Endod. 2019;45:357–63. https://doi.org/10.1016/j.joen.2019.01.003.
39. Paque F, Boessler C, Zehnder M. Accumulated hard tissue debris levels in mesial roots of mandibular molars after sequential irrigation steps. Int Endod J. 2011;44:148–53. https://doi.org/10.1111/j.1365-2591.2010.01823.
40. Malkhassian G, Manzur AJ, Legner M, Fillery ED, Manek S, Basrani BR, et al. Antibacterial efficacy of MTAD final rinse and two percent chlorhexidine gel medication in teeth with apical periodontitis: a randomized double-blinded clinical trial. J Endod. 2009;35:1483–90. https://doi.org/10.1016/j.joen.2009.08.003.
41. Ballal NV, Gandhi P, Shenoy PA, Dummer PMH. Evaluation of various irrigation activation systems to eliminate bacteria from the root canal system: a randomized controlled single blinded trial. J Dent. 2020;99:103412. https://doi.org/10.1016/j.jdent.2020.103412.
42. Sjogren U, Figdor D, Persson S, Sundqvist G. Influence of infection at the time of root filling on the outcome of endodontic treatment of teeth with apical periodontitis. Int Endod J. 1997;30:297–306. https://doi.org/10.1111/j.1365-2591.1997.tb00714.x.
43. Rocas IN, Provenzano JC, Neves MA, Siqueira JF Jr. Disinfecting effects of rotary instrumentation with either 2.5% sodium hypochlorite or 2% chlorhexidine as the main irrigant: a randomized clinical study. J Endod. 2016;42:943–7. https://doi.org/10.1016/j.joen.2016.03.01939.
44. Zandi H, Rodrigues RC, Kristoffersen AK, Enersen M, Mdala I, Orstavik D, et al. Antibacterial effectiveness of 2 root canal irrigants in root-filled teeth with infection: a randomized clinical trial. J Endod. 2016;42:1307–13. https://doi.org/10.1016/j.joen.2016.06.006.
45. Maru V, Padawe D, Naik S, et al. Assessment of bacterial load using 3.8% SDF as an irrigant in pulpectomized primary molars: a randomized controlled trial. Int. J Clin Pediatr Dent. 2022;15(S-1):S47–51.
46. Siqueira JF Jr, Rocas IN. Clinical implications and microbiology of bacterial persistence after treatment procedures. J Endod. 2008;34:1291–1301.e3. https://doi.org/10.1016/j.joen.2008.07.028.
47. Orozco EIF, Toia CC, Cavalli D, Khoury RD, Cardoso F, Bresciani E, et al. Effect of passive ultrasonic activation on microorganisms in primary root canal infection: a randomized clinical trial. J Appl Oral Sci. 2020;28:e20190100. https://doi.org/10.1590/1678-7757-2019-0100.
48. Prada I, Micó-Muñoz P, Giner-Lluesma T, Micó-Martínez P, Muwaquet-Rodríguez S, Albero-Monteagudo A. Update of the therapeutic planning of irrigation and intracanal medication in root canal treatment. A literature review. J Clin Exp Dent. 2019;11(2):e185–93. https://doi.org/10.4317/jced.55560.
49. Crozeta BM, Chaves de Souza L, Correa Silva-Sousa YT, Sousa-Neto MD, Jaramillo DE, Silva RM. Evaluation of passive ultrasonic irrigation

and GentleWave system as adjuvants in endodontic retreatment. J Endod. 2020;46(9):1279–85. https://doi.org/10.1016/j.joen.2020.06.001. Epub 2020 Jun 15.
50. Goncalves LS, Rodrigues RC, Andrade Junior CV, Soares RG, Vettore MV. The effect of sodium hypochlorite and chlorhexidine as irrigant solutions for root canal disinfection: a systematic review of clinical trials. J Endod. 2016;42:527–32. https://doi.org/10.1016/j.joen.2015.12.021.
51. Grossman LI. Endodontic practice. Philadelphia: Lea & Febiger; 1978.
52. LTC Ryan Swiss. Current trends in endodontic obturation: a web based survey comparing ADA and AAE members. Thesis. Defense Technical Information Center. https://apps.dtic.mil/sti/trecms/pdf/AD1186365.pdf. Accessed 06/01/2023.
53. Vishwanath V, Rao HM. Gutta-percha in endodontics—a comprehensive review of material science. J Conserv Dent. 2019;22(3):216–22.
54. Kombayashi T, Colmenar D, Cvach N, Bhat A, Primus C, Imai Y. Comprehensive review of current endodontic sealers. Dent Mater J. 2020;39(5):703–20. https://doi.org/10.4012/dmj.2019-288.
55. Viapiana R, Moinzadeh AT, Camilleri L, Wesselink PR, Tanomaru Filho M, Camilleri J. Porosity and sealing ability of root fillings with gutta-percha and BioRoot RCS or AH plus sealers. Evaluation by three ex vivo methods. Int Endod J. 2016;49:774–82.
56. Bouillaguet S, Shaw L, Barthelemy J, Krejci I, Wataha JC. Long-term sealing ability of Pulp Canal sealer, AH-plus, GuttaFlow and epiphany. Int Endod J. 2008;41:219–26.
57. Ørstavik D. Materials used for root canal obturation: technical, biological and clinical testing. Endod Top. 2017;12:25–38.
58. Chu CH, Lo EC, Cheung GS. Outcome of root canal treatment using Thermafil and cold lateral condensation filling techniques. Int Endod J. 2005;38:179–85.
59. Pandey P, Aggarwal H, Tikku AP, Singh A, Bains R, Mishra S. Comparative evaluation of sealing ability of gutta percha and resilon as root canal filling materials—a systematic review. J Oral Biol Craniofac Res. 2020;10(2):220–6. https://doi.org/10.1016/j.jobcr.2019.12.004. Epub 2019 Dec 30.
60. Kandemir Demirci G, Çalışkan MK. A prospective randomized comparative study of cold lateral condensation versus Core/gutta-percha in teeth with periapical lesions. J Endod. 2016;42:206–10.
61. Pirani C, Camilleri J. Effectiveness of root canal filling materials and techniques for treatment of apical periodontitis: a systematic review. Int Endod J. 2022;56:1–19. https://doi.org/10.1111/iej.13787.
62. Michanowicz AE, Michanowicz JP, Michanowicz AM, Czonstkowsky M, Zullo TP. Clinical evaluation of low-temperature thermoplasticized injectable gutta-percha: a preliminary report. J Endod. 1989;15:602–7.
63. Ozer SY, Aktener SB. Outcome of root canal treatment using soft-core and cold lateral compaction filling techniques: a randomized clinical trial. J Contemp Dent Pract. 2009;10:74–81.
64. de Figueiredo FED, Lima LF, Lima GS, Oliveira LS, Ribeiro MA, Brito-Junior M, et al. Apical periodontitis healing and postoperative pain following endodontic treatment with a reciprocating single-file, single-cone approach: a randomized controlled pragmatic clinical trial. PLoS One. 2020;15:e0227347. https://doi.org/10.1371/journal.pone.0227347. Erratum in: PLoS One. 2020 Mar 11;15(3):e0230511.
65. Sequeira-Byron P, Fedorowicz Z, Carter B, Nasser M, Alrowaili EF. Single crowns versus conventional fillings for the restoration of root-filled teeth. Cochrane Database Syst Rev. 2015;(9):CD009109. https://doi.org/10.1002/14651858.CD009109.pub3.
66. Mannocci F, Bertelli E, Sherriff M, Watson TF, Ford TR. Three-year clinical comparison of survival of endodontically treated teeth restored with either full cast coverage or with direct composite restoration. J Prosthet Dent. 2002;88(3):297–301.
67. Prakash J, Golgeri MS, Haleem S, Kausher H, Gupta P, Singh P, C SG. A comparative study of success rates of post and core treated anterior and posterior teeth using cast metal posts. Cureus. 2022;14(10):e30735. https://doi.org/10.7759/cureus.30735.
68. Bayne SC, Schmalz G. Reprinting the classic article on USPHS evaluation methods for measuring the clinical research performance of restorative materials. Clin Oral Investig. 2005;9:209–14. https://doi.org/10.1007/s00784-005-0017-0.
69. Torabinejad M, Corr R, Handysides R, Shabahang S. Outcomes of nonsurgical retreatment and endodontic surgery: a systematic review. J Endod. 2009;35(7):930–7. https://doi.org/10.1016/j.joen.2009.04.023.
70. Kang M, In Jung H, Song M, Kim SY, Kim HC, Kim E. Outcome of nonsurgical retreatment and endodontic microsurgery: a meta-analysis. Clin Oral Investig. 2015;19(3):569–82. https://doi.org/10.1007/s00784-015-1398-3. Epub 2015 Jan 18.
71. Li H, Guo Z, Li C, Ma X, Wang Y, Zhou X, Johnson TM, Huang D. Materials for retrograde filling in root canal therapy. Cochrane Database Syst Rev. 2021;(10):CD005517. https://doi.org/10.1002/14651858.CD005517.pub3. Accessed 31 Mar 2023.
72. Christiansen R, Kirkevang LL, Horested-Bindslev P, Wenzel A. Randomized clinical trial of root-end resection followed by root-end filling with mineral trioxide aggregate or smoothing of the orthograde gutta-percha root filling—1-year follow-up. Int Endod J. 2009;42(2):105–14.
73. AAE position statement: AAE guidance on the use of systemic antibiotics in endodontics. J Endod. 2017;43(9):1409–13. https://doi.org/10.1016/j.joen.2017.08.015.
74. Segura-Egea JJ, Gould K, Şen BH, Jonasson P, Cotti E, Mazzoni A, Sunay H, Tjäderhane L, Dummer PMH. Antibiotics in endodontics: a review.

Int Endod J. 2017;50(12):1169–84. https://doi.org/10.1111/iej.12741. Epub 2017 Jan 16.
75. Segura-Egea JJ, Gould K, Şen BH, Jonasson P, Cotti E, Mazzoni A, Sunay H, Tjäderhane L, Dummer PMH. European Society of Endodontology position statement: the use of antibiotics in endodontics. Int Endod J. 2018;51(1):20–5. https://doi.org/10.1111/iej.12781. Epub 2017 Jun 14.
76. Cope AL, Francis N, Wood F, Chestnutt IG. Systemic antibiotics for symptomatic apical periodontitis and acute apical abscess in adults. Cochrane Database Syst Rev. 2018;(9):CD010136. https://doi.org/10.1002/14651858.CD010136.pub3. Accessed 1 Apr 2023.
77. Agnihotry A, Fedorowicz Z, van Zuuren EJ, Farman AG, Al-Langawi JH. Antibiotic use for irreversible pulpitis. Cochrane Database Syst Rev. 2016;(2) https://doi.org/10.1002/14651858.CD004969.pub4.
78. Agnihotry A, Thompson W, Fedorowicz Z, van Zuuren EJ, Sprakel J. Antibiotic use for irreversible pulpitis. Cochrane Database Syst Rev. 2019;(5):CD004969. https://doi.org/10.1002/14651858.CD004969.pub5. Accessed 1 Apr 2023.
79. Nagle D, Reader A, Beck M, Weaver J. Effect of systemic penicillin on pain in untreated irreversible pulpitis. Oral Surg Oral Med Oral Pathol Oral Radiol Endod. 2000;90(5):636–40.
80. Ahangari Z, Nasser M, Mahdian M, Fedorowicz Z, Marchesan MA. Interventions for the management of external root resorption. Cochrane Database Syst Rev. 2015;(11):CD008003. https://doi.org/10.1002/14651858.CD008003.pub3.
81. Sondeijker CFW, Lamberts AA, Beckmann SH, Kuitert RB, van Westing K, Persoon S, Kuijpers-Jagtman AM. Development of a clinical practice guideline for orthodontically induced external apical root resorption. Eur J Orthod. 2020;42(2):115–24. https://doi.org/10.1093/ejo/cjz034.
82. Ashraf A, Pérez Alfayate R. Regenerative endodontic treatment in teeth with internal root resorption: an insight over the available literature. Int J Sci Res Dent Med Sci. 2020;2(4):131–4. https://doi.org/10.30485/ijsrdms.2020.245647.1082.
83. Rechenberg DK, Held U, Burgstaller JM, Bosch G, Attin T. Pain levels and typical symptoms of acute endodontic infections: a prospective, observational study. BMC Oral Health. 2016;16:61.
84. Management of endodontic emergencies: pulpotomy versus pulpectomy. American Association of Endodontics. 2017. https://www.aae.org/specialty/wp-content/uploads/sites/2/2017/10/COL041Fall2017EndodonticEmergencies.pdf. Accessed 07/09/2023.
85. Zanjir M, Sgro A, Lighvan NL, Yarascavitch C, Shah PS, da Costa BR, Azarpazhooh A. Efficacy and safety of postoperative medications in reducing pain after nonsurgical endodontic treatment: a systematic review and network meta-analysis. J Endod. 2020;46(10):1387–1402.e4. https://doi.org/10.1016/j.joen.2020.07.002. Epub 2020 Jul 12.
86. Smith EA, Marshall JG, Selph SS, Barker DR, Sedgley CM. Nonsteroidal anti-inflammatory drugs for managing postoperative endodontic pain in patients who present with preoperative pain: a systematic review and meta-analysis. J Endod. 2017;43:7–15.
87. Taggar T, Wu D, Khan AA. A randomized clinical trial comparing 2 ibuprofen formulations in patients with acute odontogenic pain. J Endod. 2017;43:674–8.
88. Penniston SG, Hargreaves KM. Evaluation of periapical injection of Ketorolac for management of endodontic pain. J Endod. 1996;22:55–9.
89. Chagas Carvalho Alves N, Raiane Mamede Veloso S, de Andrade Silva S, de Almeida AC, Tavares Velozo Telles C, Romeiro K, de Melo Monteiro GQ, de Albuquerque DS. Influence of occlusal reduction on pain after endodontic treatment: a systematic review and meta-analysis. Sci Rep. 2021;11(1):14019. https://doi.org/10.1038/s41598-021-93119-6.
90. Fouad AF. Are antibiotics effective for endodontic use? An evidence-based review. Endod Topics. 2002;3:52–66.
91. Bansal R, Jain A, Goyal M, Singh T, Sood H, Malviya HS. Antibiotic abuse during endodontic treatment: a contributing factor to antibiotic resistance. J Family Med Prim Care. 2019;8(11):3518–24. https://doi.org/10.4103/jfmpc.jfmpc_768_19.
92. Farzana F, Hossain SMI, Islam SMN, Rahman MA. Postoperative pain following multi-visit root canal treatment of teeth with vital and non-vital pulps. J Armed Forces Med Coll Bangladesh. 2010;6:28–31.
93. Sharma A, Sharma R, Sharma M, et al. Endodontic flare-ups: an update. Cureus. 2023;15(7):e41438. https://doi.org/10.7759/cureus.41438.
94. Udoye C, Aguwa E. Flare-up incidence and related factors in adults. J Dent Oral Hyg. 2010;2:19–22. https://academicjournals.org/journal/JDOH/article-full-text-pdf/24F538D912.
95. Gotler M, Bar-Gil B, Ashkenazi M. Postoperative pain after root canal treatment: a prospective cohort study. Int J Dent. 2012;2012:310467.
96. Magar SS Sr, Alfayyadh AY, Alruwaili KK, Almunahi HFF, Alsharari AHL, Magar SP. The determination of flare-up incidence and associated risk factors during endodontic treatment: an observational retrospective study. Cureus. 2022;14(11):e31424. https://doi.org/10.7759/cureus.31424.
97. Anagnostaki E, Mylona V, Parker S, Lynch E, Grootveld M. Systematic review on the role of lasers in endodontic therapy: valuable adjunct treatment? Dent J. 2020;8(3):63. https://doi.org/10.3390/dj8030063.
98. Chen Y, Chen XL, Zou XL, Chen SZ, Zou J, Wang Y. Efficacy of low-level laser therapy in pain management after root canal treatment or retreatment: a systematic review. Lasers Med Sci. 2019;34:1305–16.
99. Arslan H, Köseoglu S, Doganay Yildiz E, Arabaci T, Savran L, Yildiz DA, Veyisoglu G. Effect of

intracanal diode laser application and low-level laser therapy on CGRP change. Braz Oral Res. 2018;32:e125.
100. Fouad AF, Abbott PV, Tsilingaridis G, et al. International Association of Dental Traumatology guidelines for the management of traumatic dental injuries: avulsion of permanent teeth. Dent Traumatol. 2020;36(4):331–42.
101. Malmgren B, Andreasen JO, Flores MT, Robertson A, DiAngelis AJ, Andersson L, Cavalleri G, Cohenca N, Day P, Hicks ML, Malmgren O, Moule AJ, Onetto J, Tsukiboshi M. Guidelines for the management of traumatic dental injuries: 3. Injuries in the primary dentition. Pediatr Dent. 2017;39(6):420–8. https://doi.org/10.1111/j.1600-9657.2012.01146.x.
102. Treating traumatic dental injuries: updated guidelines from the AAE. J Calif Dent Assoc. 2014;42(1):14.
103. Krastl G, Weiger R, Ebeleseder K, Galler K. Present status and future directions: endodontic management of traumatic injuries to permanent teeth. Int Endod J. 2022;55(Suppl 4):1003–19. https://doi.org/10.1111/iej.13672. Epub 2021 Dec 22.
104. Kenny K, Day PF, Sharif MO, Parashos P, Lauridsen E, Feldens CA, et al. What are the important outcomes in traumatic dental injuries? An international approach to the development of a core outcome set. Dent Traumatol. 2018;34(1):4–11. https://doi.org/10.1111/edt.12367.
105. Widbiller M, Knüttel H, Meschi N, Durán-Sindreu Terol F. Effectiveness of endodontic tissue engineering in treatment of apical periodontitis: a systematic review. Int Endod J. 2022;56(Suppl 3):533. https://doi.org/10.1111/iej.13784. Epub ahead of print.
106. Murray PE, Garcia-Godoy F, Hargreaves KM. Regenerative endodontics: a review of current status and a call for action. J Endod. 2007;33:377–90.
107. Special Committee to Revise the Joint AAE/AAOMR Position Statement on Use of CBCT in Endodontics. AAE and AAOMR joint position statement: use of cone beam computed tomography in endodontics 2015 update. Oral Surg Oral Med Oral Pathol Oral Radiol. 2015;120(4):508–12. https://doi.org/10.1016/j.oooo.2015.07.033. Epub 2015 Aug 3.
108. Patel S, Brown J, Pimentel T, Kelly RD, Abella F, Durack C. Cone beam computed tomography in endodontics—a review of the literature. Int Endod J. 2019;52(8):1138–52. https://doi.org/10.1111/iej.13115. Epub 2019 Apr 9.
109. García AR. Correlation between clinical diagnosis and histopathological diagnosis in pulp pathology. Pract Odontol. 1990;11:43–6.
110. Walid L, Nabiha D, Ines K. Evaluation of a new means of pulpal diagnosis through a prospective study of 133 cases. Endodontology. 2019;31(1):21–4. https://doi.org/10.4103/endo.endo_47_18.
111. Naseri M, Khayat A, Zamaheni S, Shojaeian S. Correlation between histological status of the pulp and its response to sensibility tests. Iran Endod J. 2017;12(1):20–4. https://doi.org/10.22037/iej.2017.04.
112. The CONSORT statement. http://www.consort-statement.org/. Accessed 30 Jan 2023.
113. Lindeboom JA, Frenken JW, Valkenburg P, van den Akker HP. The role of preoperative prophylactic antibiotic administration in periapical endodontic surgery: a randomized, prospective double-blind placebo-controlled study. Int Endod J. 2005;38(12):877–81. https://doi.org/10.1111/j.1365-2591.2005.01030.x.
114. Verma A, Yadav RK, Tikku AP, Chandra A, Verma P, Bharti R, Shakya VK. A randomized controlled trial of endodontic treatment using ultrasonic irrigation and laser activated irrigation to evaluate healing in chronic apical periodontitis. J Clin Exp Dent. 2020;12(9):e821–9. https://doi.org/10.4317/jced.56368.
115. Rao NK, Kandaswamy R, Umashetty G, Rathore VP, Hotkar C, Patil BS. Post-obturation pain following one-visit and two visit root canal treatment in necrotic anterior teeth. J Int Oral Health. 2014;6(2):28–32.
116. Hilton TJ, Ferracane JL, Mancl L, et al. Comparison of CaOH with MTA for direct pulp capping: a PBRN randomized clinical trial. J Dent Res. 2013;92:S16–22.
117. Velvart P, Ebner-Zimmermann U, Ebner JP. Comparison of long-term papilla healing following sulcular full thickness flap and papilla base flap in endodontic surgery. Int Endod J. 2004;37:687–93.
118. Saltaji H, Armijo-Olivo S, Cummings GG, Amin M, da Costa BR, Flores-Mir C. Influence of blinding on treatment effect size estimate in randomized controlled trials of oral health interventions. BMC Med Res Methodol. 2018;18(1):42. Published 2018 May 18. https://doi.org/10.1186/s12874-018-0491-0.
119. Angerame D, De Biasi M, Kastrioti I, Franco V, Castaldo A, Maglione M. Application of platelet-rich fibrin in endodontic surgery: a pilot study. G Ital Endod. 2015;29:51–7.
120. Ranganathan P, Pramesh CS, Aggarwal R. Common pitfalls in statistical analysis: intention-to-treat versus per-protocol analysis. Perspect Clin Res. 2016;7(3):144–6. https://doi.org/10.4103/2229-3485.184823.
121. de Lange J, Putters T, Baas EM, van Ingen JM. Ultrasonic root-end preparation in apical surgery: a prospective randomized study. Oral Surg Oral Med Oral Pathol Oral Radiol Endod. 2007;104(6):841–5. https://doi.org/10.1016/j.tripleo.2007.06.023. Epub 2007 Sep 27.
122. Del Fabbro M, Ceresoli V, Lolato A, Taschieri S. Effect of platelet concentrate on quality of life after periradicular surgery: a randomized clinical study. J Endod. 2012;38(6):733–9. https://doi.org/10.1016/j.joen.2012.02.022. Epub 2012 Apr 13.
123. von Arx T, Jensen SS, Janner SFM, Hänni S, Bornstein MM. A 10-year follow-up study of 119 teeth treated with apical surgery and root-end filling with mineral trioxide aggregate. J Endod.

2019;45(4):394–401. https://doi.org/10.1016/j.joen.2018.12.015. Epub 2019 Mar 1.
124. Riis A, Taschieri S, Del Fabbro M, Kvist T. Tooth survival after surgical or nonsurgical endodontic retreatment: long-term follow-up of a randomized clinical trial. J Endod. 2018;44(10):1480–6. https://doi.org/10.1016/j.joen.2018.06.019. Epub 2018 Aug 25.
125. Shahravan A, Haghdoost AA, Rad M, Hashemipoor M, Sharifi M. Sample size calculation of clinical trials published in two leading endodontic journals. Iran Endod J. 2014;9(1):56–60. Epub 2013 Dec 24.
126. Bergenholtz G, Kvist T. Call for improved research efforts on clinical procedures in endodontics. Int Endod J. 2013;46(8):697–9. https://doi.org/10.1111/iej.12138.
127. Nagendrababu V, Duncan HF, Bjørndal L, Kvist T, Priya E, Jayaraman J, Pulikkotil SJ, Pigg M, Rechenberg DK, Vaeth M, Dummer PMH. PRIRATE 2020 guidelines for reporting randomized trials in Endodontics: a consensus-based development. Int Endod J. 2020;53(6):764–73. https://doi.org/10.1111/iej.13294. Epub 2020 Apr 23. Erratum in: Int Endod J. 2020;53(9):1312.
128. Lang TA, Talerico C, Siontis GCM. Documenting clinical and laboratory images in publications: the CLIP principles. Chest. 2012;141:1626–32.

5 Randomized Controlled Trials in Oral Medicine, Oral Pathology, and Oral Radiology

Stuart Taylor, Richie Kohli, Ying Wu, Lynly Beard, Harjit Singh Sehgal, and Edmond Truelove

Abbreviations

OM	Oral medicine
OP	Oral pathology
OR	Oral radiology
RCTs	Randomized controlled trials

S. Taylor (✉) · E. Truelove
Department of Oral Medicine, School of Dentistry, University of Washington, Seattle, WA, USA
e-mail: stuartt@uw.edu; edmondt@uw.edu

R. Kohli
Division of Dental Public Health, School of Dentistry, Oregon Health & Science University, Portland, OR, USA
e-mail: kohli@ohsu.edu

Y. Wu
Department of Integrative Biomedical & Diagnostic Science, School of Dentistry, Oregon Health & Science University, Portland, OR, USA
e-mail: yingw@ohsu.edu

L. Beard
Health Sciences Librarian, Health Sciences Library, University of Washington, Seattle, WA, USA
e-mail: lynly@uw.edu

H. S. Sehgal
Department of Periodontology, School of Dentistry, Oregon Health & Science University, Portland, OR, USA
e-mail: sehgal@ohsu.edu

5.1 Introduction

More than 18,000 randomized-controlled trials (RCTs) are published every year in medicine and dentistry, along with tens of thousands of other clinical studies utilizing different designs. With the resulting avalanche of findings, one would expect clear evidence for diagnostic and management strategies for most conditions. However, systematic reviews and meta-analyses of the literature often find a lack of high-level evidence available supporting one therapy or strategy over another. The lack of evidence opens the opportunity for researchers to identify and address these gaps with new work. The American Dental Association recognizes Oral and Maxillofacial Pathology, Oral and Maxillofacial Radiology, and Oral Medicine as dental specialties. These three specialties are also recognized by the dental associations of many other countries e.g., United Kingdom, Australia, India, and Canada but not in some others, e.g., Hong Kong. This chapter provides an overview, pointing out key design and implementation challenges of the published RCTs, and identifying knowledge gaps where future RCTs are warranted. The main highlights are presented in Tables 5.1 and 5.2.

R. Kohli et al. (eds.), *Randomized Controlled Trials in Evidence-Based Dentistry*,
https://doi.org/10.1007/978-3-031-47651-8_5

Table 5.1 Summary of the main findings from key randomized controlled trials in oral medicine, oral radiology, and oral pathology

• Early biopsychosocial intervention is a cost-effective measure in dealing with temporomandibular disorders (TMD) related pain.
• Autofluorescence and fluorescent probes can provide an accurate diagnosis of oral cancer, assisting the dentist during daily clinical activity, but it is not yet possible to suggest that this method may replace histopathological examination.
• There is no evidence to recommend inclusion or exclusion of screening programs for oral cancer using visual examination in the general population. In addition, no robust evidence exists that indicates whether other screening methods including toluidine blue, fluorescence imaging, or brush biopsy are either beneficial or harmful.
• Oral Lichen Planus treatment: topical corticosteroids are considered as the first-line therapy. Topical calcineurin inhibitors are offered as an alternative option.
• Cone beam computed tomography (CBCT) does not reduce the number of post-operative sensory disturbances of the inferior alveolar nerve (IAN) compared to panoramic radiography after mandibular third molar extraction.
• Burning mouth syndrome treatment: there is low-quality evidence for each short- and long-term outcome (symptom relief; changes in QoL, taste and feeling of dryness; and side effects) in different types of treatment: antidepressants and antipsychotics, antiseizure drugs, types of tranquilizers, saliva stimulants, dietary supplements, directed energy waves, physical barriers, psychological therapies, and treatments applied to the mouth surface.
• There is insufficient evidence to either claim or refute: (1) a benefit of either PRGF inserted into the post extraction alveolus during dental extractions or wound closure by primary/secondary intention after dental extractions for prophylaxis of medication-related osteonecrosis of the jaw (MRONJ); (2) a benefit for hyperbaric oxygen therapy as an adjunct to conventional therapy. Limited evidence suggests that there are higher odds of resolving MRONJ with surgical treatment compared with medical treatment.

Table 5.2 Gaps and opportunities for future randomized controlled trials in oral medicine, oral radiology, and oral pathology

Topic	Gaps and future opportunities
Detection and diagnosis	• Developing and testing comprehensive detection processes involved in the three domains of the biopsychosocial model • Natural history of oral cancer • Genetic basis of oral cancer as a prerequisite to the development of molecular markers for screening • Tools for detection of oral cancer in early stages • Efficacy and effectiveness of oral cancer screening to decrease morbidity and mortality • Evaluating the effectiveness of prevention and opportunistic screening in high-risk groups • Impact of improved dental access on decision making to seek dental care for detection of diseases in earlier stages • Effectiveness of Artificial Intelligence (AI) models for early detection of oral pathologies models
Recruitment	• Research participation for racial/ethnic minorities and other underrepresented groups such as women, low socioeconomic status populations, and older adults
Outcomes	• Impact of patient centered interventions on outcomes • Impact of CBCT reports on therapeutic decision making of patients and clinical outcomes • Impact of descriptive pathology report versus a definitive diagnosis only report on patient decision-making and outcomes • Validated tools to measure patient clinical outcomes and quality of life • Comparing different treatments to improve patient outcomes in dysplasias/pre-malignancies
Disease management	• Comparison effectiveness of different anti-viral agents on Herpes infection in the presence of modifying factors • Comparative effectiveness of different topical corticosteroid therapy in the treatment of oral lichen planus • Effectiveness of alpha-lipoic acid, tricyclic antidepressants and anticonvulsants in the management of Burning Mouth Syndrome • Effective preventive strategies for MRONJ in individuals at risk undergoing dentoalveolar surgery • Effectiveness of "drug holiday" (stopping medication) to prevent MRONJ in individuals receiving oral bisphosphonates or denosumab who require tooth extractions • Comparison of surgical versus non-surgical protocols or conservative versus aggressive surgical protocols for the stage-specific treatment of MRONJ

5.2 Key Research Questions

All providers want to help their patients improve and reduce the severity of symptoms. They would like to do this, while doing no harm. Indeed, it is often quoted as *the* central tenet of healthcare, "primum non nocere." This begs the question, who decides when a patient has improved? Who decides what is harmful? These questions about outcomes and outcome measures are challenging when designing clinical research trials, particularly in OM, OP, and OR. The discussion about outcomes and outcome measures produces interesting questions and opportunities for future research.

5.3 Choosing Outcome Measures in RCTs

Deciding upon outcome measures is challenging. Much of the work in OM aims to reduce acute and chronic pain. Within pain research in general, and in specific efforts directed at pain/TMD research in dentistry, there has been a determined effort to investigate functional measures as an outcome for therapeutic success. Pain-related activity interference [1, 2], pain disability index, and jaw use limitation scales [3] have all been suggested to measure functional improvements. However, in many RCTs, proxy outcome measures have been studied (e.g., reduction of ulcer size, inflammation size, or other measures) [4]. One fruitful avenue for future research is to gain an understanding of whether the proxy and functional measures are capturing the real *impact* of the disorder.

Specific measures, such as reduction of pain intensity, may make a particular therapy attractive to providers and patients. However, if there is no *functional* improvement for the patient across biological, psychological, and social functioning domains, has the therapy really made the patient better? The use of focused outcome measures, such as pain intensity, may be a product of treatments having weak treatment effects across multiple biopsychosocial domains in multiple patients. Or the management of the disorder being studied may have minimal impact across multiple biopsychosocial domains as measured on currently used functional measures.

5.4 Focusing on Disease Management

5.4.1 Oral Lichen Planus (OLP)

A recent Cochrane review evaluated the efficacy of corticosteroids to treat people with symptoms of OLP [5]. The authors included 35 RCTs in their review and assessed the risk of bias using the Cochrane tool [6]. Out of the 35 studies, 17 were at high risk of bias (because of no blinding, incomplete outcome data, selective reporting, or baseline imbalance) [7–23]. It is important to note that because of high variability in corticosteroid formulation, concentration, or dosage regimen among studies, it is difficult to evaluate and compare them. The review concluded that topical corticosteroids seem to be more effective than most other treatment modalities except topical tacrolimus. The benefit of topical tacrolimus over topical corticosteroids is less clear and topical tacrolimus seems to cause more adverse effects than corticosteroids. It has been reported that this drug could increase the risk of malignant transformation of oral lichen planus [24, 25].

These reviews suggest that future research studies need to address bias. For example, a validated standardized system for scoring the clinical severity of oral lichen planus is required before comparing the effectiveness of drugs within and between individuals, and across studies. Patient-reported outcome measures are needed in assessing treatment. Future trials are needed to compare different doses and treatment lengths, considering long-term relapses and adverse effects. Studies need to be appropriately powered to detect meaningful differences.

5.4.2 Burning Mouth Syndrome

Burning mouth syndrome is a common painful condition with symptoms of burning, dryness, or uncomfortable sensations in the mouth and taste change, with no obvious underlying medical or dental cause. Common treatments include drugs for anxiety, other psychological conditions, and for increasing saliva production, and protective local applications to the mouth surface. A 2016

Cochrane review [26] assessed the effectiveness and safety of different treatment interventions for symptom relief and changes in quality of life, taste, and feeling of mouth dryness. This review included 23 studies (assessing 1121 people; 83% were women), published between 1995 and 2015. The study found low-quality evidence for each short- and long-term outcome in all treatments assessed. These treatments included antidepressants and antipsychotics, antiseizure drugs, types of tranquilizers, saliva stimulants, dietary supplements, directed energy waves, physical barriers (except side effects, which was assessed as low quality), psychological therapies, and treatments applied to the mouth surface. The RCTs demonstrate considerable heterogeneity in the types of interventions and how the interventions are delivered leading to a failure to find an effectiveness treatment. Many of these trials are too short to have confidence in their findings. Studies should include at least 3 months follow-up [26]. Comparability of groups at baseline is very important especially in terms of intensity of symptoms, gender, and psychological background. Valid and reliable patient-reported outcome measures should be used for the assessment of pain intensity. Future studies should also adequately report the adverse effects of treatments as tolerability is an important factor for patients when making treatment choices [27]. There is also more research needed to understand the effect of neuropathic pain treatment and psychological therapies on burning mouth symptoms.

5.4.3 Medication-Related Osteonecrosis of the Jaw

Medication-related osteonecrosis of the jaw is a severe side-effect of certain drugs (e.g., bisphosphonates, denosumab and antiangiogenic agents) used for cancer and osteoporosis treatment. In this condition, there is progressive destruction of bone in the mandible or maxilla. It is very challenging to treat. A recent Cochrane review [28] concluded that there is insufficient evidence to either claim or refute: (1) a benefit of either plasma-rich growth factors inserted into the post-extraction alveolus during dental extraction or wound closure by primary/secondary intention after dental extractions for prevention of osteonecrosis or (2) a benefit for hyperbaric oxygen therapy as an adjunct to conventional therapy. The quality of evidence in these studies is low/very low due to limitations, e.g., participants changing groups during the study, participants not completing the study, and outcomes measured at different follow-up times. Results of studies of treatment once the condition occurs are equally equivocal. The available studies on management of jaw necrosis are of medium-to-low quality and the limited evidence suggested that there are higher odds of resolving necrosis with surgical treatment compared with medical treatment [29].

5.4.4 Sjogren's Syndrome and Oral Cancer

Diagnostic algorithms are another area where RCTs can assess clinical approaches. They have been proposed for temporomandibular disorders and other orofacial pain conditions including burning mouth syndrome, pre-malignant lesions, and Sjogren's Syndrome. One growing area is the application of artificial intelligence, machine learning, and artificial neural networks to help clinicians diagnose and manage such patients.

Primarily non-randomized studies are found on the topics of artificial intelligence and head and neck cancer [30], oral cancer [31], or Sjögren's syndrome [32], and no RCTs studying artificial intelligence were identified in oral pathology or oral radiology journals leaving a huge gap.

A systematic review of studies of the use of artificial intelligence in the diagnosis of head and neck precancerous and cancerous lesions found the overall performance of the artificial intelligence methods comparable to conventional light microscopic histopathological assessment with added advantages of a faster, more objective and more reproducible evaluation. But the integration of these methods in the digital pathology workflow requires a comprehensive evaluation of each method based on large datasets assembled across centers and disciplines. One important problem is the limited integration of dental records with medical and hospital systems. Future research opportunities include the use of deep learning methods for the development of digital biomarkers and the discovery of novel predictive features to aid in early detection of head and neck cancer and improve patient stratification. The goal is to aid the development of targeted, patient-specific diagnostics and therapeutics to reduce head and neck cancer-associated mortality [30].

Ilhan et al. [31] assessed emerging optical imaging modalities and novel artificial intelligence-based approaches to evaluate their individual and combined utility and implications for improving oral cancer detection and outcomes. They concluded that that artificial intelligence approaches combined with imaging can have a considerable impact on oral cancer outcomes, with applications ranging from low-cost screening with smartphone-based probes to algorithm-guided detection of oral lesion heterogeneity and margins using optical coherence tomography [31].

Kise et al. evaluated the diagnostic performance of a deep learning system for the detection of Sjögren's syndrome in ultrasonography (US) images, and compared it with the performance of inexperienced radiologists [32]. The authors found that deep learning systems had a high diagnostic ability for Sjögren's syndrome as compared to the performance of an inexperienced radiologist.

5.5 The Importance of Models in Designing RCTs in Oral Medicine and Related Fields

Oral medicine research has been conducted in temporomandibular disorders and orofacial pain patient populations [33–35], with a focus on the psychological and social aspects of patient experiences, in addition to the biological aspects. The model suggests that personal and environmental factors contribute to the expression of pain and dysfunction at many levels, thus interventions such as cognitive-behavioral therapy, targeted at cognitive, emotional, and behavioral levels, should be effective in modifying the expression of pain and dysfunction [36].

However, very few of the other orofacial conditions discussed in this chapter have been studied based on a biosocial model. Indeed, much of the existing research is mechanistic and has not included a clearly stated model and hypotheses. Without a clear model, it is not possible to decide which treatments to study and what outcomes should be primary.

The biopsychosocial model that has been used in temporomandibular joint disease research suggests that personal and environmental factors contribute to the expression of pain and dysfunction at many levels and that interventions such as cognitive-behavioral therapy targeted at cognitive, emotional, and behavioral levels should be studied. Similar opportunities exist in other subject areas discussed in this chapter.

The main findings from key randomized controlled trials in Oral Medicine, Oral Radiology and Oral Pathology are summarized in Table 5.1.

5.6 Design and Methodology

5.6.1 Risk of Bias

The Consolidated Standards of Reporting Trials (CONSORT) Statement facilitates assessing risk of bias and better reporting of randomized clinical trials (RCTs). The design and implementation issues related to study setting and patient population, randomization, allocation concealment, blinding, and statistical analysis have been discussed in detail in Chaps. 1 and 2. An example for these issues in oral cancer detection area is:

The most common screening method for detecting oral cancer is visual inspection. Other techniques include the use of toluidine blue, fluorescence imaging, or brush biopsy. The current evidence that a visual examination as part of a population-based screening program reduces the mortality rate of oral cancer in high-risk individuals [37] is limited to one study [38]. Even this study has a high risk of bias. For example, the authors did not include detail of sequence generation process to ensure random assignment, allocation concealment, drop-outs, and clinical standardized criteria. There was no analysis of the impact of clustering on the results and there was no blinding of the outcome assessment. The study was done in rural area in Kerala, India, with a high incidence of oral cavity cancer. Thus, its applicability to other countries with lower incidence rates is unknown. There is also no robust evidence that indicates whether other screening methods including toluidine blue, fluorescence imaging, or brush biopsy are either beneficial or harmful [37]. Further RCTs are recommended to assess the efficacy and cost-effectiveness of a visual examination as part of a population-based screening program in low, middle, and high-income countries. Future RCTs should account for the method of randomization in the analysis, do adequate allocation concealment, use standardized intervention, and have a clear follow-up procedure [37].

5.6.2 Recruitment Challenges

While planning an RCT, it is critical to recruit population that allows you to answer the question and appropriately powering the trial to allow for determining effect sizes in the specific subgroup in question. Most RCTs are conducted in research centers at universities. Participation in these studies may not be accessible to various societal groups. RCTs in such settings may not be applicable to all patients with the condition under investigation. Greater care in the design and conduct of RCTs and conducting research that demonstrates errors in conducting research where access to the widest distribution of participants could greatly improve the utility and applicability of such research outcomes.

For example, periapical cemental dysplasia is most commonly diagnosed in Black females and there is a dearth of research on the condition—why is that? Is it because it is mostly “benign”? The condition has been reported as being painful, especially in its later stages, but is often reported as being minimally symptomatic. However, there is limited data on the pain level, and is it a “benign” problem if pain arises from these lesions affecting quality of life. In such cases, the significant diagnostic error is not in the microscopic or radiographic diagnosis but in the global diagnosis which includes the pathologic process and the impact of the condition on the patient. If it is a “benign” condition, why do some clinicians confuse the condition with pulpal pathoses or worse, biopsy the condition and advocate for removing the areas within the bone. Is it because the clinician sees the word dysplasia and assumes that the bony process is progressively destructive like mucosal dysplasia? Or is it because of clinician-inherent biases associated with the patients that this condition predominantly affects? Research on factors that inform or distort clinician decision-making are not prevalent in the literature. Another important question that arises relates to conditions that affect predominantly minority populations. Has the condition, collectively been deemed unworthy of research? Is it difficult for universities to recruit the patients that this condition predominantly affects, for research? For example, an argument could be made about TMD research outcomes in Black populations in the United States. They have been under recruited, resulting in a dearth of research findings, to the point where some clinicians or researchers think that being black is postulated to be protective for the disorder. Since race is a social construct, can this really be the case, or is it that the social barriers to research for Black people in the United States are so great that there is an under-reporting and under-detection of TMD and other disorders in that population?

Recurrent aphthous ulceration is a condition that has a reasonable amount of research studying the pathophysiology. But it is not clear whether the full spectrum of contributing pathophysiologic, environmental, psychophysiological, and societal elements have been explored. Is that, in part, due to the condition predominantly affecting women versus men? In part, the discrepancy may be related to funding, with research indicating that more grant money is available for conditions that predominantly affect men, than for conditions that affect women [39].

A determined effort is needed in design of RCTs to look at how recruitment takes place.

Does the appearance of the recruiter matter? Should different recruiters and different recruiting language be used, depending upon the population that is to be recruited. Evidence suggests that these factors matter. As stated by Sugden and Moulson [40] "recruitment strategies should not be randomly selected"—it is incumbent upon researchers to seek out participants from a wide variety of groups in society. Relying on a random selection of people to appear in a clinic or research project, without actively recruiting a diverse sample of participants, is unlikely to be successful. It may be useful to develop an exhaustive list of potential diagnostic and treatment RCTs in oral medicine/oral pathology/oral radiology. However, a better first step may be to re-examine the process of design and conduct of future RCTs within OM, OP, and OR *and* dentistry in general, so that the size, scope, and design of those RCTs more effectively guides the profession in processes that improve the health and quality of life of the patients we serve.

5.6.3 Other Considerations

Since some of the trials were carried out before CONSORT introduction or before it was a requirement for publication, it is important to judiciously assess those studies.

It is also important to differentiate between trials of devices or drugs under US Food and Drug Administration (FDA) or other government authority supervision versus investigator-initiated trials that do not meet FDA/government standards. The former, for example, discourage the use of intermediate or proxy outcomes (i.e., reports by someone who is not the patient measuring concepts that are only known by the patients (e.g., symptoms) while the later may do so). Often the standards for devices or diagnostic tests are different than those for drugs. Generally, the FDA requires both disease and patient-oriented outcomes in phase 3 trials and, hence, these measures should be well planned during study design.

The FDA has approved several artificial intelligence and machine-learning systems for use in medicine, but there is an extensive (and expensive) regulatory process. The benefits within dentistry may be hard to justify, if left to market forces alone. Testing FDA approved systems for cancer of the lip, for instance, in an RCT may be an approach to begin applying systems in the orofacial region.

Artificial intelligence, machine learning, and artificial neural networks are likely to be "growth areas" in dentistry in the coming years, particularly in the spheres of oral pathology and oral radiology. The systems are only as good as the data they are developed upon. Machine learning needs large numbers of cases and samples to be effective. As discussed later, this may be problematic in a variety of areas within dentistry, particularly because patient accrual in trials is difficult and record systems are not shared across platforms and centers and medical and dental records are not integrated.

The gaps and opportunities for future randomized controlled trials in Oral Medicine, Oral Radiology, and Oral Pathology are summarized in Table 5.2.

5.7 Case Scenario Exercise

5.7.1 Case Scenario (Based on and Adapted from de Souza R, 2022 [41])

The purpose of the proposed study is to determine the effectiveness of palatal brushing in the treatment of denture-related erythematous stomatitis (DES) in complete denture wearers. This two-parallel-arm RCT will be conducted in 3 university clinics in three countries. Participants will be randomly allocated to receive (i) instructions for palatal brushing and standard oral/denture hygiene ("intervention"); or (ii) standard oral/denture hygiene instructions only ("control"). Data collection will be carried out at the baseline and at 3 and 6 months after intervention. Outcomes to be assessed include the magnitude of oral Candida carriage and the degree of inflammation of denture-bearing tissues.

Questions

1. What should be the considerations for such multi-center trial in 3 different countries?
2. During the study, some participants were lost to follow-up. How would you address this limitation?
3. From a clinical perspective, the study concluded that palatal brushing has demonstrated a net superiority in reducing clinical signs of DES. Not only did this method led to significant improvement in most participants it also established a number needed to treat of less than four patients. How would you clinically interpret number needed to treat?

Answers

1. The multicenter design of this study may result in discrepancies among study participants from different centers. Thus, subjects should be compared at baseline to ensure comparability of the study groups, and the statistical analysis should assess the influence of center on the outcomes.
2. An imputation strategy can be used to show that incomplete data has not led to biased results.
3. This means that clinician recommending palatal brushing to address DES will need to treat four patients to see an improvement in one of them, compared to standard hygiene instructions.

References

1. Miller RP, Kori S, Todd D. The Tampa scale: a measure of kinesiophobia. Clin J Pain. 1991;7(1):51–2.
2. Manfredini D, Winocur E, Ahlberg J, Guarda-Nardini L, Lobbezoo F. Psychosocial impairment in temporomandibular disorders patients. RDC/TMD axis II findings from a multicentre study. J Dent. 2010;38(10):765–72. https://doi.org/10.1016/j.jdent.2010.06.007.
3. Ohrbach R, Larsson P, List T. The jaw functional limitation scale: development, reliability, and validity of 8-item and 20-item versions. J Orofac Pain. 2008;22(3):219–30.
4. Sharma R, Pallagatti S, Aggarwal A, Sheikh S, Singh R, Gupta D. A randomized, double-blind, placebo-controlled trial on clinical efficacy of topical agents in reducing pain and frequency of recurrent aphthous ulcers. Open Dent J. 2018;12:700–13.
5. Lodi G, Manfredi M, Mercadante V, Murphy R, Carrozzo M. Interventions for treating oral lichen planus: corticosteroid therapies. Cochrane Database Syst Rev. 2020;2:CD001168. https://doi.org/10.1002/14651858.CD001168.pub3.
6. JPT H, Savović J, Page MJ, Elbers RG, JAC S. Chapter 8: Assessing risk of bias in a randomized trial. In: JPT H, Thomas J, Chandler J, Cumpston M, Li T, Page MJ, Welch VA, editors. Cochrane handbook for systematic reviews of interventions version 6.0 (updated August 2019). Cochrane; 2019. Available from www.training.cochrane.org/handbook.
7. Amanat D, Ebrahimi H, Zahedani MZ, Zeini N, Pourshahidi S, Ranjbar Z. Comparing the effects of cryotherapy with nitrous oxide gas versus topical corticosteroids in the treatment of oral lichen planus. Indian J Dent Res. 2014;25:711–6.
8. Bakhtiari S, Azari-Marhabi S, Mojahedi SM, Namdari M, Rankohi ZE, Jafari S. Comparing clinical effects of photodynamic therapy as a novel method with topical corticosteroid for treatment of oral lichen planus. Photodiagn Photodyn Ther. 2017;20:159–64.
9. Campisi G, Giandalia G, De Caro V, Di Liberto C, Arico P, Giannola LI. A new delivery system of clobetasol-17-propionate (lipid-loaded microspheres 0.025%) compared with a conventional formulation (lipophilic ointment in a hydrophilic phase 0.025%) in topical treatment of atrophic/erosive oral lichen planus. A phase IV, randomized, observer-blinded, parallel group clinical trial. Br J Dermatol. 2004;150(5):984–90.
10. Chainani-Wu N, Silverman S Jr, Reingold A, Bostrom A, Mc Culloch C, Lozada-Nur F, et al. A randomized, placebo- controlled, double-blind clinical trial of curcuminoids in oral lichen planus. Phytomedicine. 2007;14(7–8):437–46.
11. Dillenburg CS, Martins MA, Munerato MA, Marques MM, Carrard VC, Sant'Ana Filho M, et al. Efficacy of laser phototherapy in comparison to topical clobetasol for the treatment of oral lichen planus: a randomised controlled trial. J Biomed Opt. 2014;19(6):068002–9.
12. Ghabanchi J, Bahri Najafi R, Haghnegahdar S. Treatment of oral inflammatory diseases with a new mucoadhesive prednisolone table versus triamcinolone acetonide paste. Iran Red Crescent Med J. 2009;11(2):155–9.
13. Gorouhi F, Solhpour A, Beitollahi JM, Afshar S, Davari P, Hashemi P, et al. Randomized trial of pimecrolimus cream versus triamcinolone acetonide paste in the treatment of oral lichen planus. J Am Acad Dermatol. 2007;57(5):806–13.
14. Hegarty AM, Hodgson TA, Lewsey JD, Porter SR. Fluticasone propionate spray and betamethasone sodium phosphate mouthrinse: a randomized crossover study for the treatment of symptomatic oral lichen planus. J Am Acad Dermatol. 2002;47(2):271–9.
15. Hesen RR, Abuel-Ela HA, Helmy IM, El Sayed MH, Ezzatt OM. Glucosamine as a novel adjunctive ther-

apy in symptomatic oral lichen planus. J Pharm Sci Res. 2017;9:941–6.
16. Liu C, Xie B, Yang Y, Lin D, Wang C, Lin M, et al. Efficacy of intralesional betamethasone for erosive oral lichen planus and evaluation of recurrence: a randomized, controlled trial. Oral Surg Oral Med Oral Pathol Oral Radiol. 2013;116:584–90.
17. Malhotra AK, Khaitan BK, Sethuraman G, Sharma VK. Betamethasone oral mini-pulse therapy compared with topical triamcinolone acetonide (0.1%) paste in oral lichen planus: a randomized comparative study. J Am Acad Dermatol. 2008;58(4):596–602.
18. Mostafa D, Moussa E, Alnouaem M. Evaluation of photodynamic therapy in treatment of oral erosive lichen planus in comparison with topically applied corticosteroids. Photodiagn Photodyn Ther. 2017;19:56–66.
19. Pakfetrat A, Delavarian Z, Falaki F, Khorashadizadeh M, Saba M. The effect of pimecrolimus cream 1% compared with triamcinolone acetonide paste in treatment of atrophic-erosive oral lichen planus. Iran J Otorhinolaryngol. 2015;27:119–26.
20. Rodstrom PO, Hakeberg M, Jontell M, Nordin P. Erosive oral lichen planus treated with clobetasol propionate and triamcinolone acetonide in Orabase: a double-blind clinical trial. J Dermatol Treat. 1994;5(1):7–10.
21. Thomas AE, Varma B, Kurup S, Jose R, Chandy ML, Kumar SP, et al. Evaluation of efficacy of 1% curcuminoids as local application in management of oral lichen planus–interventional study. J Clin Diagn Res. 2017;11:ZC89–93.
22. Xiong C, Li Q, Lin M, Li X, Meng W, Wu Y, et al. The efficacy of topical intralesional BCG-PSN injection in the treatment of erosive oral lichen planus: a randomized controlled trial. J Oral Pathol Med. 2009;38:551–8.
23. Xu YZ, Geng Y, Liu YX, Fuan YQ, Li J. Clinical study on three-step treatment of oral lichen planus by integrated traditional and western medicine. J Mod Stomatol. 2002;16:344–6.
24. Becker JC, Houben R, Vetter CS, Bröcker EB. The carcinogenic potential of tacrolimus ointment beyond immune suppression: a hypothesis creating case report. BMC Cancer. 2006;6:7.
25. Mattsson U, Magnusson B, Jontell M. Squamous cell carcinoma in a patient with oral lichen planus treated with topical application of tacrolimus. Oral Surg Oral Med Oral Pathol Oral Radiol Endod. 2010;110(1):e19–25.
26. McMillan R, Forssell H, Buchanan JAG, Glenny AM, Weldon JC, Zakrzewska JM. Interventions for treating burning mouth syndrome. Cochrane Database Syst Rev. 2016;11:CD002779. https://doi.org/10.1002/14651858.CD002779.pub3.
27. Ioannidis JP, Evans SJ, Gøtzsche PC, O'Neill RT, Altman DG, Schulz K, et al. Better reporting of harms in randomized trials: an extension of the CONSORT statement. Ann Internal Med. 2004;141(10):781–8.
28. Beth-Tasdogan NH, Mayer B, Hussein H, Zolk O. Interventions for managing medication-related osteonecrosis of the jaw. Cochrane Database of Syst Rev. 2017;10:CD012432. https://doi.org/10.1002/14651858.CD012432.pub2.
29. El-Rabbany M, Sgro A, Lam DK, Shah PS, Azarpazhooh A. Effectiveness of treatments for medication-related osteonecrosis of the jaw: a systematic review and meta-analysis. J Am Dent Assoc. 2017;148(8):584–94.
30. Mahmood H, Shaban M, Indave BI, Santos-Silva AR, Rajpoot N, Khurram SA. Use of artificial intelligence in diagnosis of head and neck precancerous and cancerous lesions: a systematic review. Oral Oncol. 2020;110:104885. https://doi.org/10.1016/j.oraloncology.2020.104885.
31. Ilhan B, Lin K, Guneri P, Wilder-Smith P. Improving oral cancer outcomes with imaging and artificial intelligence. J Dent Res. 2020;99(3):241–8. https://doi.org/10.1177/0022034520902128.
32. Kise Y, Shimizu M, Ikeda H, Fujii T, Kuwada C, Nishiyama M, et al. Usefulness of a deep learning system for diagnosing Sjögren's syndrome using ultrasonography images. Dentomaxillofac Radiol. 2020;49(3):20190348. https://doi.org/10.1259/dmfr.20190348.
33. LeResche L, Dworkin SF. Facial expressions of pain and emotions in chronic TMD patients. Pain. 1988;35(1):71–8. https://doi.org/10.1016/0304-3959(88)90278-3.
34. Stowell AW, Gatchel RJ, Wildenstein L. Cost-effectiveness of treatments for temporomandibular disorders: biopsychosocial intervention versus treatment as usual. J Am Dent Assoc. 2007;138(2):202–8. https://doi.org/10.14219/jada.archive.2007.0137.
35. Schiffman E, Ohrbach R, Truelove E, Look J, Anderson G, Goulet JP, et al. International RDC/TMD Consortium Network, International Association for Dental Research, Orofacial Pain Special Interest Group, International Association for the Study of Pain. Diagnostic criteria for temporomandibular disorders (DC/TMD) for clinical and research applications: recommendations of the International RDC/TMD Consortium Network* and Orofacial Pain Special Interest Group. J Oral Facial Pain Headache. 2014;28(1):6–27. https://doi.org/10.11607/jop.1151.
36. Dworkin SF, Turner JA, Mancl L, Wilson L, Massoth D, Huggins KH, et al. A randomized clinical trial of a tailored comprehensive care treatment program for temporomandibular disorders. J Orofac Pain. 2002;16(4):259–76.
37. Brocklehurst P, Kujan O, O'Malley L, Ogden GR, Shepherd S, Glenny A-M. Screening programmes for the early detection and prevention of oral cancer. Cochrane Database Syst Rev. 2013;(11):CD004150. https://doi.org/10.1002/14651858.CD004150.pub4.
38. Sankaranarayanan R, Ramadas K, Thara S, Muwonge R, Thomas G, Anju G, et al. Long-term effect of visual screening on oral cancer incidence and mortality in a randomized trial in Kerala, India. Oral Oncol. 2013;49(4):314–21.

39. Mirin AA. Gender disparity in the funding of diseases by the U.S. National Institutes of Health. J Womens Health (Larchmt). 2021;30(7):956–63. https://doi.org/10.1089/jwh.2020.8682.
40. Sugden NA, Moulson MC. Recruitment strategies should not be randomly selected: empirically improving recruitment success and diversity in developmental psychology research. Front Psychol. 2015;6:523. https://doi.org/10.3389/fpsyg.2015.00523.
41. de Souza R, Chaves C, Rohani K, Bouferguene S, Barbeau J, Borie E, et al. Palatal brushing for the treatment of denture stomatitis: a multicentre randomized controlled trial. J Prosthodont Res. 2023;67(1):93–102. https://doi.org/10.2186/jpr.JPR_D_21_00258.

Randomized Controlled Trials in Oral and Maxillofacial Surgery

6

Akshay Govind, Brandon C. Maughan, and Syed Umer

6.1 Introduction

Oral and maxillofacial surgery (OMS) is arguably the broadest topic in dentistry; it consists of the intersection of dentistry and medicine, anesthesia and surgery, esthetics and function, biologic and material sciences, human behavior, and anatomy. As such, scientific articles that guide the practice of OMS may be found in multiple types of publications, including journals covering dentistry, OMS, plastic and reconstructive surgery, otolaryngology, emergency medicine, critical care, and anesthesia, to name a few. The authors organized this chapter into the following eight content-based sections:

- General medicine and oral surgery
- Outpatient anesthesia
- Dentoalveolar surgery
- Orthognathic surgery
- Facial trauma
- Pathology
- Reconstruction
- Temporomandibular disorders

These topics are presented in this order to begin broadly and grow increasingly specific. Three categories within the scope of OMS were intentionally excluded: head and neck oncology, facial cosmetic surgery, and dental implants. Oncology and cosmetic surgery were not included because only a small portion of OMS providers subspecialize in these areas, and the amount of literature on these topics is not appropriate for a textbook aimed at a dental audience. Dental implants were not included because they are discussed elsewhere in this textbook.

As the goal of this chapter is to aid the budding surgeon–scientist in designing and carrying out the studies needed in the future of oral and maxillofacial surgery, we begin by laying out the goals of randomized controlled trials (RCTs), followed by a review of existing literature in both content and quality, and we conclude by addressing gaps and common problems that exist within the literature. In doing so, we propose four concrete recommendations in methodology to optimize the yield from future studies with minimal bias.

A. Govind (✉)
Department of Oral and Maxillofacial Surgery, University of California, San Francisco, CA, USA
e-mail: agovind@alamedahealthsystem.org

B. C. Maughan
Department of Emergency Medicine, Oregon Health & Science University, Portland, OR, USA
e-mail: maughabr@ohsu.edu

S. Umer
Division of Periodontology, Oregon Health & Science University, Portland, OR, USA
e-mail: umer@ohsu.edu

R. Kohli et al. (eds.), *Randomized Controlled Trials in Evidence-Based Dentistry*,
https://doi.org/10.1007/978-3-031-47651-8_6

6.2 Goals and Prerequisites of Randomized Clinical Trials

The goal of a randomized trial is to assess the impact of an intervention (e.g., surgical technique, medication, etc.), while attempting to minimize bias from other patient characteristics that could affect the outcome(s). Some elements of RCT study design are similar to those of other study types; for instance, studies that enroll patients at multiple centers are more likely to have results that are broadly generalizable, whereas single-center investigations may have results that only reflect local practice patterns and are not generalizable to other settings. However, there are several RCT-specific design elements that can influence whether the trial is successful at achieving unbiased (or minimally biased) results. Many of these elements are reflected in the international standards established by the Consolidated Standards Of Reporting Trials (CONSORT) group for reporting of RCT results. This chapter will address some of the critical elements for reducing the risk of bias when designing and performing an RCT:

- **Randomize to equally distribute patient characteristics within an adequate sample size:** Ideally, randomization will ensure that patient characteristics—such as age, body mass index, comorbid conditions, and other relevant factors—are equally represented among patients who receive an intervention and those who do not. Randomization may be unsuccessful (i.e. intervention and control groups have different compositions) especially in trials with small numbers, which may introduce bias and lead to flawed results.
- **Blind patients to their study arm assignment:** Blind patients refer to participants not knowing their study arm assignment (i.e., intervention or control group). For instance, control-arm subjects may receive a placebo or "sham" surgery to ensure that they are unaware of group assignments. Split-mouth designs are a unique approach in dentistry in which the intervention is applied to a randomly selected half of the mouth; in this case, each subject serves as his/her own control, and patients are blinded as to which side received which treatment.
- **Aim to collect outcomes data from all enrolled patients:** Patients who complete a trial may have different baseline characteristics (i.e. demographics, comorbidities, and socioeconomic status) or other confounding variables compared to those who are lost to follow-up. Studies with a substantial amount of missing data have a higher risk of reporting biased results.
- **Blind the researchers doing outcomes assessments:** Individuals on the study team who interpret patient outcomes should also be blinded to patient assignment (i.e. control vs. intervention) since this knowledge could affect their assessments.
- **Assure clinical equipoise:** There should be true uncertainty as to what the effect is of the proposed intervention. If an intervention is known absolutely to be beneficial, it would be unethical to assign a subject to the control group. Conversely, a trial should not be conducted if an intervention is known to have a net harm greater than the standard of care. Ongoing monitoring of patient outcomes should be done throughout a trial, with very clear early results sometimes necessitating early termination of the trial. Collaboration with an Institutional Review Board is essential when developing the protocol for an RCT and carrying it out.

6.3 Study Selection

The process for inclusion in this chapter began with the lead author (AG) compiling a list of search terms relevant to each of the content sections. This can be found in Appendix. With the assistance of a medical librarian (AH), these search terms were applied to generate a preliminary list of articles that were de-duplicated and reviewed by one author (SU) to exclude studies that were not randomized trials. AG then reviewed the remaining abstracts to select for full-text review, which were analyzed for content by AG and for quality by BM.

Table 6.1 Summary statistics on eligible trials included in the chapter

	Eligible trials	Sample size		Single-center studies	Risk of bias			Study diagram
		Median	Trials <50 patients		Low	Some concerns	High	
General medicine	12	64	4 (33%)	12 (100%)	0 (0%)	10 (83%)	2 (17%)	3 (25%)
Outpatient anesthesia	11	60	4 (36%)	11 (100%)	4 (36%)	7 (64%)	0 (0%)	0 (0%)
Dentoalveolar surgery	87	46	51 (59%)	85 (98%)	5 (6%)	56 (64%)	26 (30%)	28 (32%)
Orthognathic	57	37	39 (68%)	49 (86%)	0 (0%)	44 (77%)	13 (23%)	13 (23%)
Facial trauma	29	43	15 (52%)	27 (93%)	5 (17%)	9 (31%)	15 (52%)	4 (14%)
Pathology	5	33	4 (80%)	5 (100%)	1 (20%)	2 (40%)	2 (40%)	0 (0%)
Reconstruction	16	48	9 (60%)	14 (88%)	0 (0%	14 (88%)	2 (13%)	2 (13%)
TMD	15	40	13 (87%)	14 (93%)	0 (0%)	11 (73%)	4 (27%)	1 (7%)
Overall	232	45.5	139 (60%)	217 (94%)	15 (6%)	152 (66%)	64 (28%)	51 (22%)

Of an initial set of 4587 de-duplicated titles, 435 abstracts met the criteria for initial review, which yielded 232 articles for full-text review and inclusion in this chapter. An overview of the summary statistics on the included studies is given in Table 6.1.

6.4 Quality Assessment

The quality of each study was assessed in three ways: sample size and number of enrolling institutions; risk of bias; and whether the study used a CONSORT or similar diagram.

First, the sample size and the number of enrolling institutions were used as basic measures of study precision and generalizability. There is no ideal enrollment target for a given trial; sample sizes should vary based on anticipated effect sizes, the population-level variability (i.e., standard deviation) in the primary outcome, and the desired statistical power. Nonetheless, there are recommendations regarding minimum sample sizes. Simulations of two-arm RCTs suggest that bias is notably greater in trials with samples of fewer than 50 patients (e.g., 25 patients per study arm), and a target of 70 patients has been proposed as a minimum sample size for achieving reasonable precision of results [1].

As a preliminary assessment of this aspect of quality, we report the median number of patients in the eligible studies of each content section, as well as the proportion of trials that enrolled at least 50 patients. More conservative approaches to evaluating RCT sample size could use a higher threshold (e.g., 70 patients) or identify whether a formal sample size assessment was conducted for each study.

Second, the risk of bias was assessed using four domains of potential bias from the revised Cochrane risk-of-bias tool for randomized trials (ROB2) [1]. The four domains were assessed with several questions that we adopted from the ROB2 tool, as shown below. Each domain was assigned one of three possible judgments (low risk of bias, some concerns of bias, and high risk of bias) as described by the Cochrane ROB2 algorithm, and each study received an overall risk of bias score defined by the highest risk in any of the four domains.

- **Domain 1: Risk of bias from the randomization process.** Was the allocation sequence random, and was it concealed until participants were enrolled? Were there baseline differences between groups that suggested a problem with randomization? Techniques such as alternating assignment or assignment based on dates (e.g., birth date) are predictable and are not truly random; assignment techniques such as computer-generated random number lists, drawing envelopes, or flipping coins are preferred. Even if the approach to assignment is random, study arms may nonetheless differ in critical ways (e.g., age, comorbidities, etc.) that could introduce bias.

- **Domain 2: Risk of bias due to deviations from the intended interventions.** Were study participants or experimenters aware of assigned interventions during the trial? Were there deviations from the intended interventions? Were these deviations likely to have affected the outcome? Even if subjects were appropriately randomized, could adherence to study protocols differ if they or the staff were aware of the assigned study arm.
- **Domain 3: Risk of bias due to missing outcome data.** Were data for this outcome available for all (or nearly all) participants who were randomized? If no, could the result have been biased because of this missing data? Is it likely that certain data were missing because of the value (i.e. result) of those data? Study results could be biased if participants in a certain study arm were systematically less likely to complete study follow-up.
- **Domain 4: Risk of bias in measurement of the outcome.** Was the method of outcome measurement appropriate? Could the measurement of the outcome have differed between groups? Were assessors aware of the interventions received by study participants? If so, could this knowledge have influenced their assessment of the outcome? Despite appropriate randomization and full collection of outcome data, results could still be biased if outcome assessments were measured differently based on the study arm or if outcome assessors were not blinded to patient assignment.

Third, we report whether each study included a diagram of participants' enrollment, randomization, receipt of interventions, and completion of follow-up. The CONSORT diagram is the most widely used standard and is highly recommended for inclusion in reporting of all randomized trials, but we also gave credit for using other similar diagrams if they met most CONSORT criteria (e.g., a diagram that included enrollment, allocation, and follow-up but failed to address data analysis). Reporting these basic characteristics assist readers in interpreting the overall study quality and generalizability of its results.

6.5 Topic-Specific Content Review

6.5.1 General Medicine and Oral Surgery

This section addresses study questions relating to the types of precautions or modifications to oral surgery that should be undertaken when treating a patient with a general health condition. The main questions of interest are how to safely perform oral surgery on a patient with systemic disease, including control of pain, bleeding, and optimization of wound healing (Table 6.2).

Content summary: RCTs support the use of local measures for hemostasis rather than altering the dose of anticoagulants. There is some evidence consistent with the trend that optimization of oral health decreases other systemic health sequelae. There is a paucity of evidence from RCTs on the safety profiles of oral surgery on patients with cardiovascular, kidney, or liver disease.

Quality assessment: The General Medicine category was one of two categories in which more than half the studies enrolled at least 50 patients. All trials were single-center studies. The majority of studies (83%) had some concerns regarding the risk of bias, while the remaining studies had a high risk of bias.

6.5.1.1 Opportunities for Future Study

Randomized controlled trials that study the intersection of oral surgery with general medical conditions can be challenging due to tension between internal and external validities. For example, the answer to a dental research question in a population of healthy patients may not necessarily be true among patients with certain medical conditions. Conducting research on patients who both have specific medical conditions and require certain dental treatment provides a challenge in recruitment for adequate sample size, and the risk of the interventions may be uncertain based on the systemic diseases themselves.

Table 6.2 Select content from RCTs covering general medicine and oral surgery

Topic	Key findings	Supporting studies	Journal types
Warfarin	• There is no advantage to stopping warfarin or reducing therapeutic International normalised ratio, INR goal for tooth extractions [2]. Use of local measures is supported for post-op bleeding control [3]. TXA[a] soaked gauze reduces time to immediate hemostasis [4]	Al-Mubarak (2007) [2], Sacco (2007) [3], Queiroz (2018) [4]	Dental, OMS
Antiplatelets	• Local measures can be used to control bleeding after dental extractions in patients taking aspirin [5, 6]. There is no indication to stop aspirin for dental extractions [7]	Giudice (2019) [5], Medeiros (2011) [6], Brennan (2008) [7]	Implants, OMS, Dental Research
Critical care	• Dental treatment is effective in preventing lower respiratory tract infections in critically ill patients [8]	Bellissimo-Rodrigues (2014) [8]	Infection control & Epidemiology
Diabetes Mellitus	• Extraction of teeth with advanced periodontitis in patients with Type 2 Diabetes (DM2) improves glycemic control [9]	Khader (2010) [9]	Periodontal Research
Medication-related osteonecrosis of the jaw	• Patients on zoledronic acid should be monitored by dentists every 12 weeks to reduce the risk of developing medication-related osteonecrosis of the jaw (MRONJ) [10]	Mucke (2016) [10]	Craniomaxillofacial Surgery

[a]*TXA* tranexamic acid

From both an ethical and a practical standpoint, one cannot randomize subjects to a given state of health. As a result, sample sizes analyzing oral surgery topics must be large enough to represent multiple different states of health in the population. Appropriate studies would then analyze the primary exposures and outcomes and stratify the results based on the medical conditions of interest to examine for an effect. Baseline characteristics of the subjects in the study arms should include commonly used metrics to assess the disease under investigation (e.g., CHADS-2 score for anticoagulation, Hb A1c for diabetes, or eGFR for chronic kidney disease).

Some specific topics that would be useful to the dental community include local anesthetic vasoconstrictor concentration in patients with cardiovascular disease, use of antibiotics following extractions in patients with diabetes, and drug holidays and incidence of medication-related osteonecrosis of the jaw (MRONJ) in the setting of oral bisphosphonate use. Because MRONJ is a relatively rare outcome, this study in particular would need to have a large enough sample size to pick up a difference in incidence of disease. This should undoubtedly be a multi-center study. Partnerships with the companies that make these medications and/or groups that research osteoporosis outcomes should be considered to maximize reach when designing such a study.

6.5.2 Outpatient Anesthesia

Oral and maxillofacial surgeons in the United States routinely perform, as a single operator, surgery and anesthesia simultaneously. This practice is central to the model of provision of care to a population where rates of severe dental phobia have been estimated at 10–20% of the adult population [11] (Table 6.3).

Content summary: In children, PO administration of 0.7 mg/kg of midazolam is supported in combination with inhaled nitrous oxide for anxiolysis. Pediatric outpatient IV anesthesia for oral surgery is not well described in RCTs. In adults and seniors, IV midazolam improves comfort and satisfaction and reduces hemodynamic changes during dental extractions. During an IV anesthetic, opioids may be delivered by infusion or in boluses. Propofol and ketamine can be used with success, alone or in combination.

Quality assessment: The Anesthesia section had the best (i.e., lowest) overall risk of bias among all categories examined (36% low risk

Table 6.3 Select content from RCTs covering outpatient anesthesia

Topic	Key findings	Supporting studies	Journal types
Geriatrics	• In older patients, use of nitrous oxide or intravenous, IV midazolam produces fewer changes in heart rate (HR) and blood pressure (BP) during dental extractions than local anesthesia alone [12, 13]	Shao (2013)[a] [12], Zhao (2007) [13]	Medical
Pediatric oral sedation	• The most effective oral pre-medication for children ages 5–8 prior to nitrous oxide/oxygen is 0.7 mg/kg midazolam PO [14]	Baygin (2010) [14]	Anesthesiology
IV sedation	• When combining drugs in a single syringe, the optimal ratio of propofol: ketamine is 10:1 for continuous IV infusion [14]	Baygin (2010) [14]	Anesthesiology
Benzodiazepines	• Use of IV Midazolam as a single agent improves comfort and satisfaction in adult patients compared to local anesthesia alone [15]	Wan (2007) [15]	Stomatology
Opioids	• During a propofol infusion, either boluses of fentanyl or infusion of alfentanil provide acceptable hemodynamics and patient satisfaction [16] • Remifentanil 0.1 mcg/kg/min leads to higher patient and surgeon satisfaction than 0.05 mcg/kg/min [17]	Kwak (2006) [16], Torun (2017) [17]	OMS

[a]Abstract only reviewed

and 64% some concerns). These results likely reflected a relatively high proportion of double-blinded studies that performed well in regard to both randomization and outcome assessment. Double-blinded and placebo-controlled trials are more practical to perform in studies of administered medications, in contrast to studies of surgical interventions. As in the General Medicine section, the majority of eligible Anesthesia studies included at least 50 patients. However, all eligible trials in this category were single-center studies, and none included a study diagram such as CONSORT.

6.5.2.1 Opportunities for Future Study

Delivery of safe and effective anesthesia is based on real-time response to the physiology and behavior of the patient. This includes airway interventions, dosing and timing of medications, and appropriate preparation for office safety.

Although in usual practice, oral and maxillofacial surgeons practice under the single-provider model, using a two-provider model for research would allow the surgeon to be blinded to the anesthetic regimen and thus more accurately describe its level of success without risk of bias.

The outcomes of the greatest importance in anesthesia are quite rare: death or serious injury, typically resulting from a pulmonary or cardiovascular complication. As such, randomized controlled trials do not make the best model for assessing these outcomes. It is, however, quite reasonable to create a trial comparing one medication regimen to another. Appropriate outcomes to consider include depth of sedation, need for airway interventions, post-operative satisfaction of the surgeon and patient, as well as any side effects such as nausea, vomiting, or post-operative delirium.

The consideration to include of CONSORT or similar diagram is worth particular mention in this section, thus adding a representation of enrollment, study arm allocation, analysis, and follow-up for the reader to process visually.

6.5.3 Dentoalveolar Surgery

Dentoalveolar surgery is the mainstay of oral and maxillofacial surgery and consists primarily of tooth extractions and modification of the bone and soft tissues of the oral cavity. The content outlined below relates to intraoperative techniques, medications to reduce symptoms, and predictors of post-operative outcomes (Table 6.4).

Content summary: RCTs in this section tend to focus on the third molar surgery, as the case

Table 6.4 Select content from RCTs covering dentoalveolar surgery

Topic	Key findings	Supporting studies	Journal types
Periodontal status of 2nd molar after 3rd molar surgery	• There is not a single flap design that optimizes this outcome [18, 19]. Simple suture technique is appropriate [20] • In mesioangular or horizontal impactions, there is some benefit to placing a resorbable membrane [21], root planning [22], and bone grafting obvious defects [22]	Chaves (2008) [19], Laurito (2016) [20], Cetinkaya (2009) [21], Cortell-Balester (2015) [22], Ge (2017) [23]	Dental hygiene, Craniofacial Surgery, OMS, Implant dentistry
Adjuncts in 3rd molar sockets	• There is no support for routine placement of platelet-rich-plasma (PRP) or platelet-rich-fibrin (PRF) into third molar sockets [23–26]. There is a modest benefit of dry socket prevention in smokers [27]	Gurbuzer (2008) [24], Sammartino (2009) [25], Afat (2018) [26], Daugela (2018) [27], Unsal (2018) [28]	OMS, Dentistry, Clinical Practice
Bone removal technique	• Drills are superior to chisels in operating time and post-operative complications for 3rd molar surgery [28, 29]	Guo (2012)[a] [29], Yang (2015) [30]	Stomatology
Lingual nerve retraction	• Lingual retraction carries 3.4 times the risk of transient lingual nerve injury (8.94%) but it is typically reversible. Buccal flap only technique carries lingual nerve injury rate of 2.63% but is more likely to be permanent [30]	Shad (2015) [31]	Medical
Coronectomy	• In patients with 3rd molar roots radiographically close to the IA nerve, extraction yields higher incidence of nerve injury than coronectomy. Pain and dry socket are lower in coronectomy group. No difference in infection rate. Reoperation secondary to root exposure is higher in coronectomy group [31]	Leung (2009) [32]	OMS
Pain control following dental extractions	• Combination treatment with non-steroidal anti-inflammatory drug (NSAID) plus acetaminophen provides better analgesia than either drug alone [32]. Addition of codeine does not improve analgesia [33] • Non-selective NSAIDs and selective Cox-2 inhibitors are equally effective [34] • Peri-operative administration of oral pregabalin or NSAID (oral or IV) improves post-operative pain [35, 36] • Submucosal tramadol 1 mg/kg improves post-operative pain through 48 h [37] • After extraction of an average of 3.15 teeth, the mean number of opioid pills consumed is 13 (without dry socket) and 18 (with dry socket) [38]	Akural (2009) [33], Best (2017) [34], Benetello (2007) [35], Olmedo-Gaya (2016) [36], Pektas (2007) [37], Gonul (2015) [38], Maughan (2016) [39]	Therapeutics, OMS, Medical Research, OMS, Medicine, Drug Dependence
Antibiotics	• Evidence from RCTs is mixed for the routine use of antibiotics for 3rd molar surgery. The following studies do not support its use [39–43]. The following studies do [44–47]. Methods are heterogeneous	Rabi (2018) [40], Xue (2014) [41], Adde (2012) [42], Ataoglu (2008) [43], Milani (2015) [44], Monaco (2009) [45], Arteagoitia (2005) [46], Halpern (2007) [47], Lopez-Cedrun (2011) [48]	Dentistry, Stomatology, OMS,

(continued)

Table 6.4 (continued)

Topic	Key findings	Supporting studies	Journal types
Suturing	• Sutures worsen post-operative edema, trismus, and pain. They should be used to approximate wounds only when necessary [48, 49] • Triangular 3rd molar flaps may be closed with a single suture [50] • Monofilament sutures accumulate less bacteria than braided sutures [51]	Ricard (2015) [49], Xavier (2008) [50], Gay-Escoda (2015) [51], Asher (2019) [52]	Stomatology, Dentistry, OMS, Oral Investigations
Steroids	• Perioperative use of steroids improves post-operative pain, swelling, difficulty eating/speaking, missed school/work. 4–8 mg of dexamethasone, given systemically by injection or orally is supported [52–59] • Steroids alone are not superior to NSAIDs [60]. Steroids and NSAIDs together are better than either alone [61, 62]	Al-Dajani (2017) [53], Ilhan (2014) [54], Vicentini (2018) [55], Warraich (2013) [56], Alcantara (2014) [57], Antunes (2011) [58], Mico-Llorens (2006) [59], Kocer (2014) [60], Sotto-Maior (2011) [61], Barbalho (2017) [62], Lima (2018) [63]	OMS, Medical, Pharmacology, Craniofacial Surgery,
Local anesthesia	• Gow-Gates technique has higher anesthetic success rate (97.15% vs. 89.10%) and lower complication rate than Halstead technique [63]	Hu (2015)[a] [64]	Stomatology
Chlorhexidine gel	• Chlorhexidine gel may reduce the incidence of alveolar osteitis [64, 65]	Torres-Lagares (2006) [70], Torres-Lagares (2010) [71]	OMS

[a]Abstract only reviewed

volume in oral surgery makes this quite reliable to study. For the administration of mandibular anesthesia, the Gow-Gates technique is superior to the Halstead technique. There is not a single flap design or suturing technique that is optimal in all cases. Lingual nerve retraction carries a higher risk of transient nerve injury but a lower risk of permanent nerve injury than buccal flap only, and obesity is a risk factor for adverse effects in third molar surgery.

NSAIDs and acetaminophen together perform better for post-operative pain control than either drug alone; the addition of codeine does not improve analgesia. Patients who undergo multiple tooth extractions can be expected to use an average of 13 tablets of opioid medication per 3.15 teeth removed. Evidence is mixed on routine use of antibiotics, while steroids reliably improve post-operative pain and swelling.

Quality assessment: The large collection of articles on dentoalveolar surgery represents over one-third of all literature reviewed for this chapter (87 of 232 studies). The risk of bias was low in 6%, moderate (some concerns) in 64%, and high in 30%, similar to our overall sample. Of these 87 studies, 51 (59%) had a sample size of under 50 subjects, and only 2 (2%) were multicenter studies. Almost one-third of trials (28 studies, 32%) included some type of study diagram to illustrate enrollment, receipt of study intervention, and follow-up.

6.5.3.1 Opportunities for Future Study

Antibiotics and steroids have been described both in RCTs and in observational studies. It is true that those at higher risk for infection (older patients, deeper tooth impactions, longer surgery time, smokers, and poor local wound care) should be prescribed antibiotics and that steroids seem to improve post-operative course without interfering with wound healing. Future studies on this topic should aim to elucidate the risk–benefit calculations clinicians should undergo when deciding who should be prescribed these medications around oral surgery.

Important areas for future study include what exactly should be placed into a third molar socket in the subset of patients likely to have periodontal defects (patients older than 26 with mesioangular or horizontal impactions).

As there is only one RCT on lingual nerve retraction and there is great interest in how to minimize permanent lingual nerve injuries, it is prudent to perform more studies similar to that of Shad 2015 [31]. Likewise for inferior alveolar nerve injury, more studies similar to Leung 2009 [32] examining coronectomy versus extraction would be appropriate.

Dentoalveolar surgery provides many opportunities for RCTs. There is a high volume of this type of surgery performed in both private practice and institutional settings, and future studies should be carried out in both realms. The split-mouth study design lends itself well to this topic. Specifically, this involves using each subject as his/her own control, comparing an experimental intervention on one side to a control on the other. A key feature should be blinding the researcher doing the outcomes assessment as to which side received which treatment. A particular advantage of this design is that it removes the need for there to be equal baseline characteristics among groups of subjects.

6.5.4 Orthognathic Surgery

Orthognathic surgery is always a multidisciplinary field, particularly involving OMS, orthodontics, anesthesia, along with involvement from cleft teams, when indicated. The literature outlined includes topics such as hardware choices, medication management, treatment planning, and minimization of bleeding (Table 6.5).

Content summary: Three-day courses of antibiotics seem to be optimal following orthognathic surgery. Computer-aided surgical planning is more accurate than traditional model surgery. A single dose of pregabalin improves post-operative pain control. Multiple pharmacologic options exist for the stabilization of hemodynamics and hypotensive anesthesia. The use of TXA is supported to reduce blood loss during bimaxillary

Table 6.5 Select content from RCTs covering orthognathic surgery

Topic	Key findings	Supporting studies	Journal types
Stability	• 5-year stability favors maxillary distraction osteogenesis (DO) to one-stage orthognathic surgery in cleft patients [66] • Bilateral sagittal split osteotomy (BSSO) vs. mandibular DO in Class II advancements show similar amounts of relapse, slightly favoring DO [67] • Intraoral vertical ramus osteotomy (IVRO) + coronoidectomy is more stable at 1 year than IVRO alone in mandibular setbacks [68]	Cheung (2006) [72], Ow (2010) [73], Talesh (2011) [74]	Plastic Surgery, OMS,
Steroids	• Dexamethasone 15 mg is not superior to 5 mg in reducing facial swelling, nausea, or vomiting [69]. Steroids do not influence neurosensory disturbances after orthognathic surgery [70, 71]	Lin (2017) [75], Semper-Hogg (2017) [76], Widar (2015) [77]	Plastic Surgery, Medicine, OMS
Antibiotics	• Three-day courses of post-operative antibiotics are more effective at preventing surgical site infections than 1-day courses, which are more effective than just a single dose [72–74]. There is not a benefit of extending the course longer [75, 76]	Danda (2010) [78], Wahab (2013) [79], Davis (2017) [80], Ghantous (2019) [81], Kang (2009) [82]	OMS, Craniofacial Surgery, Medicine
Computer-aided treatment planning	• This technique reduces neurosensory disturbances in IVRO [77] • In bimaxillary surgery, virtual surgical planning (VSP) is more accurate than traditional model surgery [78, 79]	Al-Ahmad (2013) [83], Schneider (2019) [84], Hanafy (2020) [85]	Medical Robotics, Clinical Oral Investigations, Stomatology

(continued)

Table 6.5 (continued)

Topic	Key findings	Supporting studies	Journal types
Pain control	• A single pre-operative dose of pregabalin improves post-operative pain, reduces opioid consumption, and lowers nausea/vomiting [80]	Ahiskalioglu (2016) [86]	OMS
Intraoperative medication management	• Remifentanil 0.75 mcg/kg/min stabilizes hemodynamics during Le Fort I osteotomy [81] • There is not a single best pharmacologic protocol for induced hypotension during orthognathic surgery [82–85]. Clonidine, sodium nitroprusside, nitroglycerin, remifentanil, enalapril, and dexmedetomidine are all supported • Dexmedetomidine 1 mcg/kg for 10 min during emergence reduces cough, tachycardia, and pain. Agitation is not reduced, and time to eye opening is longer [86]	Abukawa (2015) [87], Farah (2008) [88], Yoshikawa (2009) [89], Mohammadi (2016) [90], Kim (2015) [91], Ham (2014) [92]	OMS, Anesthesiology, Medicine
Bleeding	• Use of tranexamic acid (TXA) 10–20 mg/kg during bimaxillary surgery reduces blood loss. The higher doses do not yield more benefit [87, 88]. There is not a benefit of adding TXA to irrigating fluid [89]. There may be a higher benefit in women than in men [90] • Use of gauze strips soaked with 100 mg cocaine and 2 ml 1:1000 adrenaline placed in the nasal floor at the time of Le Fort I osteotomy reduces blood loss [91] • Hypotensive anesthesia during Le Fort I osteotomy reduces blood loss compared to normotension and hemodilution. Field quality/visibility is also superior [92] • Remifentanil 0.1 mcg/kg/min reduces blood loss during bimaxillary surgery compared to propofol 50 mcg/kg/min [93]	Apipan (2018)` [93], Choi (2009) [94], Kaewpradub (2011) [95], Secher (2018) [96], de Lange (2008) [97], Ervens (2010) [98], Eshghpour (2018) [99]	OMS
Resorbable hardware	• Resorbable screws can be effectively used in fixating BSSO mandibular advancements, but are more likely to require post-operative use of elastics due to rotation around the screws [94] • Maxillary stability after Le Fort I osteotomy fixated with absorbable plates is comparable to that of titanium plates when postoperative maxillomandibular fixation (MMF) is used [95]	Yu (2014) [100], Ueki (2012) [101]	OMS
Intraoperative technique	• Cutting a sagittal split with a piezoelectric can be faster than with a combination of Lindemann bur and microsaw but does not offer an advantage in preventing neurosensory disturbances [96] • Distraction osteogenesis for mandibular advancement does not have a better rate of neurosensory disturbance compared to conventional advancement [97, 98]. Wound infections may be more prevalent in the DO group [98] • Intraoperative awakening to check occlusion during bimaxillary surgery seems to help identify errors in condylar positioning not noted with manipulation under general anesthesia [99, 100]	Kohnke (2017) [102], Baas (2015) [103], Ow (2010) [104], Politi (2007) [105], Toro (2007) [106]	OMS
Local anesthesia	• Use of regional blocks during bimaxillary surgery reduces the amount of medication necessary to achieve hypotensive anesthesia. This facilitates intraoperative BP control and decreases blood loss [101, 102]	Chen (2016) [107], Espitalier (2011) [108]	OMS, Craniomaxillofacial Surgery

surgery. Resorbable hardware can be effective, and the use of local anesthesia regional blocks reduces the amount of medication necessary to achieve hypotensive anesthesia. Steroids do not influence neurosensory disturbances.

Quality assessment: The collection of articles on orthognathic surgery (57 studies) has a large proportion of studies (39 trials, 68%) with a sample size under 50 patients. The risk of bias among trials in this section (low 0%, some concerns 77%, and high 23%) is slightly higher than the overall set of studies reviewed, although it included the largest proportion (14%, 8 trials) of multi-center studies.

6.5.4.1 Opportunities for Future Study

Various cephalometric analyses have been developed, including those by Steiner, Downs, McNamara, Wits, and Ricketts. These analyses help quantify dentofacial abnormalities, and randomizing by which analyses are used to plan treatment followed by assessments of standardized post-operative photographs may be a useful study design to consider. Today's age of 3D treatment planning will almost certainly yield updates in facial analysis that can and should be compared to the tools from the 2D era.

The use of tranexamic acid is well supported to reduce blood loss during this type of surgery. Likewise, more studies should be performed to elucidate which medications should be used in which contexts for intraoperative control of hemodynamics.

There is considerable discussion among orthognathic surgeons about whether to use plates, positional screws, or lag screws to fixate the mandible after sagittal split osteotomies. Appropriate outcomes to analyze include OR time, stability of the jaw movements, and changes over time in the mandibular condyles, the last of which may take several years to study.

Lastly, although there is not much benefit to comparing traditional stone model surgery to computer-aided planning for bimaxillary surgery, there are multiple subtleties of computer-aided planning that can be studied, including a comparison of intraoral scanners to scanned dental models taken with impression material. Likewise, multiple approaches can be taken to splint design—for instance, the use of a palatal strap for multi-piece Le Fort osteotomies.

Orthognathic surgery is as much an art as it is a science. In the end, careful analysis of the above-mentioned factors will help surgeons to find the harmony of dental occlusion, facial projection, and esthetics.

6.5.5 Facial Trauma

Management of the patient with facial trauma may involve coordination among emergency physicians, dentists, surgeons, and even law enforcement officials. Acutely, decisions must be made about airway management, medication administration, and timing of surgery relative to the trauma. This produces a tremendous amount of variability in patterns of injuries and timing of surgery, and thus yields heterogeneity in the body of literature on the topic (Table 6.6).

Content summary: The use of antibiotics intraoperatively for facial trauma is well supported. There is likely a modest effect of post-operative antibiotics, although an optimal length of therapy is not known. Shorter periods of maxillomandibular fixation (2 weeks) may be effective for routine fractures treated in a closed fashion. Multiple different fixation techniques for the treatment of mandibular fractures are supported in the literature. Zygomaticomaxillary complex fractures may have better outcomes with 3-point fixation than 2-point. Steroids improve post-operative course in orbital fracture repair, and the transconjunctival approach is superior to the subciliary approach in terms of post-operative scleral show and ectropion.

Quality assessment: Compared to other categories, the 29 eligible trials in the Facial Trauma category had the largest proportion of studies (52%) with a high overall risk of bias. One potential explanation for this limitation is that blinding is very difficult in many of these studies; many also had a relatively high risk of potential bias due to either subpar execution or poor description of randomization techniques. The Facial Trauma

Table 6.6 Select content from RCTs covering facial trauma

Topic	Key findings	Supporting studies	Journal types
Airway management	• In panfacial fractures, submental intubation is faster than elective tracheostomy and less likely to require scar revision [103]	Emara (2019) [111]	OMS
Antibiotics	• There is a clear benefit to using intraoperative antibiotics in open treatment of mandible fractures, particularly when tooth bearing segments are involved [104] • In patients with mandible fractures treated with open reduction and internal fixation (ORIF), who received pre-operative and intra-operative antibiotics, there is a trend toward a modest added benefit of post-operative antibiotics [105] • In midface and orbital fractures treated with ORIF, a 1-day course is as effective as a 5-day course of postoperative prophylactic antibiotics at preventing wound infections [106, 107]	Chole (1987) [112], Miles (2006) [113], Zix (2013) [114], Soong (2014) [115]	Otolaryngology, OMS
Bioresorbable hardware	• Bioresorbable plates have higher rates of breakage of screws and plates than titanium plates for mandible fractures [108]. These studies were underpowered to draw conclusions about fracture healing [108, 109] • A single optimal polymer out of which to make bioresorbable hardware for zygoma fractures is not supported, and many perform as well as titanium in fracture healing and complication rate. Smoking is a risk factor for complications in bioresorbable groups [110] • Use of bioresorbable plates does not reduce the need for plate removal in facial trauma [111]	Ahmed (2013) [116], Bhatt (2010) [117], Wittwer (2006) [118], Gareb (2017) [119]	Physicians and Surgeons, OMS, Science and medicine
Closed reduction of mandible fractures	• Closed reduction of mandible fractures using maxillomandibular fixation (MMF) for 2 weeks followed by maintenance of an arch bar for an additional 4 weeks performed as well as 6 weeks of MMF. The 2-week MMF group had earlier improvement in mouth opening [112] • Longer MMF groups have more weight loss, worse oral hygiene, but faster bony healing [113] • Oral health-related quality of life is not significantly different whether mandible fractures are treated with MMF vs. ORIF [114]	Al-Belasy (2005) [120], Adeyemi (2012) [121], Shetty (2008) [122]	OMS
Mandibular condylar process fractures	• Subcondylar fractures can be treated with equal success using two straight mini-plates or one delta-shaped plate. The delta plate can be adapted in less time than the two mini-plates [115] • Unilateral high condylar fractures with joint effusion may be treated with equal 12-month outcomes with MMF or arthrocentesis/betamethasone injection. Range of motion and joint pain at 1 and 3 months are less in the arthrocentesis/joint injection group [116]	Ahuja (2018) [123], Nogami (2014) [124]	OMS, Oral rehabilitation

Table 6.6 (continued)

Topic	Key findings	Supporting studies	Journal types
ORIF mandible fractures (dentate segment)	• Symphyseal fractures can be treated effectively with two lag screws or two mini-plates [117] • When treating mandibular fractures with mini-plates, there is no difference between locking and non-locking plates in terms of pain, swelling, infection, hardware failure, or mobility • Bite force at 6 weeks and 3 months is greater in the locking plate group [118]	Agnihotri (2014) [125], Agarwal (2011) [126]	OMS
ORIF mandibular angle fractures	• The ladder-style lateral border miniplate performs as well as the Champy style miniplate in terms of fracture healing and complications [119] • Champy style miniplate vs. miniplate placed flat against lateral ramus/body with transbuccal trocar in angle fractures: plate removal is required more often in intraoral (Champy) approach. Transbuccal plate has lower infection rate [120] • 3rd molar in the line of fracture was not a predictor of post-op complications in angle fractures [120]. When randomizing to retention or removal of 3rd molar in angle fractures, fracture healing is not affected • Nerve injury rates are higher when the molar is removed [121]	Al-Moraissi (2015) [127], Laverick (2012) [128], McNamara (2016) [129]	OMS
Zygomaticomaxillary complex fractures	• Decreased malar height and vertical dystopia are more common with 2-point (ZF, ZM) than with 3-point (ZF, ZM, IO) [122]	Rana (2012) [130]	Trials
Orbital fractures	• Use of perioperative steroids decreases post-operative pain and improves eye opening [123, 124] • Fibrin sealant is superior to buried 6-0 vicryl sutures for conjunctival wound closure in terms of time to wound healing, post-operative pain, and periorbital ecchymosis [125] • Transconjunctival approach is superior to subciliary approach in terms of postoperative scleral show and ectropion [126]	Kormi (2017) [131], Flood (1999) [132], You (2016) [133], El-Anwar (2017) [134]	OMS

category was similar to the overall sample in regard to the proportion of trials that were conducted in a single center (94%) and the proportion of studies that enrolled fewer than 50 patients (52%).

6.5.5.1 Opportunities for Future Study

Both anecdotally and as described in observational studies, facial trauma can be treated in a variety of different ways. There are principles to which one must adhere, and then there are a number of variations on each theme. This includes surgical approach, fixation style, and order of treatment of injuries, to name a few variables. Coordination of multi-center trials would be best done at tertiary care centers that treat large volumes and varieties of cases, in order to get adequate sample sizes for study despite the heterogeneity in injury patterns. In fact, the use of cluster randomization, where the randomization is done at the level of the center rather than the patient, may be well applied in this scenario. There is a risk of limited external validity, however, if the cases treated and described at tertiary care centers do not reflect the types of cases seen in the general community.

The background of a facial trauma surgeon may be in OMS, plastic surgery, otolaryngology, or even ophthalmology in some cases. The training in each field has overlap, but trends and specific foci may be somewhat different. For instance, the oral surgeon may be more likely to use the dental occlusion as a guide for facial reconstruction than the oculoplastic surgeon, who may use the intercanthal distance.

6.5.6 Pathology

As mentioned in the introduction to this chapter, the authors have chosen to exclude malignant pathology from this chapter. Randomized controlled trials on benign pathologic entities of the mouth and jaws are extremely rare, despite how common many of these lesions are, including mucoceles, fibromas, pyogenic granulomas, and other such soft tissue lesions. This is largely because simple excision is curative and carries minimal morbidity, thus not requiring an RCT to guide treatment. The existing literature to date leaves a strong desire for RCTs on benign bony cysts and tumors of the jaws (Table 6.7).

Content summary: The reviewed studies on benign bony pathology are mixed as to whether any bone grafting should be done on a defect after the removal of a pathologic lesion. The addition of BMP-2 and L-PRF to debridement sites in MRONJ is beneficial. There were no studies on osteomyelitis of the jaws, treatment of ameloblastomas, or odontogenic keratocysts, all commonly seen disease processes for oral and maxillofacial surgeons.

Quality assessment: The Pathology section appeared to have trials of generally similar quality as other categories, but other conclusions about study quality are difficult for this category as there were only five eligible studies.

6.5.6.1 Opportunities for Future Study

Future studies should explore various treatment modalities for the odontogenic keratocyst. It is a common enough lesion (13.8% of odontogenic tumors) [131] with a high enough recurrence potential (16–30%) [132] that multiple surgeons and authors have debated the best way to minimize recurrence potential and surgical morbidity. While en bloc resection removes the lesion reliably, it has a significant impact on quality of life, while simple enucleation yields high recurrence rates. Peripheral ostectomy, cryotherapy, topical 5-FU, or some combination of these modalities has been studied in the observational literature and warrants comparisons with RCT design. The same holds true for ameloblastoma; however, its higher rate of aggressive activity may make it more complicated to study. A challenging hurdle in these types of studies will be follow-up, as the time to recurrence may be years.

Osteomyelitis of the mandible is often treated with some combination of debridement and antibiotics. The ideal length of antibiotics is not known, nor is the optimal timing of surgery in

Table 6.7 Select content from RCTs covering oral and maxillofacial pathology

Topic	Key findings	Supporting studies	Journal types
MRONJ	• Addition of bone morphogenetic protein 2 (BMP-2) to leukocyte-platelet-rich fibrin (L-PRF) after intraoral debridement and primary closure improves wound healing [127]	Park (2017) [135]	OMS
Submandibular gland excision	• A submental approach provides a superior cosmetic outcome compared to a submandibular approach without increasing operation time or complication rates [128]	Roh (2008) [136]	Oral Oncology
Bony fill after enucleation of cysts of the jaws	• Evidence is mixed as to the effect of simultaneous bone grafting and guided bone regeneration (GBR) on bony fill after enucleation of intrabony cysts of the jaws [129, 130]	Ludovichetti (2018) [137], Santamaria (1998) [138]	Stomatology, OMS

relationship to antibiotics. Multiple details about types of soft tissue closure and adjuvant therapies (such as PRP, PRF, and BMP-2) can be studied as well. Other common pathologic entities without clear regimens for medical treatment include lichen planus, aphthous ulcers, and fungal infections.

6.5.7 Reconstruction

Content summary: The included studies on alveolar cleft grafting call into question the conventional practice of iliac crest bone grafts alone, as the use of barrier membranes and/or BMP-2 is supported. The ideal technique is still not known but should balance bone fill, morbidity, and material cost/handling properties. If an iliac crest graft is done, the use of an indwelling catheter-based infiltration of local anesthetic is effective for donor-site pain relief. The use of computer-aided surgical planning, lingual nerve repair cuffs, and venous couplers are also supported. The optimal number of implants in a fibula-neomandibular prosthesis is not known (Table 6.8).

Quality assessment: While none of the 16 reconstruction trials were assigned a low overall risk of bias, the category also included a relatively lower proportion of trials with a high overall risk of bias (12.5%) compared to most other categories. As with most other categories, a majority of trials in this category were single-center studies (87.5%) and enrolled fewer than 50 patients (60%).

6.5.7.1 Opportunities for Future Study

Pogrel's landmark study in 1997 [148] supported the use of non-vascularized bone grafts in mandibular defects up to 9 cm; however, as more surgeons have become comfortable with vascularized mandible reconstruction, there has been a trend toward vascularized bone grafts for continuity defects greater than 4–5 cm. In this intermediate-sized range of mandibular reconstruction, it may be prudent to create a multi-center RCT examining patient satisfaction, donor site morbidity, hospital stay, cost, and esthetic and functional outcomes for implant-based dental rehabilitation in defects between 3 and 9 cm reconstructed with vascularized versus non-vascularized bone grafts.

One of the central questions in reconstruction uniquely facing oral and maxillofacial surgeons is how best to get a patient from a continuity defect of the jaws to restored dental occlusion. Even in observational literature, studies evaluating this topic have only a small fraction of subjects completing dental rehabilitation. In the United States, bone grafting a continuity defect is often covered by medical insurers. The endosseous implants are rarely covered, and the dental prostheses are almost never covered. Further, the number of dentists/prosthodontists who can restore these difficult cases is quite small, and the process is quite time consuming and expensive. RCTs in this field, while potentially logistically difficult and expensive, would be very meaningful. Studying non-vascularized versus vascularized grafts, implant placement at the time of vascularized free flap versus delayed, and different types of prosthetic designs would help guide the field tremendously. Partnerships with companies interested in testing specific restorative materials may be a way to bring these important studies to reality.

6.5.8 Temporomandibular Disorders (TMD)

Temporomandibular disorders include pain and dysfunction involving the bones, articular disc, or musculature of the jaw. Outcomes of interest are primarily related to reduction of pain and increase in range of motion (Table 6.9).

TMJOA temporomandibular joint osteoarthritis, *PRP* platelet-rich plasma, *HA* hyaluronic acid, *TMD* temporomandibular disorder, *VAS* visual analog scale, *MIO* maximal incisal opening, *ROM* range of motion

Content summary: There have been multiple small studies on intra-articular injections, showing promise with multiple techniques. More studies with careful inclusion criteria are necessary to see if one regimen proves supreme. For all TMD, multi-modal therapy with habit/behavior modification is beneficial. There is a modest effect of

Table 6.8 Select content from RCTs covering reconstruction

Topic*	Key findings	Supporting studies	Journal types
Alveolar cleft grafting	• Alveolar cleft reconstruction with iliac crest bone graft and BMP-2 yield similar effect on nasal symmetry [133] • Iliac bone plus plasma-rich growth factors yield higher volume of regenerated bone at 6 months compared to freeze-dried bone allograft and plasma-rich growth factors (PRGF) [134] • Use of a barrier membrane + iliac bone (GBR technique) reduces bone resorption and improves osteogenesis as compared to iliac crest alone [135]	Alonso (2014) [141], Shirani (2017) [142], Xiao (2016) [143]	Plastic Surgery, Craniomaxillofacial surgery, OMS
Surgical guides	• Preoperative planning and use of a surgical guide improve oral health-related quality of life compared to freehand reconstruction for mandibular dental prostheses on a microvascular free fibula reconstruction [136] • Mirroring only the resected portion of the mandible is more effective than mirroring the entire hemimandible when designing a reconstruction plate [137]	Brandao (2016) [144], Khalifa (2016) [145]	Prosthetic Dentistry, OMS
Lingual nerve repair	• For lingual nerve repairs, use of a cuff is superior to direct neurorrhaphy [138]	Fujita (2014) [146]	OMS
Free flap survival	• Couplers should be used rather than hand-sewing venous anastomoses. They are faster and have a trend toward lower thrombosis rates [139] • Magnetic resonance angiography (MRA) is an acceptable alternative to digital subtraction angiography in preoperative planning of free fibula flap reconstruction [140]	Senthil Murugan (2018) [147], Klein (2013) [148]	OMS, Microsurgery
Non-vascularized bone grafting	• Iliac crest on-lay graft on edentulous mandible has comparable amounts of resorption and bone quality at 3 months whether it is covered with bioresorbable membrane or periosteum [141]	Heberer (2009) [149]	Oral Implants

Table 6.8 (continued)

Pain control following anterior iliac crest harvest	• A single dose of bupivacaine does not reliably reduce postoperative pain and gait disturbance [142] • Use of an indwelling catheter-based infiltration of bupivacaine or levobupivacaine is effective for pain relief in the pediatric and adult populations [143, 144] • Femoral nerve block causes motor nerve blockade and delays ambulation • In pediatric populations, IV ketorolac provides comparable analgesia to the bupivacaine infusion [145]	Barkhuysen (2010) [150], Kumar Raja (2014) [151], Coulthard (2008) [152], Hayes (2011) [153]	OMS, General Surgery, Cleft Palate-Craniofacial
Implants placed into microvascular free flap	• Neomandibular (fibula) prostheses placed on two implants have higher marginal bone loss than those placed on four implants [146], but the quality of life outcomes is comparable [147]	Kumar (2016) [154], Kumar (2016) [155]	Craniomaxillofacial Surgery

*Reconstruction is a broad topic in itself in oral and maxillofacial surgery. It includes use of bone grafts, rotational or free vascularized flaps containing bone, muscle, and/or skin, dental implants, and prostheses for teeth, ears, and noses. Computer-aided surgical planning has revolutionized how all of these are performed In the 21st century.

Table 6.9 Select content from RCTs covering temporomandibular disorders

Topic	Key findings	Supporting studies	Journal types
TMJ Osteoarthritis (TMJOA)	• In patients with TMJOA, two injections of sodium hyaluronate was superior to corticosteroid in pain relief and range of motion [149]. Platelet-rich plasma (PRP) performs better than hyaluronic acid (HA) [150] • Joint injection with morphine provides superior pain relief to injection with bupivacaine or saline [151]	Bjornland (2007) [157], Hegab (2015) [158], Ziegler (2010) [159]	Oral rehabilitation, OMS

(continued)

Table 6.9 (continued)

Topic	Key findings	Supporting studies	Journal types
Myofascial pain	• Counseling for TMD (habits/behavior modification) was effective in improving headache. The addition of an occlusal appliance did not offer additional therapeutic effect [152] • Trigger point injections with local anesthetic (three times in 2 days) in combination with splint therapy is more effective than splint therapy alone in Visual Analogue Scale (VAS) pain scores [153]	Costa (2015) [160], Ozkan (2011) [161]	Facial Pain and Headache, Pain
Botulinum toxin	• There is likely a modest effect of botulinum toxin on pain and range of motion for patients with myofascial pain [154–158], although some studies did not find an effect [159, 160] • Dry needling and botulinum toxin both have an effect on VAS pain [161] • Botulinum toxin also decreases bite force [162]	Von Lindern (2003) [162], Guarda-Nardini (2014) [163], Kurtoglu (2008) [164], Venancio (2009) [165], Guarda-Nardini (2014) [166], Ernberg (2011) [167], Nixdorf (2002) [168], Kutuk (2019) [169], Zhang (2016) [170]	OMS, Craniomaxillofacial, Pain,
Arthrocentesis	• Arthrocentesis + PRP performs comparably to arthrocentesis + HA for TMJOA in terms of pain and range of motion (ROM) [163] • VAS pain and maximum interincisal opening (MIO) ROM are comparable for use of arthrocentesis + PRP and arthrocentesis alone for TMJ OA • There is some radiographic evidence that the PRP group shows more reparative remodeling and less progression of degeneration [163]	Comert Kilic (2016), Comert Kilic (2015) [171]	OMS

trigger point injections on myofascial pain, whether dry needling, local anesthetic, or botulinum toxin is used. PRP is a promising adjunct for joint injection alone or in combination with arthrocentesis. The literature to date has no RCTs on open temporomandibular joint surgery.

Quality assessment: The eligible trials of TMD were generally small, with 87% of the trials enrolling fewer than 50 patients. The overall risk of bias was higher than average in our sample; 73% of studies received a rating of some concerns of bias and the remaining 27% were rated as having a High risk of bias. Randomization and outcome assessment were the most common sources of potential bias.

6.5.8.1 Opportunities for Future Study

Non-invasive and minimally invasive treatment of TMD is performed by enough providers that it is quite reasonable to design a medium- to large-scale, multi-center study with strict criteria on pre-intervention pain scores and/or maximal incisal opening (MIO). Prior studies have been quite heterogeneous in these inclusion criteria, thus making the impact of the tested intervention difficult to appreciate. Certainly, all studies on the topic should be in conjunction with the behavioral therapy that is well supported. There are relatively few surgeons who perform full-scope open TMJ surgery, and many of them have camps to which they belong (in terms of preferred treatment). In addition, it is very difficult to decide on the appropriate control groups, as there is not really a standard of care for TMD as a whole. It may be reasonable to randomize one accepted treatment versus another, although there is heterogeneity in how these procedures are performed from surgeon to surgeon. TMJ open surgery is likely the most difficult area of oral and maxillofacial surgery to study well, but careful attention to inclusion and exclusion criteria and outcomes assessments are the keys to steady improvement of the literature on the topic.

6.6 Recommendations Based on Common Weaknesses from the Existing Literature

Our examination of RCTs in oral and maxillofacial surgery identified several concerns regarding overall study quality. We have four recommendations for future dental and surgical investigators to improve the quality of literature in this field:

1. Improve enrollment techniques:

   Investigators conducting an RCT should be purposeful about prespecifying and reaching RCT enrollment goals, and they should make robust efforts to enroll patients at more than one institution. More than one-fifth of studies in this review (51/232, 22%) enrolled fewer than 25 patients, and the vast majority of trials (217/232, 94%) were single-center studies. While RCT sample size requirements may vary based on anticipated effect size, treatment response variability, and other factors, Teare [2] has suggested that studies with fewer than 70 subjects are especially challenging to interpret regarding the reliability and generalizability of results. In some studies, it is difficult to randomize individual patients to an intervention, such as the adoption of clinical guidelines or standard of care across a practice, hospital, or health system. Investigations of new interventions that affect an entire practice or hospital—such as a new practice guideline or staffing model—may suffer from "contamination" in which clinicians are knowingly or unknowingly influenced by the aspects of the new intervention, even when treating patients assigned to the control group. In this context, a study design that randomizes entire clinics or hospital floors to an intervention (e.g., such as cluster randomized trials or stepped-wedge randomized trials) may be more effective at measuring the effect of these interventions.
2. Clearly demonstrate whether patients receive their assigned interventions and complete follow-up:

   RCTs must clearly state whether patients received the assigned interventions and whether they completed follow-up. Even if randomization is successful, RCTs can be biased if patients deviate from the intended assignment (e.g., a patient randomized to the intervention arm may decline the intervention and opt for conventional treatment) or if patients are lost to follow-up. These elements are two of the key elements in the CONSORT diagram.

3. Researcheres who assess patients' outcomes must be blinded to study assignments:

   Dental and maxillofacial surgery RCTs should use blinded observers to assess patient outcomes. This requirement is especially critical for subjective outcomes such as nerve function, pain control, or quality of an anesthetic that could be influenced by an individual's knowledge of each patient's study assignment. Only 15% of RCTs reviewed in this chapter (excluding split-mouth studies) clearly stated that outcome assessors were unaware of patients' student assignment.
4. Improve reporting of key RCT elements:

   For instance, authors must report the methods used to randomize study participants and describe whether randomization was successful. Excluding the split-mouth designs ($n = 31$), only 23% of studies in the review clearly stated the randomization methods used, and only 29% reported whether there were baseline differences between control and intervention groups (e.g., failure of randomization). Similarly, a few studies explicitly described whether patients received their assigned interventions or whether all patients completed follow-up. Many studies did not describe whether the individuals who assessed study outcomes were blinded to the study hypothesis or patient assignment. These and other fundamental methodological aspects of randomized trials are addressed by the CONSORT standards, which were first published in 1996 and were most recently updated in 2010 [164], yet only 20% of RCTs in our review reported a CONSORT or similar diagram. Improving the reporting of these elements in dental and maxillofacial surgery RCTs is a simple recommendation for authors to do when writing the manuscript.

6.6.1 Communicating Research Findings to Relevant Audiences

As the scope of oral and maxillofacial surgery has overlap with many other fields (in both dentistry and medicine), target journals for publication vary among the different content areas. It is worth reminding the reader that the topic of dental implants was omitted from this chapter but remains one of great importance to the oral and maxillofacial surgeon, the periodontist, and the restorative dentist alike. Plastic surgeons will be particularly interested in literature on facial trauma, reconstruction, and orthognathic surgery (especially involving patients with cleft lip and palate). Otolaryngologists may benefit from studies on pathologic entities of the jaws. General dentists and primary-care physicians will base many management decisions on literature regarding general medicine and oral surgery as well as dentoalveolar surgery. Anesthesiologists will gain important peri-operative management lessons from the literature on orthognathic surgery, facial trauma, and dentoalveolar surgery. Emergency physicians will gain acute management insight from the literature particularly on facial trauma and infections, and lastly pain specialists and orthopedists may have an interest in our literature on temporomandibular disorders. When considering publishing in a journal aimed at a different specialty, authors should write the manuscript in such a way as to familiarize the target audience with the appropriate amount of background information as well as the direct relevance to the reader's field.

Journals on oral and maxillofacial surgery may be found at the state, national, and international levels, with an ever-increasing presence of online publication platforms. Authors should consider reviewing journals' editorial policies and target those that meet international standards for adherence to CONSORT and also require researchers to register clinical trials before they are started. Data transparency and sharing are growing increasingly important as well, and authors should make their data easy to follow, with the long-term goal of their trials being accurately included in meta-analytic work in the future.

6.7 Conclusions

Investigators can take several steps to improve the quality of future RCTs in dentistry and oral surgery. The most straightforward way to improve generalizability would be to increase sample size and utilize multicenter designs to build a broader study population. Researchers and journal editors could improve also the quality of future RCTs by requiring manuscripts to include more details regarding fundamental aspects of the methodology. Less than half of RCTs in this review included sufficient detail regarding the nature of patient randomization, such as how the assignment was performed (e.g., what was the basis of randomization) and whether there were baseline differences in the study arms after randomization. Including these data in future studies will substantially enhance the quality of RCTs in dentistry and oral surgery, and it will allow clinicians to make more informed decisions about incorporating study results into their practices.

Lastly, the hierarchy of evidence lists randomized controlled trials as the gold standard for individual studies, but not every topic is realistically studied in this way. Other study designs may still be indicated when studying outcomes that are rare or take a very long time to assess, in diseases with a known best simple treatment, or for studying exposures that would be unethical to assign a subject (including harmful effects of proposed interventions). The aspiring clinician–scientist who is designing an RCT in oral and maxillofacial surgery must consider the physiology and the logistics of a given disease or intervention in combination with the points discussed throughout this chapter to recruit a broad and representative study population and standardize the fundamentals of methodology that allow the researchers to truly compare the intervention to the control in the purest way.

6.8 Case Scenario Exercise

6.8.1 Case Scenario 1

Questions

1. Discuss the methodological strengths and limitations of the following study. Does it meet the criteria to be considered a randomized controlled trial?

Adapted from deCarvalho RW, do Egito Vasconcelos BC. High weight standard and removal of third molars: a prospective randomized study. Oral Surgery, Oral Medicine, Oral Pathology and Oral Radiology. 2015;120(5):554–61.[18].

Group 1: Consists of subjects who are overweight (BMI 25.0–29.9 kg/m^2). Age 25.1 ± 2.2 years. F:M = 3:1. 280 surgeries.

Group 2: Consists of subjects who are normal weight (BMI 18.5–24.9 kg/m^2). Age 21.6 ± 1.6 years. F:M = 3:1. 280 surgeries.

Intervention: Surgical removal of impacted mandibular third molars

Predictor variables being tested: gender, age, BMI, pathology associated with the impacted molar, radiographic classifications of the impacted molar.

Outcome being assessed: adverse intraoperative events.

Results: Adverse events were found in 29.3% of surgeries in overweight patients and only 10.7% of normal-weight patients.

Authors' conclusions: Overweight patients have three times greater risk of morbidity during the removal of impacted mandibular third molars than patients with normal weight.

Answers

1. The key observation the reader should make is that a randomized controlled trial should randomize participants in otherwise similar groups to receive one intervention or another. In this study, the same intervention was applied to two fundamentally different groups. Given that the two groups were chosen based on a predictor variable being tested, this is actually not a randomized controlled trial, and it may have been better not to use the word in the title of the study.

   The authors were thoughtful to consider the fact that intraoperative morbidity in third molar surgery has many contributing variables. This meant their sample size had to be large enough to be able to meaningfully run analyses that accounted for the multiple predictors. They were appropriate in having the same number of surgeries in the two groups as well as a similar gender makeup. Age >25 is a known risk factor for both difficulty in third molar surgery and for periodontal pathology. In these two study groups, the age distribution was significantly different, increasing the risk of confounding the results. Stratification by age group is one way to further explore these relationships.

The authors' conclusion that the overweight group was more likely to have intraoperative morbidity is correct; however, the differences in baseline characteristics (age) of the groups do not allow for isolation of the effect of BMI, and the level of evidence from this study would be that of an observational study rather than that of a randomized controlled trial.

6.8.2 Case Scenario 2

Questions

1. You have been asked to design a randomized controlled trial on orthognathic surgery outcomes comparing two treatment planning methods: traditional model surgery and computer-aided virtual surgical planning.

   In the following categories, describe the considerations the you must take in designing the study:

   (a) How would you describe the general study design?
   (b) What are appropriate Inclusion/exclusion criteria? What baseline characteristics of the study groups are acceptable?
   (c) How do you determine an acceptable sample size?
   (d) What outcome measures should be used, and how should they be determined?

Answers

(a) The general study design would take two groups of patients undergoing orthognathic surgery. One group would be treatment planned using traditional stone model surgery, and the other group would be treatment planned virtually using a computer software system. The outcome of interest should be measured reliably in both groups, and these may include pre-operative, intra-operative, or post-operative measures.

(b) We are trying to isolate the role of the treatment planning method (model surgery vs. virtual planning), so we want our study population to be free from other systemic diseases that could influence outcomes. We want to have roughly equal distributions in the two groups of patients with indications for orthognathic surgery (e.g. one-jaw vs. two-jaw surgery, angle classification of malocclusion). The more restrictive we are with the inclusion criteria, the more internal validity the study has, but the smaller the population to whom the study applies (external validity). For instance, we may want to perform different studies on patients with and without a history of cleft lip and palate, as this is known to make orthognathic surgery much more difficult.

(c) Determining the acceptable sample size depends on four things:

   1. Incidence of the outcome(s) being measured: If an outcome occurs rarely, a larger sample size is necessary in order to capture cases
   2. Variance in outcomes: If there is a large variance in outcomes, larger sample size is necessary in order to gain statistical significance in the differences between groups
   3. Treatment effect size: If the treatment effect is small, larger sample sizes will be necessary to detect a difference between groups
   4. Acceptable error in detecting a difference between groups: Alpha and Beta type errors of 5% and 20%, respectively, are the standard in medical literature

   Sample size should be maximized to detect meaningful differences between groups; however, creating a larger study inherently increases the cost and time necessary to complete the study. Data from observational studies should be utilized to anticipate the variables mentioned above while designing the trial.

(d) Previous literature on the topic should be reviewed also to help determine what outcomes to measure. In addition to providing results of our own trials, we should aim to produce raw data that can then be analyzed further in meta-analyses. Outcomes of interest in this study may be pre-operative (time and cost of the treatment planning method), intraoperative (operating time, surgical difficulty), or post-operative (patient satisfaction/quality of life measures, analysis of post-operative skeletal and soft tissue results using standardized photographs and calibrated reviewers).

Acknowledgment Andrew Hamilton—Librarian.

Appendix: Literature Search Terms

General Medicine and Oral Surgery

- Diabetes and recovery from oral surgery (tooth extractions, bone grafts, and implants)
- Cardiovascular disease and oral surgery
- Kidney and liver disease and oral surgery
- Bleeding disorders/anticoagulant medications
- Steroid use and oral surgery
- Medication-related osteonecrosis of the jaw

Outpatient Anesthesia

- Outcomes in single-operator surgeon-anesthetist model vs. two operator model (surgeon and anesthetist)
- Medication usage (which meds) in outpatient oral surgery
- Illicit drug use and in-office anesthetic
- Airway interventions
- ASA (American Society of Anesthesiologists) status
- Oral surgery compared to the rest of dentistry

Dentoalveolar Surgery (Third Molars, Impacted Teeth)

- Management of impacted non-third molars
- Management of impacted third molars
- Coronectomy
- Nerve injuries (lingual and inferior alveolar)

Orthognathic Surgery

- Le Fort osteotomy (maxilla)
- Sagittal split osteotomy (mandible)
- Virtual surgical planning versus traditional model surgery (done with CT scan)
- Traditional dental impressions (stone) versus scanning
- Splint making—3D printing
- Timing of surgery (related to growth of child/teen)
- Cleft (presence or absence) and how this influences management

Common Diagnoses

- Maxillary hypoplasia
- Mandibular hypoplasia or hyperplasia
- Apertognathia
- Open bite
- Deep bite
- Retrognathia

Facial Trauma

- Mandible fracture
- Le Fort fractures
- Orbital fractures
- Zygomaticomaxillary complex fractures
- Frontal sinus fractures
- Traumatic malocclusion
- Dental trauma—tooth avulsion, luxation, etc.
- Lip injuries—dog bites
- Facial lacerations

Pathology

- Osteoradionecrosis
- Actinomycosis
- Osteomyelitis mandible

Ameloblastoma

- Odontogenic keratocyst (aka keratocystic odontogenic tumor)

- Mandible cyst
- Maxilla cyst
- Enucleation versus marsupialization versus excision

Reconstruction—Minor and Major

Vascularized (fibula, scapula, deep circumflex iliac artery (DCIA), radial forearm, pectoralis major, latissimus dorsi, submental island), versus non-vascularized (costochondral, tibia, anterior iliac crest, posterior iliac crest, mandibular ramus)

Temporomandibular Joint Disorders

Osteoarthritis = Degenerative Joint Disease
Crepitus (sign)
Disc abnormalities—anterior disc displacement with or without reduction—plication, discectomy (c and k), temporalis flap, auricular conchal cartilage, cadaver cartilage
Open lock
Closed lock
Anterior dislocation of the mandibular condyle
LeClerq, Dautrey, eminectomy, eminoplasty
Arthroscopy, arthrocentesis
Steroid injection, trigger point injection
Occlusal guards (stents)
Occlusal adjustment
Medications (muscle relaxants, NSAIDs, tricyclic antidepressants (TCA), opioids, PRP = platelet-rich plasma)
Myofascial pain
Botulinum toxin and myofascial pain

References

1. Teare MD, Dimairo M, Shephard N, Hayman A, Whitehead A, Walters SJ. Sample size requirements to estimate key design parameters from external pilot randomised controlled trials: a simulation study. Trials. 2014;15(1):264.
2. Al-Mubarak S, Al-Ali N, Abou-Rass M, Al-Sohail A, Robert A, Al-Zoman K, et al. Evaluation of dental extractions, suturing and INR on postoperative bleeding of patients maintained on oral anticoagulant therapy. Br Dent J. 2007;203(7):E15. discussion 410-1
3. Sacco R, Sacco M, Carpenedo M, Mannucci PM. Oral surgery in patients on oral anticoagulant therapy: a randomized comparison of different intensity targets. Oral Surg Oral Med Oral Pathol Oral Radiol Endod. 2007;104(1):e18–21.
4. Queiroz S, Silvestre VD, Soares RM, Campos GBP, Germano AR, da Silva JSP. Tranexamic acid as a local hemostasis method after dental extraction in patients on warfarin: a randomized controlled clinical study. Clin Oral Investig. 2018;22(6):2281–9.
5. Giudice A, Esposito M, Bennardo F, Brancaccio Y, Buti J, Fortunato L. Dental extractions for patients on oral antiplatelet: a within-person randomised controlled trial comparing haemostatic plugs, advanced-platelet-rich fibrin (A-PRF+) plugs, leukocyte- and platelet-rich fibrin (L-PRF) plugs and suturing alone. Int J Oral Implantol. 2019;12(1):77–87.
6. Medeiros FB, de Andrade AC, Angelis GA, Conrado VC, Timerman L, Farsky P, et al. Bleeding evaluation during single tooth extraction in patients with coronary artery disease and acetylsalicylic acid therapy suspension: a prospective, double-blinded, and randomized study. J Oral Maxillofac Surg. 2011;69(12):2949–55.
7. Brennan MT, Valerin MA, Noll JL, Napenas JJ, Kent ML, Fox PC, et al. Aspirin use and post-operative bleeding from dental extractions. J Dent Res. 2008;87(8):740–4.
8. Bellissimo-Rodrigues WT, Menegueti MG, Gaspar GG, Nicolini EA, Auxiliadora-Martins M, Basile-Filho A, et al. Effectiveness of a dental care intervention in the prevention of lower respiratory tract nosocomial infections among intensive care patients: a randomized clinical trial. Infect Control Hosp Epidemiol. 2014;35(11):1342–8.
9. Khader YS, Al Habashneh R, Al Malalheh M, Bataineh A. The effect of full-mouth tooth extraction on glycemic control among patients with type 2 diabetes requiring extraction of all remaining teeth: a randomized clinical trial. J Periodontal Res. 2010;45(6):741–7.
10. Mucke T, Deppe H, Hein J, Wolff KD, Mitchell DA, Kesting MR, et al. Prevention of bisphosphonate-related osteonecrosis of the jaws in patients with prostate cancer treated with zoledronic acid - A prospective study over 6 years. J Craniomaxillofac Surg. 2016;44(10):1689–93.
11. Milgrom P, Newton JT, Boyle C, Heaton LJ, Donaldson N. The effects of dental anxiety and

irregular attendance on referral for dental treatment under sedation within the National Health Service in London: the effects of dental anxiety and irregular attendance on referral for dental treatment. Community Dent Oral Epidemiol. 2010;38(5):453–9.
12. Shao Y, Wang XH, Su RX, Dong YC, Li G. Application of nitrous oxide/oxygen inhalation sedation in tooth extraction of elderly patients with hypertension. Shanghai Kou Qiang Yi Xue/Shanghai J Stomatol. 2013;22(3):302–4.
13. Zhao JZ, Wan K, Jing Q, Chen X. Blood pressure changes of elderly hypertensive patients during dental extraction under sedation with continuous intravenous infusion of midazolam. Chin Med Sci J. 2007;22(2):132–5.
14. Baygin O, Bodur H, Isik B. Effectiveness of premedication agents administered prior to nitrous oxide/oxygen. Eur J Anaesthesiol. 2010;27(4):341–6.
15. Wan K, Jing Q, Liu DY, Zhao JZ, Chen X, Dong YL. Evaluation of midazolam intravenous sedated patient's comfort degree in mandibular third molar surgery. Chung-Hua Kou Chiang i Hsueh Tsa Chih Chinese J Stomato. 2007;42(9):568–9.
16. Kwak HJ, Kim JY, Kwak YL, Park WS, Lee KC. Comparison of a bolus of fentanyl with an infusion of alfentanil during target-controlled propofol infusion in third molar extraction under conscious sedation. J Oral Maxillofac Surg. 2006;64(11):1577–82.
17. Torun AC, Yilmaz MZ, Ozkan N, Ustun B, Koksal E, Kaya C. Sedative-analgesic activity of remifentanil and effects of preoperative anxiety on perceived pain in outpatient mandibular third molar surgery. Int J Oral Maxillofac Surg. 2017;46(3):379–84.
18. de Carvalho RW, do Egito Vasconcelos BC. High weight standard and removal of third molars: a prospective randomized study. Oral Surg Oral Med Oral Pathol Oral Radiol. 2015;120(5):554–61.
19. Chaves AJ, Nascimento LR, Costa ME, Franz-Montan M, Oliveira-Junior PA, Groppo FC. Effects of surgical removal of mandibular third molar on the periodontium of the second molar. Int J Dent Hyg. 2008;6(2):123–8.
20. Laurito D, Lollobrigida M, Graziani F, Guerra F, Vestri A, De Biase A. Periodontal effects of a transposed versus a conventional flap in mandibular third molar extractions. J Craniofac Surg. 2016;27(3):708–11.
21. Cetinkaya BO, Sumer M, Tutkun F, Sandikci EO, Misir F. Influence of different suturing techniques on periodontal health of the adjacent second molars after extraction of impacted mandibular third molars. Oral Surg Oral Med Oral Pathol Oral Radiol Endod. 2009;108(2):156–61.
22. Cortell-Ballester I, Figueiredo R, Valmaseda-Castellon E, Gay-Escoda C. Effects of collagen resorbable membrane placement after the surgical extraction of impacted lower third molars. J Oral Maxillofac Surg. 2015;73(8):1457–64.
23. Ge J, Yang C, Zheng J, Hu Y. Autogenous bone grafting for treatment of osseous defect after impacted mandibular third molar extraction: a randomized controlled trial. Clin Implant Dent Rel Res. 2017;19(3):572–80.
24. Gurbuzer B, Pikdoken L, Urhan M, Suer BT, Narin Y. Scintigraphic evaluation of early osteoblastic activity in extraction sockets treated with platelet-rich plasma. J Oral Maxillofac Surg. 2008;66(12):2454–60.
25. Sammartino G, Tia M, Gentile E, Marenzi G, Claudio PP. Platelet-rich plasma and resorbable membrane for prevention of periodontal defects after deeply impacted lower third molar extraction. J Oral Maxillofac Surg. 2009;67(11):2369–73.
26. Afat IM, Akdogan ET, Gonul O. Effects of leukocyte- and platelet-rich fibrin alone and combined with hyaluronic acid on pain, edema, and trismus after surgical extraction of impacted mandibular third molars. J Oral Maxillofac Surg. 2018;76(5):926–32.
27. Daugela P, Grimuta V, Sakavicius D, Jonaitis J, Juodzbalys G. Influence of leukocyte- and platelet-rich fibrin (L-PRF) on the outcomes of impacted mandibular third molar removal surgery: a split-mouth randomized clinical trial. Quintessence Int. 2018;49(5):377–88.
28. Unsal H, GN HE. Evaluation of the effect of platelet-rich fibrin on the alveolar osteitis incidence and periodontal probing depth after extracting partially erupted mandibular third molars extraction. Niger J Clin Pract. 2018;21(2):201–5.
29. Guo ZZ, Zhang H, Li Y, Li X, Liu Y, Wang Y, et al. Comparative study of complications among routine method,high speed turbine handpiece and piezosurgery device after extraction of impacted wisdom teeth. Shanghai Kou Qiang Yi Xue/Shanghai J Stomatol. 2012;21(2):208–10.
30. Yang YY, Du SN, Lv ZK. Evaluation of the results of high-speed handpiece and minimally invasive extraction in impacted mandibular third molar extraction. Shanghai Kou Qiang Yi Xue/Shanghai J Stomatol. 2015;24(4):489–92.
31. Shad S, Shah SM, Alamgir AMM. Frequency of lingual nerve injury in mandibular third molar extraction: a comparison of two surgical techniques. J Ayub Med Coll. 2015;27(3):580–3.
32. Leung YY, Cheung LK. Safety of coronectomy versus excision of wisdom teeth: a randomized controlled trial. Oral Surg Oral Med Oral Pathol Oral Radiol Endod. 2009;108(6):821–7.
33. Akural EI, Jarvimaki V, Lansineva A, Niinimaa A, Alahuhta S. Effects of combination treatment with ketoprofen 100 mg + acetaminophen 1000 mg on postoperative dental pain: a single-

dose, 10-hour, randomized, double-blind, active- and placebo-controlled clinical trial. Clin Ther. 2009;31(3):560–8.
34. Best AD, De Silva RK, Thomson WM, Tong DC, Cameron CM, De Silva HL. Efficacy of codeine when added to paracetamol (acetaminophen) and ibuprofen for relief of postoperative pain after surgical removal of impacted third molars: a double-blinded randomized control trial. J Oral Maxillofac Surg. 2017;75(10):2063–9.
35. Benetello V, Sakamoto FC, Giglio FP, Sakai VT, Calvo AM, Modena KC, et al. The selective and non-selective cyclooxygenase inhibitors valdecoxib and piroxicam induce the same postoperative analgesia and control of trismus and swelling after lower third molar removal. Braz J Med Biol Res. 2007;40(8):1133–40.
36. Olmedo-Gaya MV, Manzano-Moreno FJ, Galvez-Mateos R, Gonzalez-Rodriguez MP, Talero-Sevilla C, Vallecillo-Capilla M. Oral pregabalin for postoperative pain relief after third molar extraction: a randomized controlled clinical trial. Clin Oral Investig. 2016;20(7):1819–26.
37. Pektas ZO, Sener M, Bayram B, Eroglu T, Bozdogan N, Donmez A, et al. A comparison of pre-emptive analgesic efficacy of diflunisal and lornoxicam for postoperative pain management: a prospective, randomized, single-blind, crossover study. Int J Oral Maxillofac Surg. 2007;36(2):123–7.
38. Gonul O, Satilmis T, Bayram F, Gocmen G, Sipahi A, Goker K. Effect of submucosal application of tramadol on postoperative pain after third molar surgery. Head Face Med. 2015;11:35.
39. Maughan BC, Hersh EV, Shofer FS, Wanner KJ, Archer E, Carrasco LR, et al. Unused opioid analgesics and drug disposal following outpatient dental surgery: a randomized controlled trial. Drug Alcohol Depend. 2016;168:328–34.
40. Rabi A, Maheshwari R, Srinivasan B, Warad LP, Suvarna CC, Tank KS. Effectiveness of antimicrobial therapy after extraction of impacted mandibular third molar: a randomized clinical trial. J Contemp Dent Pract. 2018;19(1):81–5.
41. Xue P, Hou R, Shang L, Ma Y, Wu F, Zhang S. Effect of antibiotics on postoperative inflammatory complications after surgical extraction of the impacted mandibular third molar. Chung-Hua Kou Chiang i Hsueh Tsa Chih Chinese J Stomato. 2014;49(10):603–6.
42. Adde CA, Soares MS, Romano MM, Carnaval TG, Sampaio RM, Aldarvis FP, et al. Clinical and surgical evaluation of the indication of postoperative antibiotic prescription in third molar surgery. Oral Surg Oral Med Oral Pathol Oral Radiol. 2012;114(Suppl. 5):S26–31.
43. Ataoglu H, Oz GY, Candirli C, Kiziloglu D. Routine antibiotic prophylaxis is not necessary during operations to remove third molars. Br J Oral Maxillofac Surg. 2008;46(2):133–5.
44. Milani BA, Bauer HC, Sampaio-Filho H, Horliana AC, Perez FE, Tortamano IP, et al. Antibiotic therapy in fully impacted lower third molar surgery: randomized three-arm, double-blind, controlled trial. Oral Maxillofac Surg. 2015;19(4):341–6.
45. Monaco G, Tavernese L, Agostini R, Marchetti C. Evaluation of antibiotic prophylaxis in reducing postoperative infection after mandibular third molar extraction in young patients. J Oral Maxillofac Surg. 2009;67(7):1467–72.
46. Arteagoitia I, Diez A, Barbier L, Santamaria G, Santamaria J. Efficacy of amoxicillin/clavulanic acid in preventing infectious and inflammatory complications following impacted mandibular third molar extraction. Oral Surg Oral Med Oral Pathol Oral Radiol Endod. 2005;100(1):e11–8.
47. Halpern LR, Dodson TB. Does prophylactic administration of systemic antibiotics prevent postoperative inflammatory complications after third molar surgery? J Oral Maxillofac Surg. 2007;65(2):177–85.
48. Lopez-Cedrun JL, Pijoan JI, Fernandez S, Santamaria J, Hernandez G. Efficacy of amoxicillin treatment in preventing postoperative complications in patients undergoing third molar surgery: a prospective, randomized, double-blind controlled study. J Oral Maxillofac Surg. 2011;69(6):e5–14.
49. Ricard AS, Nau O, Veyret A, Majoufre-Lefebvre C, Laurentjoye M. Comparison between closure and absence of closure after removal of fully impacted mandibular third molar: a prospective randomized study. Rev Stomatol Chir Maxillofac Chir Orale. 2015;116(1):12–7.
50. Xavier RL, Vasconcelos BC, Caubi AF, Porto GG, Maurette MA. Passive drainage through the vestibular oblique incision in impacted inferior third molar surgery: a preliminary study. Acta Odontol Latinoam. 2008;21(1):57–63.
51. Gay-Escoda C, Gomez-Santos L, Sanchez-Torres A, Herraez-Vilas JM. Effect of the suture technique on postoperative pain, swelling and trismus after removal of lower third molars: a randomized clinical trial. Med Oral Patol Oral Cir Bucal. 2015;20(3):e372–7.
52. Asher R, Chacartchi T, Tandlich M, Shapira L, Polak D. Microbial accumulation on different suture materials following oral surgery: a randomized controlled study. Clin Oral Investig. 2019;23(2):559–65.
53. Al-Dajani M. Can preoperative intramuscular single-dose dexamethasone improve patient-centered outcomes following third molar surgery? J Oral Maxillofac Surg. 2017;75(8):1616–26.
54. Ilhan O, Agacayak KS, Gulsun B, Koparal M, Gunes N. A comparison of the effects of methylprednisolone and tenoxicam on pain, edema, and trismus after impacted lower third molar extraction. Med Sci Monit. 2014;20:147–52.
55. Vicentini CB, Ramacciato JC, Groppo FC, Teixeira RG, Motta RHL. Clinical evaluation of two dexamethasone regimens in the extractions of impacted

third molars-a randomized clinical trial. Oral Maxillofac Surg. 2018;22(2):177–83.
56. Warraich R, Faisal M, Rana M, Shaheen A, Gellrich NC, Rana M. Evaluation of postoperative discomfort following third molar surgery using submucosal dexamethasone - a randomized observer blind prospective study. Oral Surg Oral Med Oral Pathol Oral Radiol. 2013;116(1):16–22.
57. Alcantara CE, Falci SG, Oliveira-Ferreira F, Santos CR, Pinheiro ML. Pre-emptive effect of dexamethasone and methylprednisolone on pain, swelling, and trismus after third molar surgery: a split-mouth randomized triple-blind clinical trial. Int J Oral Maxillofac Surg. 2014;43(1):93–8.
58. Antunes AA, Avelar RL, Martins Neto EC, Frota R, Dias E. Effect of two routes of administration of dexamethasone on pain, edema, and trismus in impacted lower third molar surgery. Oral Maxillofac Surg. 2011;15(4):217–23.
59. Mico-Llorens JM, Satorres-Nieto M, Gargallo-Albiol J, Arnabat-Dominguez J, Berini-Aytes L, Gay-Escoda C. Efficacy of methylprednisolone in controlling complications after impacted lower third molar surgical extraction. Eur J Clin Pharmacol. 2006;62(9):693–8.
60. Kocer G, Yuce E, Tuzuner Oncul A, Dereci O, Koskan O. Effect of the route of administration of methylprednisolone on oedema and trismus in impacted lower third molar surgery. Int J Oral Maxillofac Surg. 2014;43(5):639–43.
61. Sotto-Maior BS, Senna PM, de Souza Picorelli Assis NM. Corticosteroids or cyclooxygenase 2-selective inhibitor medication for the management of pain and swelling after third-molar surgery. J Craniofac Surg. 2011;22(2):758–62.
62. Barbalho JC, Vasconcellos RJ, de Morais HH, Santos LA, Almeida RA, Rebelo HL, et al. Effects of co-administered dexamethasone and nimesulide on pain, swelling, and trismus following third molar surgery: a randomized, triple-blind, controlled clinical trial. Int J Oral Maxillofac Surg. 2017;46(2):236–42.
63. Lima TC, Bagordakis E, Falci SGM, Dos Santos CRR, Pinheiro MLP. Pre-emptive effect of dexamethasone and diclofenac sodium associated with codeine on pain, swelling, and trismus after third molar surgery: a split-mouth, randomized, triple-blind, controlled clinical trial. J Oral Maxillofac Surg. 2018;76(1):60–6.
64. Hu YP, Jin GF. Clinical study of modified Gow-Gates technique of inferior alveolar nerve block in impacted mandibular third molar extraction. Shanghai Kou Qiang Yi Xue/Shanghai J Stomatol. 2015;24(3):373–7.
65. Eshghpour M, Ahrari F, Takallu M. Is low-level laser therapy effective in the management of pain and swelling after mandibular third molar surgery? J Oral Maxillofac Surg. 2016;74(7):1322.e1–8.
66. Ferrante M, Petrini M, Trentini P, Perfetti G, Spoto G. Effect of low-level laser therapy after extraction of impacted lower third molars. Lasers Med Sci. 2013;28(3):845–9.
67. Pol R, Ruggiero T, Gallesio G, Riso M, Bergamasco L, Mortellaro C, et al. Efficacy of anti-inflammatory and analgesic of superpulsed low level laser therapy after impacted mandibular third molars extractions. J Craniofac Surg. 2016;27(3):685–90.
68. Lopez-Ramirez M, Vilchez-Perez MA, Gargallo-Albiol J, Arnabat-Dominguez J, Gay-Escoda C. Efficacy of low-level laser therapy in the management of pain, facial swelling, and postoperative trismus after a lower third molar extraction. A preliminary study. Lasers Med Sci. 2012;27(3):559–66.
69. Sierra SO, Deana AM, Bussadori SK, da Mota AC, Motta LJ, Ferrari RA, et al. Effect of low-intensity laser treatment on pain after extraction of impacted mandibular third molars: a randomised, controlled, clinical trial. Br J Oral Maxillofac Surg. 2015;53(10):996–1000.
70. Torres-Lagares D, Infante-Cossio P, Gutierrez-Perez JL, Romero-Ruiz MM, Garcia-Calderon M, Serrera-Figallo MA. Intra-alveolar chlorhexidine gel for the prevention of dry socket in mandibular third molar surgery. A pilot study. Med Oral Patol Oral y Cir Bucal. 2006;11(2):E179–84.
71. Torres-Lagares D, Gutierrez-Perez JL, Hita-Iglesias P, Magallanes-Abad N, Flores-Ruiz R, Basallote-Garcia M, et al. Randomized, double-blind study of effectiveness of intra-alveolar application of chlorhexidine gel in reducing incidence of alveolar osteitis and bleeding complications in mandibular third molar surgery in patients with bleeding disorders. J Oral Maxillofac Surg. 2010;68(6):1322–6.
72. Cheung LK, Chua HD, Hagg MB. Cleft maxillary distraction versus orthognathic surgery: clinical morbidities and surgical relapse. Plast Reconstr Surg. 2006;118(4):996–1008. discussion 9
73. Ow A, Cheung LK. Bilateral sagittal split osteotomies and mandibular distraction osteogenesis: a randomized controlled trial comparing skeletal stability. Oral Surg Oral Med Oral Pathol Oral Radiol Endod. 2010;109(1):17–23.
74. Talesh KT, Motamedi MH, Yazdani J, Ghavimi A, Ghoreishizadeh A. Prevention of relapse following intraoral vertical ramus osteotomy mandibular setback: can coronoidotomy help? Oral Surg Oral Med Oral Pathol Oral Radiol Endod. 2011;111(5):557–60.
75. Lin HH, Kim SG, Kim HY, Niu LS, Lo LJ. Higher dose of dexamethasone does not further reduce facial swelling after orthognathic surgery: a randomized controlled trial using 3-dimensional photogrammetry. Ann Plast Surg. 2017;78(3 Suppl. 2):S61–S9.
76. Semper-Hogg W, Fuessinger MA, Dirlewanger TW, Cornelius CP, Metzger MC. The influence of dexamethasone on postoperative swelling and neurosensory disturbances after orthognathic surgery: a randomized controlled clinical trial. Head Face Med. 2017;13(1):19.

77. Widar F, Kashani H, Alsen B, Dahlin C, Rasmusson L. The effects of steroids in preventing facial oedema, pain, and neurosensory disturbances after bilateral sagittal split osteotomy: a randomized controlled trial. Int J Oral Maxillofac Surg. 2015;44(2):252–8.
78. Danda AK, Wahab A, Narayanan V, Siddareddi A. Single-dose versus single-day antibiotic prophylaxis for orthognathic surgery: a prospective, randomized, double-blind clinical study. J Oral Maxillofac Surg. 2010;68(2):344–6.
79. Wahab PU, Narayanan V, Nathan S, Madhulaxmi. Antibiotic prophylaxis for bilateral sagittal split osteotomies: a randomized, double-blind clinical study. Int J Oral Maxillofac Surg. 2013;42(3):352–5.
80. Davis CM, Gregoire CE, Davis I, Steeves TW. Prevalence of surgical site infections following orthognathic surgery: a double-blind, randomized controlled trial on a 3-day versus 1-day postoperative antibiotic regimen. J Oral Maxillofac Surg. 2017;75(4):796–804.
81. Ghantous Y, Araidy S, Yaffe V, Mirochnik R, El-Raziq MA, El-Naaj IA. The efficiency of extended postoperative antibiotic prophylaxis in orthognathic surgery: a prospective, randomized, double-blind, placebo-controlled clinical trial. J Craniomaxillofac Surg. 2019;47(2):228–32.
82. Kang SH, Yoo JH, Yi CK. The efficacy of postoperative prophylactic antibiotics in orthognathic surgery: a prospective study in Le Fort I osteotomy and bilateral intraoral vertical ramus osteotomy. Yonsei Med J. 2009;50(1):55–9.
83. Al-Ahmad HT, Saleh MWM, Hussein AM. Evaluation of an innovative computer-assisted sagittal split ramus osteotomy to reduce neurosensory alterations following orthognathic surgery: a pilot study. Int J Med Robot + Compu Assist Surg. 2013;9(2):134–41.
84. Schneider D, Kämmerer P, Hennig M, Schön G, Thiem D, Bschorer R. Customized virtual surgical planning in bimaxillary orthognathic surgery: a prospective randomized trial. Clin Oral Investig. 2019;23(7):3115–22.
85. Hanafy M, Akoush Y, Abou-Elfetouh A, Mounir RM. Precision of orthognathic digital plan transfer using patient-specific cutting guides and osteosynthesis versus mixed analogue–digitally planned surgery: a randomized controlled clinical trial. Int J Oral Maxillofac Surg. 2020;49(1):62–8.
86. Ahiskalioglu A, Ince I, Aksoy M, Yalcin E, Ahiskalioglu EO, Kilinc A. Effects of a single-dose of pre-emptive pregabalin on postoperative pain and opioid consumption after double-jaw surgery: a randomized controlled trial. J Oral Maxillofac Surg. 2016;74(1):53.e1–7.
87. Abukawa H, Matsuo A, Watanabe M, Kono M, Satomi T, Chikazu D. A randomized trial to identify the most effective dose of remifentanil during Le Fort I osteotomy. J Oral Maxillofac Surg. 2015;73(6):1073–7.
88. Farah GJ, de Moraes M, Filho LI, Pavan AJ, Camarini ET, Previdelli IT, et al. Induced hypotension in orthognathic surgery: a comparative study of 2 pharmacological protocols. J Oral Maxillofac Surg. 2008;66(11):2261–9.
89. Yoshikawa F, Kohase H, Umino M, Fukayama H. Blood loss and endocrine responses in hypotensive anaesthesia with sodium nitroprusside and nitroglycerin for mandibular osteotomy. Int J Oral Maxillofac Surg. 2009;38(11):1159–64.
90. Mohammadi F, Marashi M, Tavakoli I, Khakbaz O. Effects of oral clonidine premedication on hemodynamic status in bimaxillary orthognathic surgery: a double-blind randomized clinical trial. J Craniomaxillofac Surg. 2016;44(4):436–9.
91. Kim NY, Yoo YC, Chun DH, Lee HM, Jung YS, Bai SJ. The effects of oral atenolol or enalapril premedication on blood loss and hypotensive anesthesia in orthognathic surgery. Yonsei Med J. 2015;56(4):1114–21.
92. Ham SY, Kim JE, Park C, Shin MJ, Shim YH. Dexmedetomidine does not reduce emergence agitation in adults following orthognathic surgery. Acta Anaesthesiol Scand. 2014;58(8):955–60.
93. Apipan B, Rummasak D, Narainthonsaenee T. The effect of different dosage regimens of tranexamic acid on blood loss in bimaxillary osteotomy: a randomized, double-blind, placebo-controlled study. Int J Oral Maxillofac Surg. 2018;47(5):608–12.
94. Choi WS, Irwin MG, Samman N. The effect of tranexamic acid on blood loss during orthognathic surgery: a randomized controlled trial. J Oral Maxillofac Surg. 2009;67(1):125–33.
95. Kaewpradub P, Apipan B, Rummasak D. Does tranexamic acid in an irrigating fluid reduce intraoperative blood loss in orthognathic surgery? A double-blind, randomized clinical trial. J Oral Maxillofac Surg. 2011;69(6):e186–9.
96. Secher JJ, Sidelmann JJ, Ingerslev J, Thorn JJ, Pinholt EM. The effect of tranexamic acid and gender on intraoperative bleeding in orthognathic surgery-a randomized controlled trial. J Oral Maxillofac Surg. 2018;76(6):1327–33.
97. de Lange J, Baas EM, Horsthuis RB, Booij A. The effect of nasal application of cocaine/adrenaline on blood loss in Le Fort I osteotomies. Int J Oral Maxillofac Surg. 2008;37(1):21–4.
98. Ervens J, Marks C, Hechler M, Plath T, Hansen D, Hoffmeister B. Effect of induced hypotensive anaesthesia vs isovolaemic haemodilution on blood loss and transfusion requirements in orthognathic surgery: a prospective, single-blinded, randomized, controlled clinical study. Int J Oral Maxillofac Surg. 2010;39(12):1168–74.
99. Eshghpour M, Samieirad S, Attar AS, Kermani H, Seddigh S. Propofol versus remifentanil: which one is more effective in reducing blood loss during orthognathic surgery? A randomized clinical trial. J Oral Maxillofac Surg. 2018;76(9):1882.e1–7.

100. Yu S, Bloomquist D. Can resorbable screws effectively be used in fixating bilateral sagittal split osteotomies for mandibular advancement? A randomized controlled trial. J Oral Maxillofac Surg. 2014;72(11):2273–7.
101. Ueki K, Okabe K, Moroi A, Marukawa K, Sotobori M, Ishihara Y, et al. Maxillary stability after Le Fort I osteotomy using three different plate systems. Int J Oral Maxillofac Surg. 2012;41(8):942–8.
102. Kohnke R, Kolk A, Kluwe L, Ploder O. Piezosurgery for sagittal split osteotomy: procedure duration and postoperative sensory perturbation. J Oral Maxillofac Surg. 2017;75(9):1941–7.
103. Baas EM, Bierenbroodspot F, de Lange J. Bilateral sagittal split osteotomy versus distraction osteogenesis of the mandible: a randomized clinical trial. Int J Oral Maxillofac Surg. 2015;44(2):180–8.
104. Ow A, Cheung LK. Bilateral sagittal split osteotomies versus mandibular distraction osteogenesis: a prospective clinical trial comparing inferior alveolar nerve function and complications. Int J Oral Maxillofac Surg. 2010;39(8):756–60.
105. Politi M, Toro C, Costa F, Polini F, Robiony M. Intraoperative awakening of the patient during orthognathic surgery: a method to prevent the condylar sag. J Oral Maxillofac Surg. 2007;65(1):109–14.
106. Toro C, Robiony M, Costa F, Sembronio S, Politi M. Conscious analgesia and sedation during orthognathic surgery: preliminary results of a method of preventing condylar displacement. Br J Oral Maxillofac Surg. 2007;45(5):378–81.
107. Chen YA, Rivera-Serrano CM, Chen C, Chen YR. Pre-surgical regional blocks in orthognathic surgery: prospective study evaluating their influence on the intraoperative use of anaesthetics and blood pressure control. Int J Oral Maxillofac Surg. 2016;45(6):783–6.
108. Espitalier F, Remerand F, Dubost AF, Laffon M, Fusciardi J, Goga D. Mandibular nerve block can improve intraoperative inferior alveolar nerve visualization during sagittal split mandibular osteotomy. J Craniomaxillofac Surg. 2011;39(3):164–8.
109. Howley C, Ali N, Lee R, Cox S. Use of the alar base cinch suture in Le Fort I osteotomy: is it effective? Br J Oral Maxillofac Surg. 2011;49(2):127–30.
110. Ritto FG, Medeiros PJ, de Moraes M, Ribeiro DP. Comparative analysis of two different alar base sutures after Le Fort I osteotomy: randomized double-blind controlled trial. Oral Surg Oral Med Oral Pathol Oral Radiol Endod. 2011;111(2):181–9.
111. Emara T, El-Anwar M, Omara T, Anany A, Elawa I, Rabea M. Submental intubation versus tracheostomy in maxillofacial fractures. Oral Maxillofac Surg. 2019;23(3):337–41.
112. Chole RA, Yee J. Antibiotic prophylaxis for facial fractures. A prospective, randomized clinical trial. Arch Otolaryngol--Head Neck Surg. 1987;113(10):1055.
113. Miles BA, Potter JK, Ellis E 3rd. The efficacy of postoperative antibiotic regimens in the open treatment of mandibular fractures: a prospective randomized trial. J Oral Maxillofac Surg. 2006;64(4):576–82.
114. Zix J, Schaller B, Iizuka T, Lieger O. The role of postoperative prophylactic antibiotics in the treatment of facial fractures: a randomised, double-blind, placebo-controlled pilot clinical study. Part 1: Orbital fractures in 62 patients. Br J Oral Maxillofac Surg. 2013;51(4):332–6.
115. Soong PL, Schaller B, Zix J, Iizuka T, Mottini M, Lieger O. The role of postoperative prophylactic antibiotics in the treatment of facial fractures: a randomised, double-blind, placebo-controlled pilot clinical study. Part 3: Le Fort and zygomatic fractures in 94 patients. Br J Oral Maxillofac Surg. 2014;52(4):329–33.
116. Ahmed W, Ali Bukhari SG, Janjua OS, Luqman U, Shah I. Bioresorbable versus titanium plates for mandibular fractures. J Coll Phys Surg Pak. 2013;23(7):480–3.
117. Bhatt K, Roychoudhury A, Bhutia O, Trikha A, Seith A, Pandey RM. Equivalence randomized controlled trial of bioresorbable versus titanium miniplates in treatment of mandibular fracture: a pilot study. J Oral Maxillofac Surg. 2010;68(8):1842–8.
118. Wittwer G, Adeyemo WL, Yerit K, Voracek M, Turhani D, Watzinger F, et al. Complications after zygoma fracture fixation: is there a difference between biodegradable materials and how do they compare with titanium osteosynthesis? Oral Surg Oral Med Oral Pathol Oral Radiol Endod. 2006;101(4):419.
119. Gareb B, van Bakelen NB, Buijs GJ, Jansma J, de Visscher J, Hoppenreijs TJM, et al. Comparison of the long-term clinical performance of a biodegradable and a titanium fixation system in maxillofacial surgery: a multicenter randomized controlled trial. PLoS ONE. 2017;12(5):e0177152.
120. Al-Belasy FA. A short period of maxillomandibular fixation for treatment of fractures of the mandibular tooth-bearing area. J Oral Maxillofac Surg. 2005;63(7):953–6.
121. Adeyemi MF, Adeyemo WL, Ogunlewe MO, Ladeinde AL. Is healing outcome of 2 weeks intermaxillary fixation different from that of 4 to 6 weeks intermaxillary fixation in the treatment of mandibular fractures? J Oral Maxillofac Surg. 2012;70(8):1896–902.
122. Shetty V, Atchison K, Leathers R, Black E, Zigler C, Belin TR. Do the benefits of rigid internal fixation of mandible fractures justify the added costs? Results from a randomized controlled trial. J Oral Maxillofac Surg. 2008;66(11):2203–12.
123. Ahuja SA, Galinde J, Asnani U, Mistry YA. Comparative evaluation of clinical outcomes using delta plates and conventional miniplates for internal fixation of mandibular condylar fractures in adults. J Oral Maxillofac Surg. 2018;76(6):1255–66.
124. Nogami S, Yamauchi K, Kataoka Y, Takano H, Yamashita Y, Takahashi T. Clinical comparison between arthrocentesis and conventional conserva-

tive treatment with maxillomandibular fixation for unilateral high condylar fractures. J Oral Rehabil. 2014;41(2):141–7.
125. Agnihotri A, Prabhu S, Thomas S. A comparative analysis of the efficacy of cortical screws as lag screws and miniplates for internal fixation of mandibular symphyseal region fractures: a randomized prospective study. Int J Oral Maxillofac Surg. 2014;43(1):22–8.
126. Agarwal M, Mohammad S, Singh RK, Singh V. Prospective randomized clinical trial comparing bite force in 2-mm locking plates versus 2-mm standard plates in treatment of mandibular fractures. J Oral Maxillofac Surg. 2011;69(7):1995–2000.
127. Al-Moraissi EA, Mounair RM, El-Sharkawy TM, El-Ghareeb TI. Comparison between three-dimensional and standard miniplates in the management of mandibular angle fractures: a prospective, randomized, double-blind, controlled clinical study. Int J Oral Maxillofac Surg. 2015;44(3):316–21.
128. Laverick S, Siddappa P, Wong H, Patel P, Jones DC. Intraoral external oblique ridge compared with transbuccal lateral cortical plate fixation for the treatment of fractures of the mandibular angle: prospective randomised trial. Br J Oral Maxillofac Surg. 2012;50(4):344–9.
129. McNamara Z, Findlay G, O'Rourke P, Batstone M. Removal versus retention of asymptomatic third molars in mandibular angle fractures: a randomized controlled trial. Int J Oral Maxillofac Surg. 2016;45(5):571–4.
130. Rana M, Warraich R, Tahir S, Iqbal A, Von See C, Eckardt AM, et al. Surgical treatment of zygomatic bone fracture using two points fixation versus three point fixation—a randomised prospective clinical trial. Trials. 2012;13:36.
131. Kormi E, Snäll J, Koivusalo A-M, Suominen AL, Thorén H, Törnwall J. Analgesic effect of perioperative systemic dexamethasone on blowout fracture surgery. J Oral Maxillofac Surg. 2017;75(6):1232–7.
132. Flood TR, McManners J, Attar AE, Moos KF. Randomized prospective study of the influence of steroids on postoperative eye-opening after exploration of the orbital floor. Br J Oral Maxillofac Surg. 1999;37(4):312–5.
133. You HJ, Son ST, Kim DY, Han SK. A prospective randomized study comparing fibrin sealant versus suture for conjunctival wound closure in orbital wall fracture surgery. Int J Oral Maxillofac Surg. 2016;45(11):1418–23.
134. El-Anwar M, Elsheikh E, Hussein A, Tantawy A, Abdelbaki Y. Transconjunctival versus subciliary approach to the infraorbital margin for open reduction of zygomaticomaxillary complex fractures: a randomized feasibility study. Oral Maxillofac Surg. 2017;21(2):187–92.
135. Park JH, Kim JW, Kim SJ. Does the addition of bone morphogenetic protein 2 to platelet-rich fibrin improve healing after treatment for medication-related osteonecrosis of the jaw? J Oral Maxillofac Surg. 2017;75(6):1176–84.
136. Roh JL. Removal of the submandibular gland by a submental approach: a prospective, randomized, controlled study. Oral Oncol. 2008;44(3):295–300.
137. Ludovichetti FS, De Biagi M, Bacci C, Bressan E, Sivolella S. Healing of human critical-size alveolar bone defects secondary to cyst enucleation: a randomized pilot study with 12 months follow-up. Minerva Stomatol. 2018;67(4):148–55.
138. Santamaría J, García AM, de Vicente JC, Landa S, López-Arranz JS. Bone regeneration after radicular cyst removal with and without guided bone regeneration. Int J Oral Maxillofac Surg. 1998;27(2):118–20.
139. Avelar RL, Primo BT, Pinheiro-Nogueira CB, Studart-Soares EC, de Oliveira RB, Romulo de Medeiros J, et al. Worldwide incidence of odontogenic tumors. J Craniofac Surg. 2011;22(6):2118–23.
140. Bande CR, Prashant MC, Sumbh B, Pandilwar PK. Prevalence, treatment and recurrence of odontogenic keratocyst in Central India. J Maxillofac Oral Surg. 2010;9(2):146–9.
141. Alonso N, Risso GH, Denadai R, Raposo-Amaral CE. Effect of maxillary alveolar reconstruction on nasal symmetry of cleft lip and palate patients: a study comparing iliac crest bone graft and recombinant human bone morphogenetic protein-2. J Plast Reconstruct Aesthet Surg. 2014;67(9):1201–8.
142. Shirani G, Abbasi AJ, Mohebbi SZ, Moharrami M. Comparison between autogenous iliac bone and freeze-dried bone allograft for repair of alveolar clefts in the presence of plasma rich in growth factors: a randomized clinical trial. J Craniomaxillofac Surg. 2017;45(10):1698–703.
143. Xiao WL, Zhang DZ, Chen XJ, Yuan C, Xue LF. Osteogenesis effect of guided bone regeneration combined with alveolar cleft grafting: assessment by cone beam computed tomography. Int J Oral Maxillofac Surg. 2016;45(6):683–7.
144. Brandao TB, Vechiato Filho AJ, Prado Ribeiro AC, Gebrim EM, Bodard AG, da Silva DP, et al. Evaluation of use of acrylic resin-based surgical guide in the function and quality of life provided by mandibular prostheses with microvascular free fibula flap: a four-year, randomized, controlled trial. J Prosthet Dent. 2016;116(3):457–63.e2.
145. Khalifa GA, Abd El Moniem NA, Elsayed SA, Qadry Y. Segmental mirroring: does it eliminate the need for intraoperative readjustment of the virtually pre-bent reconstruction plates and is it economically valuable? J Oral Maxillofac Surg. 2016;74(3):621–30.
146. Fujita S, Tojyo I, Yamada M, Go Y, Matsumoto T, Kiga N. Outcome following lingual nerve repair with vein graft cuff: a preliminary report. J Oral Maxillofac Surg. 2014;72(7):1433.e1–7.
147. Senthil Murugan M, Ravi P, Mohammed Afradh K, Tatineni V, Krishnakumar Raja VB. Comparison of the efficacy of venous coupler and hand-sewn

anastomosis in maxillofacial reconstruction using microvascular fibula free flaps: a prospective randomized controlled trial. Int J Oral Maxillofac Surg. 2018;47(7):854–7.
148. Klein S, Van Lienden KP, Van' T Veer M, Smit JM, Werker PMN. Evaluation of the lower limb vasculature before free fibula flap transfer. A prospective blinded comparison between magnetic resonance angiography and digital subtraction angiography. Microsurgery. 2013;33(7):539–44.
149. Heberer S, Ruhe B, Krekeler L, Schink T, Nelson JJ, Nelson K. A prospective randomized split-mouth study comparing iliac onlay grafts in atrophied edentulous patients: covered with periosteum or a bioresorbable membrane. Clin Oral Implants Res. 2009;20(3):319–26.
150. Barkhuysen R, Meijer GJ, Soehardi A, Merkx MA, Borstlap WA, Berge SJ, et al. The effect of a single dose of bupivacaine on donor site pain after anterior iliac crest bone harvesting. Int J Oral Maxillofac Surg. 2010;39(3):260–5.
151. Kumar Raja D, Anantanarayanan P, Christabel A, Manikandhan R, Elavazhagan N, Naveen KJ. Donor site analgesia after anterior iliac bone grafting in paediatric population: a prospective, triple-blind, randomized clinical trial. Int J Oral Maxillofac Surg. 2014;43(4):422–7.
152. Coulthard P, Oliver R, Afridi KAK, Jackson-Leech D, Adamson L, Worthington H. The efficacy of local anaesthetic for pain after iliac bone harvesting: a randomised controlled trial. (report). Int J Surg. 2008;6(1):57.
153. Hayes JA, Forrest CR, Walsh W, Pétroz GC, Adeli K, Bissonnette B. Continuous bupivacaine infusion post-iliac crest bone graft harvesting in pediatric cleft surgery: role and comparison with ketorolac. Cleft Palate Craniofac J. 2011;48(5):532–7.
154. Kumar VV, Ebenezer S, Kammerer PW, Jacob PC, Kuriakose MA, Hedne N, et al. Implants in free fibula flap supporting dental rehabilitation—implant and peri-implant related outcomes of a randomized clinical trial. J Craniomaxillofac Surg. 2016;44(11):1849–58.
155. Kumar VV, Jacob PC, Ebenezer S, Kuriakose MA, Kekatpure V, Baliarsing AS, et al. Implant supported dental rehabilitation following segmental mandibular reconstruction- quality of life outcomes of a prospective randomized trial. J Craniomaxillofac Surg. 2016;44(7):800–10.
156. Pogrel MA, Podlesh S, Anthony JP, Alexander J. A comparison of vascularized and nonvascularized bone grafts for reconstruction of mandibular continuity defects. J Oral Maxillofac Surg. 1997;55(11):1200–6.
157. Bjornland T, Gjaerum AA, Moystad A. Osteoarthritis of the temporomandibular joint: an evaluation of the effects and complications of corticosteroid injection compared with injection with sodium hyaluronate. J Oral Rehabil. 2007;34(8):583–9.
158. Hegab AF, Ali HE, Elmasry M, Khallaf MG. Platelet-rich plasma injection as an effective treatment for temporomandibular joint osteoarthritis. J Oral Maxillofac Surg. 2015;73(9):1706–13.
159. Ziegler CM, Wiechnik J, Muhling J. Analgesic effects of intra-articular morphine in patients with temporomandibular joint disorders: a prospective, double-blind, placebo-controlled clinical trial. J Oral Maxillofac Surg. 2010;68(3):622–7.
160. Costa YM, Porporatti AL, Stuginski-Barbosa J, Bonjardim LR, Speciali JG, Rodrigues Conti PC. Headache attributed to masticatory myofascial pain: clinical features and management outcomes. J Oral Facial Pain Headache. 2015;29(4):323–30.
161. Ozkan F, Cakir Ozkan N, Erkorkmaz U. Trigger point injection therapy in the management of myofascial temporomandibular pain. Agri Dergisi. 2011;23(3):119–25.
162. von Lindern JJ, Niederhagen B, Bergé S, Appel T. Type A botulinum toxin in the treatment of chronic facial pain associated with masticatory hyperactivity. J Oral Maxillofac Surg. 2003;61(7):774–8.
163. Guarda-Nardini L, Manfredini D, Salamone M, Salmaso L, Tonello S, Ferronato G. Efficacy of botulinum toxin in treating myofascial pain in bruxers: a controlled placebo pilot study. Cranio. 2014;26(2):126–35.
164. Kurtoglu C, Gur OH, Kurkcu M, Sertdemir Y, Guler-Uysal F, Uysal H. Effect of botulinum toxin-A in myofascial pain patients with or without functional disc displacement. J Oral Maxillofac Surg. 2008;66(8):1644–51.
165. de Abreu VR, Guedes Pereira Alencar F, Zamperini C. Botulinum toxin, lidocaine, and dry-needling injections in patients with myofascial pain and headaches. Cranio. 2014;27(1):46–53.
166. Guarda-Nardini L, Stecco A, Stecco C, Masiero S, Manfredini D. Myofascial pain of the jaw muscles: comparison of short-term effectiveness of botulinum toxin injections and fascial manipulation technique. Cranio. 2014;30(2):95–102.
167. Ernberg M, Hedenberg-Magnusson B, List T, Svensson P. Efficacy of botulinum toxin type A for treatment of persistent myofascial TMD pain: a randomized, controlled, double-blind multicenter study. Pain. 2011;152(9):1988–96.
168. Nixdorf DR, Heo G, Major PW. Randomized controlled trial of botulinum toxin A for chronic myogenous orofacial pain. Pain (Amsterdam). 2002;99(3):465–73.
169. Kutuk SG, Ozkan Y, Kutuk M, Ozdas T. Comparison of the efficacies of dry needling and botox methods in the treatment of myofascial pain syndrome affecting the temporomandibular joint. J Craniofac Surg. 2019;30(5):1556–9.
170. Zhang LD, Liu Q, Zou DR, Yu LF. Occlusal force characteristics of masseteric muscles after intramuscular injection of botulinum toxin A(BTX - A) for treatment of temporomandibular disorder. Br J Oral Maxillofac Surg. 2016;54(7):736–40.

171. Comert Kilic S, Gungormus M, Sumbullu MA. Is arthrocentesis Plus platelet-rich plasma superior to arthrocentesis alone in the treatment of temporomandibular joint osteoarthritis? A randomized clinical trial. J Oral Maxillofac Surg. 2015;73(8):1473–83.

Further Reading

Schulz KF, Altman DG, Moher D. CONSORT 2010 statement: updated guidelines for reporting parallel group randomised trials. PLoS Med. 2010;7(3):e1000251.

Santos-Paul MA, Neves IL, Neves RS, Ramires JA. Local anesthesia with epinephrine is safe and effective for oral surgery in patients with type 2 diabetes mellitus and coronary disease: a prospective randomized study. Clinics (Sao Paulo). 2015;70(3):185–9.

Tsukamoto M, Koyama S, Esaki K, Hitosugi T, Yokoyama T. Low-dose carperitide (alpha-human A-type natriuretic peptide) alleviates hemoglobin concentration decrease during prolonged oral surgery: a randomized controlled study. J Anesth. 2017;31(3):325–9.

Arpaci AH, Isik B, Ilhan E, Erdem E. Association of postoperative nausea and vomiting incidence with neutrophil-lymphocyte ratio in ambulatory maxillofacial surgery. J Oral Maxillofac Surg. 2017;75(7):1367–71.

Efeoglu C, Sipahi Calis A, Karasu Z, Koca H, Boyacioglu H. Prospective randomized single-blind study of post-operative bleeding after minor oral surgery in patients with cirrhosis. Turk J Gastroenterol. 2019;30(2):171–6.

Abrams R, Morrison JE, Villasenor A, Hencmann D, Da Fonseca M, Mueller W. Safety and effectiveness of intranasal administration of sedative medications (ketamine, midazolam, or sufentanil) for urgent brief pediatric dental procedures. Anesth Prog. 1993;40(3):63–6.

Cheung CW, Ying CL, Chiu WK, Wong GT, Ng KF, Irwin MG. A comparison of dexmedetomidine and midazolam for sedation in third molar surgery. Anaesthesia. 2007;62(11):1132–8.

Watts AK, Thikkurissy S, Smiley M, McTigue DJ, Smith T. Local anesthesia affects physiologic parameters and reduces anesthesiologist intervention in children undergoing general anesthesia for dental rehabilitation. Pediatr Dent. 2009;31(5):414–9.

Goktay O, Satilmis T, Garip H, Gonul O, Goker K. A comparison of the effects of midazolam/fentanyl and midazolam/tramadol for conscious intravenous sedation during third molar extraction. J Oral Maxillofac Surg. 2011;69(6):1594–9.

Taguchi T, Fukuda K, Sekine H, Kakizawa T. Intravenous sedation and hemodynamic changes during dental implant surgery. Int J Oral Maxillofac Implants. 2011;26(6):1303–8.

Cillo JE Jr. Analysis of propofol and low-dose ketamine admixtures for adult outpatient dentoalveolar surgery: a prospective, randomized, positive-controlled clinical trial. J Oral Maxillofac Surg. 2012;70(3):537–46.

Nooh N, Sheta SA, Abdullah WA, Abdelhalim AA. Intranasal atomized dexmedetomidine for sedation during third molar extraction. Int J Oral Maxillofac Surg. 2013;42(7):857–62.

El-Sharrawy E, Yagiela JA. Anesthetic efficacy of different ropivacaine concentrations for inferior alveolar nerve block. Anesth Prog. 2006;53(1):3–7.

Metin M, Tek M, Sener I. Comparison of two chlorhexidine rinse protocols on the incidence of alveolar osteitis following the surgical removal of impacted third molars. J Contemp Dent Pract. 2006;7(2):79–86.

Santos CF, Modena KC, Giglio FP, Sakai VT, Calvo AM, Colombini BL, et al. Epinephrine concentration (1:100,000 or 1:200,000) does not affect the clinical efficacy of 4% articaine for lower third molar removal: a double-blind, randomized, crossover study. J Oral Maxillofac Surg. 2007;65(12):2445–52.

Kirk DG, Liston PN, Tong DC, Love RM. Influence of two different flap designs on incidence of pain, swelling, trismus, and alveolar osteitis in the week following third molar surgery. Oral Surg Oral Med Oral Pathol Oral Radiol Endod. 2007;104(1):e1–6.

Calvo AM, Sakai VT, Giglio FP, Modena KC, Colombini BL, Benetello V, et al. Analgesic and anti-inflammatory dose-response relationship of 7.5 and 15 mg meloxicam after lower third molar removal: a double-blind, randomized, crossover study. Int J Oral Maxillofac Surg. 2007;36(1):26–31.

Aimetti M, Romano F. Use of resorbable membranes in periodontal defects treatment after extraction of impacted mandibular third molars. Minerva Stomatol. 2007;56(10):497–508.

Pozos-Guillen A, Martinez-Rider R, Aguirre-Banuelos P, Perez-Urizar J. Pre-emptive analgesic effect of tramadol after mandibular third molar extraction: a pilot study. J Oral Maxillofac Surg. 2007;65(7):1315–20.

Gharaibeh TM, Al-Nimri KS. Postoperative pain after surgical exposure of palatally impacted canines: closed-eruption versus open-eruption, a prospective randomized study. Oral Surg Oral Med Oral Pathol Oral Radiol Endod. 2008;106(3):339–42.

Brennan MT, Hong C, Furney SL, Fox PC, Lockhart PB. Utility of an international normalized ratio testing device in a hospital-based dental practice. J Am Dent Assoc. 2008;139(6):697–703.

Malmquist JP, Clemens SC, Oien HJ, Wilson SL. Hemostasis of oral surgery wounds with the HemCon dental dressing. J Oral Maxillofac Surg. 2008;66(6):1177–83.

Limeres J, Sanroman JF, Tomas I, Diz P. Patients' perception of recovery after third molar surgery following postoperative treatment with moxifloxacin versus amoxicillin and clavulanic acid: a randomized, double-blind, controlled study. J Oral Maxillofac Surg. 2009;67(2):286–91.

Kosger H, Polat HB, Demirer S, Ozdemir H, Ay S. Periodontal healing of marginal flap versus paramarginal flap in palatally impacted canine surgery: a prospective study. J Oral Maxillofac Surg. 2009;67(9):1826–31.

Gacic B, Todorovic L, Kokovic V, Danilovic V, Stojcev-Stajcic L, Drazic R, et al. The closure of oroantral communications with resorbable PLGA-coated beta-TCP root analogs, hemostatic gauze, or buccal flaps: a prospective study. Oral Surg Oral Med Oral Pathol Oral Radiol Endod. 2009;108(6):844–50.

De Menezes SA, Cury PR. Efficacy of nimesulide versus meloxicam in the control of pain, swelling and trismus following extraction of impacted lower third molar. Int J Oral Maxillofac Surg. 2010;39(6):580–4.

Daniels SE, Bandy DP, Christensen SE, Boice J, Losada MC, Liu H, et al. Evaluation of the dose range of etoricoxib in an acute pain setting using the postoperative dental pain model. Clin J Pain. 2011;27(1):1–8.

Ostenfeld T, Price J, Albanese M, Bullman J, Guillard F, Meyer I, et al. A randomized, controlled study to investigate the analgesic efficacy of single doses of the cannabinoid receptor-2 agonist GW842166, ibuprofen or placebo in patients with acute pain following third molar tooth extraction. Clin J Pain. 2011;27(8):668–76.

Trindade PA, Giglio FP, Colombini-Ishikiriama BL, Calvo AM, Modena KC, Ribeiro DA, et al. Sublingual ketorolac and sublingual piroxicam are equally effective for postoperative pain, trismus, and swelling management in lower third molar removal. Oral Surg Oral Med Oral Pathol Oral Radiol. 2012;114(1):27–34.

Marques J, Pie-Sanchez J, Figueiredo R, Valmaseda-Castellon E, Gay-Escoda C. Effect of the local administration of betamethasone on pain, swelling and trismus after impacted lower third molar extraction. A randomized, triple blinded, controlled trial. Med Oral Patol Oral Cir Bucal. 2014;19(1):e49–54.

Eshghpour M, Mortazavi H, Mohammadzadeh Rezaei N, Nejat A. Effectiveness of green tea mouthwash in postoperative pain control following surgical removal of impacted third molars: double blind randomized clinical trial. Daru: J Faculty Pharm Tehran Univ Med Sci. 2013;21(1):59.

Gutta R, Koehn CR, James LE. Does ketorolac have a preemptive analgesic effect? A randomized, double-blind, control study. J Oral Maxillofac Surg. 2013;71(12):2029–34.

Alvira-Gonzalez J, Gay-Escoda C. Compliance of postoperative instructions following the surgical extraction of impacted lower third molars: a randomized clinical trial. Med Oral Patol Oral Cir Bucal. 2015;20(2):e224–30.

Cagiran E, Eyigor C, Sezer B, Uyar M. Preemptive analgesic efficacy of dexketoprofen trometamol on impacted third molar surgery. Agri Dergisi. 2014;26(1):29–33.

Costa FW, Soares EC, Esses DF, Silva PG, Bezerra TP, Scarparo HC, et al. A split-mouth, randomized, triple-blind, placebo-controlled study to analyze the pre-emptive effect of etoricoxib 120 mg on inflammatory events following removal of unerupted mandibular third molars. Int J Oral Maxillofac Surg. 2015;44(9):1166–74.

Haraji A, Rakhshan V. Chlorhexidine gel and less difficult surgeries might reduce post-operative pain, controlling for dry socket, infection and analgesic consumption: a split-mouth controlled randomised clinical trial. J Oral Rehabil. 2015;42(3):209–19.

Dereci O, Tuzuner-Oncul AM, Kocer G, Yuce E, Askar M, Ozturk A. Efficacy of immediate postoperative intramasseteric dexamethasone injection on postoperative swelling after mandibular impacted third molar surgery: a preliminary split-mouth study. J Pak Med Assoc. 2016;66(3):320–3.

Elo JA, Sun HH, Dong F, Tandon R, Singh HM. Novel incision design and primary flap closure reduces the incidence of alveolar osteitis and infection in impacted mandibular third molar surgery. Oral Surg Oral Med Oral Pathol Oral Radiol. 2016;122(2):124–33.

Rocha-Neto AM, Nogueira EF, Borba PM, Laureano-Filho JR, Vasconcelos BC. Application of dexamethasone in the masseter muscle during the surgical removal of lower third molars. J Craniofac Surg. 2017;28(1):e43–e7.

Sivalingam VP, Panneerselvam E, Raja KV, Gopi G. Does topical ozone therapy improve patient comfort after surgical removal of impacted mandibular third molar? A randomized controlled trial. J Oral Maxillofac Surg. 2017;75(1):51.e1–9.

Cristalli MP, La Monaca G, De Angelis C, Pranno N, Annibali S. Efficacy of preoperative administration of paracetamol-codeine on pain following impacted mandibular third molar surgery: a randomized, split-mouth, placebo-controlled, double-blind clinical trial. Pain Res Manag. 2017;2017:9246352.

Zupelari-Goncalves P, Weckwerth GM, Calvo AM, Simoneti LF, Dionisio TJ, Brozoski DT, et al. Efficacy of oral diclofenac with or without codeine for pain control after invasive bilateral third molar extractions. Int J Oral Maxillofac Surg. 2017;46(5):621–7.

Pippi R, Santoro M, Cafolla A. The use of a chitosan-derived hemostatic agent for postextraction bleeding control in patients on antiplatelet treatment. J Oral Maxillofac Surg. 2017;75(6):1118–23.

Asutay F, Yolcu U, Gecor O, Acar AH, Ozturk SA, Malkoc S. An evaluation of effects of platelet-rich-fibrin on postoperative morbidities after lower third molar surgery. Niger J Clin Pract. 2017;20(12):1531–6.

Acar AH, Kazancioglu HO, Erdem NF, Asutay F. Is horizontal mattress suturing more effective than simple interrupted suturing on postoperative complications and primary wound healing after impacted mandibular third molar surgery? J Craniofac Surg. 2017;28(7):e657–e61.

Oladega AA, James O, Adeyemo WL. Cyanoacrylate tissue adhesive or silk suture for closure of surgical wound following removal of an impacted mandibular third molar: a randomized controlled study. J Craniomaxillofac Surg. 2019;47(1):93–8.

Akinbade AO, Ndukwe KC, Owotade FJ. Comparative analgesic effects of ibuprofen, celecoxib and tramadol after third molar surgery: a randomized double blind controlled trial. J Contemp Dent Pract. 2018;19(11):1334–40.

Maulina T, Diana H, Cahyanto A, Amaliya A. The efficacy of curcumin in managing acute inflammation pain on the post-surgical removal of impacted third molars patients: a randomised controlled trial. J Oral Rehabil. 2018;45(9):677–83.

Gorecki P, Rainsford KD, Taneja P, Bulsara Y, Pearson D, Saund D, et al. Submucosal diclofenac for acute postoperative pain in third molar surgery: a randomized, controlled clinical trial. J Dent Res. 2018;97(4):381–7.

Jadhao VA, Rao A, Hande P, Mahajani M, Raktade PP, Gedam R, et al. The efficiency of three irrigating solutions after surgical removal of impacted mandibular third molars: a cross-sectional study. J Contemp Dent Pract. 2018;19(9):1147–51.

Degala S, Bathija NA. Evaluation of the efficacy of simvastatin in bone regeneration after surgical removal of bilaterally impacted third molars-a split-mouth randomized clinical trial. J Oral Maxillofac Surg. 2018;76(9):1847–58.

Saka B, Petsch I, Hingst V, Härtel J. The influence of pre- and intraoperative positioning of the condyle in the centre of the articular fossa on the position of the disc in orthognathic surgery. A magnetic resonance study. Br J Oral Maxillofac Surg. 2004;42(2):120.

Takazakura D, Ueki K, Nakagawa K, Marukawa K, Shimada M, Shamiul A, et al. A comparison of postoperative hypoesthesia between two types of sagittal split ramus osteotomy and intraoral vertical ramus osteotomy, using the trigeminal somatosensory-evoked potential method. Int J Oral Maxillofac Surg. 2007;36(1):11–4.

Tang ZL, Wang X, Yi B, Li ZL, Liang C, Wang XX. Effects of the preoperative administration of Yunnan Baiyao capsules on intraoperative blood loss in bimaxillary orthognathic surgery: a prospective, randomized, double-blind, placebo-controlled study. Int J Oral Maxillofac Surg. 2009;38(3):261–6.

Ueki K, Hashiba Y, Marukawa K, Okabe K, Nakagawa K, Alam S, et al. Evaluation of bone formation after sagittal split ramus osteotomy with bent plate fixation using computed tomography. J Oral Maxillofac Surg. 2009;67(5):1062–8.

Kang MG, Yun KI, Kim CH, Park JU. Postoperative condylar position by sagittal split ramus osteotomy with and without bone graft. J Oral Maxillofac Surg. 2010;68(9):2058–64.

Chua HD, Hagg MB, Cheung LK. Cleft maxillary distraction versus orthognathic surgery—which one is more stable in 5 years? Oral Surg Oral Med Oral Pathol Oral Radiol Endod. 2010;109(6):803–14.

Aizenbud D, Ciceu C, Hazan-Molina H, Abu-El-Naaj I. Relationship between inferior alveolar nerve imaging and neurosensory impairment following bilateral sagittal split osteotomy in skeletal Class III cases with mandibular prognathism. Int J Oral Maxillofac Surg. 2012;41(4):461–8.

Al-Delayme R, Al-Khen M, Hamdoon Z, Jerjes W. Skeletal and dental relapses after skeletal class III deformity correction surgery: single-jaw versus double-jaw procedures. Oral Surg Oral Med Oral Pathol Oral Radiol. 2013;115(4):466–72.

Fuhrer-Valdivia A, Noguera-Pantoja A, Ramirez-Lobos V, Sole-Ventura P. Low-level laser effect in patients with neurosensory impairment of mandibular nerve after sagittal split ramus osteotomy. Randomized clinical trial, controlled by placebo. Med Oral Patol Oral Cir Bucal. 2014;19(4):e327–34.

Gasperini G, Rodrigues de Siqueira IC, Rezende CL. Does low-level laser therapy decrease swelling and pain resulting from orthognathic surgery? Int J Oral Maxillofac Surg. 2014;43(7):868–73.

Chen YW, Chiu YW, Chen CY, Chuang SK. Botulinum toxin therapy for temporomandibular joint disorders: a systematic review of randomized controlled trials. Int J Oral Maxillofac Surg. 2015;44(8):1018–26.

Baas EM, Bierenbroodspot F, de Lange J. Skeletal stability after bilateral sagittal split osteotomy or distraction osteogenesis of the mandible: a randomized clinical trial. Int J Oral Maxillofac Surg. 2015;44(5):615–20.

van Bakelen NB, Vermeulen KM, Buijs GJ, Jansma J, de Visscher JGAM, Hoppenreijs TJM, et al. Cost-effectiveness of a biodegradable compared to a titanium fixation system in maxillofacial surgery: a multicenter randomized controlled trial. PLoS ONE. 2015;10(7):e0130330.

Shetty V, Sriram SG. Effectiveness of intravenous haemocoagulase on haemorrhage control in bi-maxillary orthognathic surgery—a prospective, randomised, controlled, double-blind study. J Craniomaxillofac Surg. 2015;43(10):2000–3.

Vieira CL, Vasconcelos BC, Leao JC, Laureano Filho JR. Effect of the use of combination uridine triphosphate, cytidine monophosphate, and hydroxycobalamin on the recovery of neurosensory disturbance after bilateral sagittal split osteotomy: a randomized, double-blind trial. Int J Oral Maxillofac Surg. 2016;45(2):186–93.

Eshghpour M, Shaban B, Ahrari F, Erfanian M, Shadkam E. Is low-level laser therapy effective for treatment of neurosensory deficits arising from sagittal split ramus osteotomy? J Oral Maxillofac Surg. 2017;75(10):2085–90.

Schmitt ARM, Ritto FG, de Azevedo J, Medeiros PJD, de Mesquita MCM. Efficacy of gastric aspiration in reducing postoperative nausea and vomiting after orthognathic surgery: a double-blind prospective study. J Oral Maxillofac Surg. 2017;75(4):701–8.

Mohajerani SH, Tabeie F, Bemanali M, Tabrizi R. Effect of low-level laser and light-emitting diode on inferior alveolar nerve recovery after sagittal split osteotomy of the mandible: a randomized clinical trial study. J Craniofac Surg. 2017;28(4):e408–e11.

Berger M, Nova I, Kallus S, Ristow O, Freudlsperger C, Eisenmann U, et al. Can electromagnetic-navigated maxillary positioning replace occlusional splints in orthognathic surgery? A clinical pilot study. J Craniomaxillofac Surg. 2017;45(10):1593–9.

Lateef TA, Al-Anee AM, Agha MTF. Evaluation the efficacy of hilotherm cooling system in reducing postoperative pain and edema in maxillofacial traumatized patients and orthognathic surgeries. J Craniofac Surg. 2018;29(7):e697–706.

Tabrizi R, Pourdanesh F, Jafari S, Behnia P. Can platelet-rich fibrin accelerate neurosensory recovery following sagittal split osteotomy? A double-blind, split-mouth, randomized clinical trial. Int J Oral Maxillofac Surg. 2018;47(8):1011–4.

Troedhan A. Piezotome genioplasty reduces postsurgical morbidity and enhances patient satisfaction: a randomized clinical trial. J Oral Maxillofac Surg. 2018;76(7):1564.e1–e12.

Randomized Controlled Trials in Orthodontics

7

Dalya Al-Moghrabi, Nikolaos Pandis, and Padhraig S. Fleming

7.1 Introduction

Randomized controlled trials (RCTs) are directed at improving clinical practice and informing decision making founded upon reliable and trusted evidence. Properly designed RCTs are paramount to achieve internal validity. Data from robust trials with low risk of bias may in turn contribute to synthesis of evidence within meta-analyses leading to increased precision of estimates of effect of interventions. However, flaws in trial methodology may contribute to research waste, inflated effect sizes, and possibly erroneous inferences [1, 2]. An appreciation of appropriate study design and the use of relevant outcomes are paramount within all areas of dentistry including orthodontics in order to ensure optimal research outputs and evidence-informed decisions.

There has been a marked increase in the number of RCTs in orthodontics over the past three decades (Fig. 7.1). In particular, a 17-fold increase in orthodontic randomized trials was observed from 1992 to 2018 [3]. The majority (71%) of orthodontic RCTs published between 2003 and 2007 were published in four leading journals: *The American Journal of Orthodontics and Dentofacial Orthopedics, Angle Orthodontist, European Journal of Orthodontics and Journal of Orthodontics* [4]. As such, the quantity of high-level studies is undeniably increasing; it is therefore perhaps more important now than ever that awareness of optimal trial methodology, execution, and reporting exists.

We discuss 10 key design and implementation considerations relevant to the contemporary orthodontic literature. We also highlight areas of future research in orthodontics that appear to be particularly pressing.

D. Al-Moghrabi
Department of Preventive Dental Sciences, College of Dentistry, Princess Nourah bint Abdulrahman University, Riyadh, Saudi Arabia
e-mail: dhalmoghrabi@pnu.edu.sa

N. Pandis
Department of Orthodontics and Dentofacial Orthopedics, School of Dental Medicine, Medical Faculty, University of Bern, Bern, Switzerland

P. S. Fleming (✉)
Division of Public and Child Dental Health, Dublin Dental University Hospital, The University of Dublin, Trinity College Dublin, Dublin, Ireland
e-mail: padhraig.fleming@dental.tcd.ie

R. Kohli et al. (eds.), *Randomized Controlled Trials in Evidence-Based Dentistry*,
https://doi.org/10.1007/978-3-031-47651-8_7

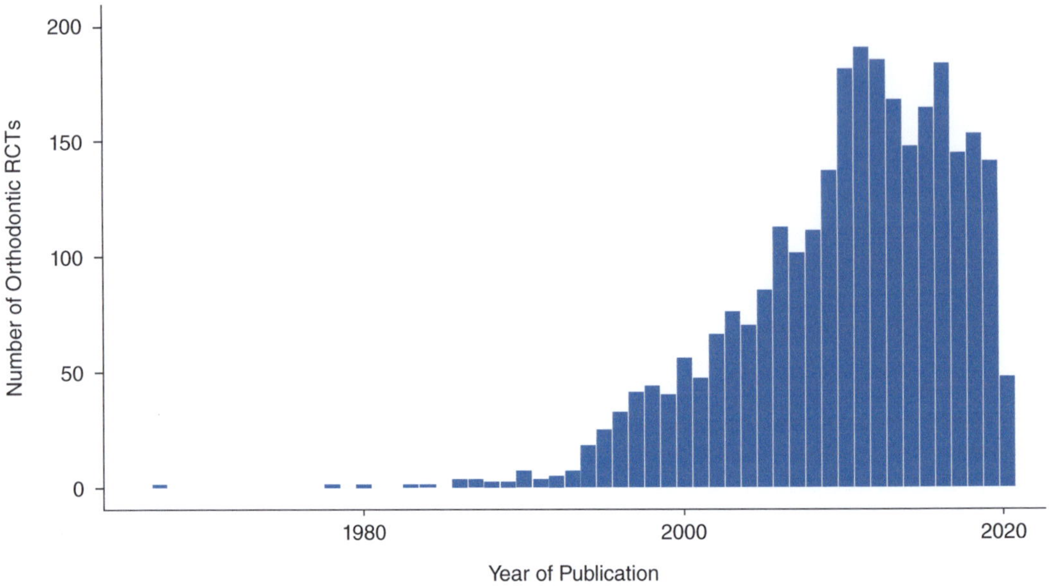

Fig. 7.1 Number of randomized controlled trials (RCTs) in orthodontics published in recent decades (up to July 2020)

7.2 Critical Analysis of Orthodontic Trials: 10 Considerations

In this section, we discuss aspects related to the research questions, as well as highlighting design, methodological, and reporting issues (Fig. 7.2). An appreciation of these issues may contribute to better use of resources and, therefore, limit research waste.

7.2.1 Research Questions

Evidence-based clinical practice relies on research, which is driven by clinically relevant questions aiming to ascertain meaningful and appropriate outcome variables and measures reflecting relevant benefits and potential harms of an intervention. Useful orthodontic research and optimal use of resources is, therefore, predicated on assessment of relevant research questions, particularly set against a backdrop of limited research funding within the specialty.

7.2.1.1 Focus of Research

A number of key orthodontic RCTs have been published to address important clinical questions providing robust evidence to underpin key treatment decisions (Table 7.1; Box 7.1). The focus of the majority of published RCTs in orthodontics has been on evaluation of the effectiveness of interventions and comparative assessment of different appliances, with a limited number of RCTs focusing on improving patient experiences during treatment and care provision (Table 7.1). Certain orthodontic topics have been researched more than others, with the majority of clinical trials published between 1989 and 1998 in three orthodontic journals involving an assessment on bonding materials (21.9%), growth modification (21.3%), and oral hygiene practices (9.0%) [5]. Furthermore, 45% of RCTs published over a 5-year period (2012–2016) involved an evaluation of marketed orthodontic products, indicating undue emphasis on clinical assessment of advertised products, and the effects of intrusion of market forces on clinical practice and research [6]. On

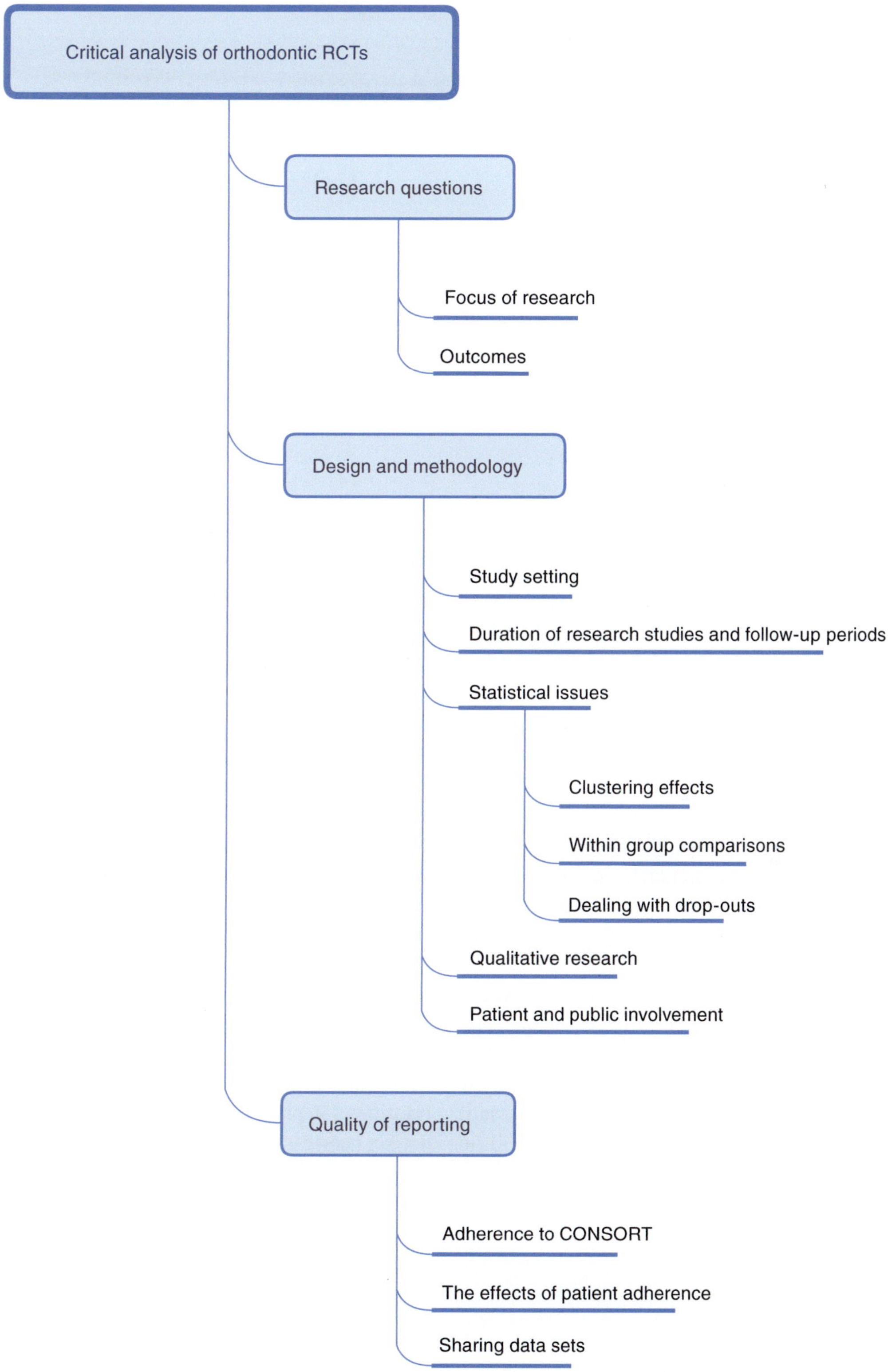

Fig. 7.2 Key aspects concerning randomized controlled trial (RCT) design and execution in orthodontics

Table 7.1 Key randomized controlled trials in the orthodontic literature

Topic			Study
Growth modification	Class II		Tulloch et al. (1998) [10], O'Brien et al. (2009) [11], Parekh et al. (2019) [12]
	Class III		Mandall et al. (2010) [13], Mandall et al. (2012) [14], Mandall et al. (2016) [15]
Fixed appliance mechanics	Space closure		Dixon et al. (2002) [16]
	Archwire sequence		Mandall et al. (2006) [17]
	The use of lacebacks		Usmani et al. (2002) [18], Irvine et al. (2004) [19]
	Bracket type	Mode of ligation	Fleming et al. (2010) [20]
		Slot size	Yassir (2019) [18]
		Bracket customization	Penning et al. (2017) [21]
Adhesives			Manning et al. (2006) [22], Banks and Thiruvenkatachari (2007) [23]
Anchorage			Sandler et al. (2008) [24], Stivaros et al. (2010) [25], Sandler et al. (2014) [26]
Retention	Fixed vs removable		Al-Moghrabi et al. (2016) [27], Forde et al. (2018) [28]
	Vacuum-formed retainer vs Hawley		Rowland et al. (2007) [29]
	Wear regime		Gill et al. (2007) [30], Shawesh et al. (2010) [31]
Vibrational forces			Woodhouse et al. (2015) [32]
Prevention and treatment of white spot lesions			Robertson et al. (2011) [33], Huang et al. (2013) [34]
Oral hygiene reinforcement during orthodontic treatment			Li et al. (2016) [35], Alkadhi et al. (2017) [36]
Patient knowledge and retention of orthodontic-related information			Al-Silwadi et al. (2015) [37]
Sleep apnea oral appliance			Engleman et al. (2002) [38]
Interceptive treatment of palatally displaced canine			Naoumova et al. (2015) [39]
Surgical exposure of palatally displaced canine			Parkin et al. (2013) [40]

the corollary, it is evident that further high-quality research is particularly pressing in other areas such as the relative merits of extraction vs. non-extraction treatment and various appointment intervals.

Prioritization of orthodontic research would help to provide a framework for researchers and funding agencies for allocation of relatively scarce research funds. This could be done by engaging both the public and professional groups using Priority Setting Partnerships (PSPs) in keeping with previous approaches [7, 8]. PSPs have been used to help in identification of the leading priorities in oral health and dental research including themes such as prevention of oral disease, access to dental care, and patient–clinician communication [8]. Furthermore, The Cochrane Oral Health Group developed a core portfolio to prioritize Cochrane Reviews in oral health and orthodontics [9]. However, research priorities for primary orthodontic research have not yet been established.

Box 7.1 Summary of the Main Findings from Key Randomized Controlled Trials in Orthodontics

- Functional appliance therapy for Class II malocclusion produced a temporary acceleration of mandibular growth rate with little if any sustained skeletal effect [10, 11] but was associated with significant dentoalveolar improvement [12]. This information has been instrumental in informing treatment decisions and rationalizing the use of growth modification, particularly in juvenile patients.
- Early treatment of increased overjet is rarely suggested and is reserved for cases with increased risk of dental trauma [41]. Again, this information has been derived from multicenter studies indicating comparable outcomes with early versus later treatment in the management of Class II malocclusion [11].
- Protraction facemask therapy for Class III has limited sustained skeletal effect, can be used to achieve occlusal correction, and is successful in the reduction of subjective need for surgery [15]. The latter was based on a clinical trial with 6-year follow-up involving objective analysis of cephalometric data coupled with subjective impressions relating to the need for orthognathic surgery involving a panel of experts [15].
- Fixed appliance mechanics, prescription, and design:
  - NiTi springs shown to be more effective in terms of rate of space closure when compared with active ligature and powerchain [16]. However, the latter is the most cost-effective [16].
  - There is no ideal archwire sequence [17], with equivocal evidence pertaining to the effect of lacebacks on anchorage balance [18, 19].
  - In terms of orthodontic brackets, little to no difference was found in the effectiveness of different types in terms of mode of ligation [20], slot size [42], and customization [21].
- No difference in bond failure rate between self-etching primer and conventional acid etch and primer [22, 23].
- Anchorage support:
  - No significant difference exists between mid-palatal implants and headgear in terms of orthodontic treatment outcomes as judged by peer assessment rating scores [24].
  - Temporary anchorage devices, Nance palatal arch, and headgear offer similar levels of anchorage support [26].
  - There appears to be no significant difference in terms of effectiveness between Nance palatal arch and Transpalatal arch (TPA) during initial alignment phase [25].
- With regard to orthodontic retainers, fixed retention offers a greater stability of alignment of mandibular incisors when compared to Essix-type retainers, especially in the long term [28, 43].
- Application of vibrational stimuli does not accelerate rate of tooth movement during the alignment phase in 4-premolar extraction cases [32].
- The use of a form of Casein Phosphopeptide Amorphous Calcium Phosphate (CPP-ACP; MI Paste Plus) or fluoride varnish was similar to control in terms of regression of white spot lesions following debond of active appliances [34]. However, the former was more effective in preventing new white spot lesions during treatment when compared to a placebo paste [33].
- There is equivocal evidence on the effect of receipt of mobile application on oral hygiene in orthodontic patients [35, 36]. However, provision of orthodontic information using YouTube videos has proven effective in improving knowledge retention [37].
- In terms of management of obstructive sleep apnea, mandibular repositioning

splints have proven inferior to continuous positive airway pressure (CPAP) for treatment of sleep apnea/hypopnea syndrome [38].

- Extraction of primary canines is considered an effective interceptive approach in the treatment of palatally displaced canines [39] resulting in improvement in the position of canines up to 15 months following the procedure.
- When open and closed surgical exposures of palatally displaced canines are compared, there are no significant differences in terms of the periodontal health in the short-term [40], as well as surgical morbidity [44]. As such, there appears to be equipoise between these with the specific choice of technique governed by local factors including the depth of impaction and location relative to adjacent teeth.

7.2.1.2 Outcomes

Patient values are integral to evidence-based practice [45]; moreover, it is important that holistic and relevant assessments of the relative merits and demerits of orthodontic interventions are considered in clinical research. Research outputs focusing on patient perspectives have been overlooked in one-third of orthodontic RCTs published over a 3-year period (up to 2015), with similar findings observed in dental research more broadly [46]. The majority of outcomes assessed in orthodontic RCTs appear to relate to morphologic features of malocclusion with excessive focus on cephalometric outcomes and relatively little reference to patient-centered outcomes including effects on quality of life and social interactions [47]. The latter is particularly important in orthodontics, in which typical mean duration of treatment is 20 months [48], with reported negative experiences and impact on daily and social activities, impairment of quality of life and pain with different orthodontic appliances being recognized issues which may impact both on the overall experience and the treated result [49–51]. Therefore, it is imperative that diverse outcomes reflecting aspects and attributes important to patients are selected in order to ensure that research outputs are relevant to practicing clinicians and prospective patients [47].

The lack of an agreed set of outcome variables and measures in orthodontics has also resulted in the inability to assimilate primary data from clinical trials due to insufficient homogeneity in meta-analysis with 73% of 157 systematic reviews published over a 14-year period (2000–2014) lacking meta-analysis [52]. Furthermore, a median of just four studies were included within these meta-analyses, while systematic reviews within medicine have a median of 15 trials [52]. Recently, there has been an appreciation of the need to standardize outcomes in healthcare research to facilitate data synthesis and, therefore, increase precision and robustness of systematic review findings, prompting a drive to produce core outcome sets spanning a range of medical and dental interventions and conditions [53].

7.2.2 Design and Methodology

A number of issues related to study design are discussed in this section. Addressing these issues may ultimately increase the applicability, robustness, and relevance of findings of orthodontic RCTs.

7.2.2.1 Study Setting

The generalizability of trial findings hinges on the diversity of the sample and clinical settings. Larger and therefore more diverse sample could be attained in multicentered trials [54]. However, based on a meta-epidemiologic overview, 72% of orthodontic clinical trials were single-centered [54], risking possible overestimation of effect sizes and limited external validity [55]. Based on this analysis of 217 orthodontic randomized studies published between 2013 and 2017, clinical trials conducted in a university hospital exceeded those based in specialist practice by a factor of seven [54]. The nature of participants and their characteristics tend to be similar within the same setting. This may have implications for compliance, in particular. For example, significantly longer median wear time of removable appliances was found in private practice compared to the university hospital setting [56]. This is potentially important as research conducted in university and hospital settings, which forms the mainstay of orthodontic research, may involve participants who are being treated in a publicly funded or heavily subsidized system. Furthermore, funded orthodontic treatment carried out in university hospitals in the UK is restricted to children and young people with severe malocclusion [57].

Practice-based research involves testing of the effectiveness of treatment or interventions in real-word clinical practice, therefore, helping to bridge the translational gap between research and clinical practice [55]. Undertaking practice-based research in orthodontics has been encouraged [58] with establishment of the National Dental Practice-Based Research Network in the USA supported by the National Institute of Dental and Craniofacial Research. This funding led to the publication of practice-based trials in orthodontics concerning the management of white spot lesions [34] and open bite correction [59]. This involvement of practice-based specialist orthodontists and general dentists may ultimately assist in providing more relevant and generalizable research outputs [54].

7.2.2.2 Duration of Research Studies and Follow-Up Periods

Our understanding of orthodontic treatment effects is mainly reliant on short-term studies often confined to the initial stages of treatment [60]. Many of these have used surrogate outcome measures, such as the rate of initial alignment or orthodontic space closure, as an indication of the likely effect of an intervention on overall treatment duration. Only 9% of orthodontic trials published over a 4-year period (up to 2016) involved an assessment of outcomes following the whole treatment [60]. Moreover, very few orthodontic RCTs have spanned periods of 5 years or more [11, 61]. Short-term follow-up is particularly limited in the evaluation of orthodontic retention. This is exemplified by findings related to stability related to two types of retainers changing over time with longer follow-up periods revealing a benefit of fixed rather than removable designs [43, 62]. Additionally, longer follow-up of participants wearing protraction facemask facilitated a clearer understanding of sustainability of treatment success at 15-month [13], 3-year [14], and 6-year follow-up [15]. While undertaking long-term RCTs is an arduous task and is associated with increased cost, as well as the inevitable high drop-out rate [43], this more holistic approach may allow sufficient time for the manifestation of disease or impact of interventions, and identification of harms.

7.2.2.3 Statistical Issues

Meta-epidemiologic analyses of orthodontic trials have highlighted a number of statistical issues in published trials. A common issue in orthodontics is the failure to account for clustering effects with more than 75% of orthodontic studies being deficient in this respect [63]. Clustering effects arise when data are gathered from one sample at different time points, or due to multiple observations obtained within individuals. As a result, the clustered data are likely to be correlated resulting in lack of independency in observations, as is the case with orthodontic attachment failure. Therefore, clustering effects should be accounted for statistically in both sample size estimation and data analysis [64, 65]. Neglecting to account for clustering effects can result in false positive results and, therefore, incorrect interpretation and conclusion [65].

Another statistical issue highlighted in the orthodontic literature pertains to the conduct of inferential comparisons within rather than between groups. Such comparisons are likely to result in false positive result as a result of "natural or temporal" changes of the outcome, and due to the increased number of tests undertaken [66]. Common examples of this include the assessment of treatment related changes (e.g., overjet reduction) with two appliances leading to a conclusion that both are equally effective, while failing to account for key differential changes between the treatment interventions. Within orthodontics, only one quarter of studies based their interpretation solely on between-group comparisons, with the majority of studies including both between-group and within-group comparisons [67].

Drop-out is common in orthodontic clinical trials and is typically of the order of 13% of those recruited, as a result of premature discontinuation of treatment or withdrawal from the study [68]. However, higher drop-out rates were noted in studies with prolonged follow-ups particularly with no active treatment being provided [43, 61]. Drop-out is less likely, however, in short-term analyses, particularly involving those with fixed rather than removable appliances in place. Those who drop-out might exhibit different characteristics or experience different outcomes leading to their discontinuation. For example, patients with high motivation towards orthodontic treatment are likely to be more adherent to appliance wear [69, 70]. Therefore, ignoring the drop-outs in the analysis may risk analyzing the outcome based on only the more successful participants.

Exclusion of drop-outs from the analysis might influence the results and hampers the statistical power of the study risking erroneous inferences [71]. Therefore, analysis of the results on an intention-to-treat basis is considered more appropriate than per protocol analysis; however, the former was conducted only in 13% of orthodontic RCTs published over a 20-year period [68]. Proper handling of missing data entails accounting for and compensating of missing values to obtain a complete data set [72]. Additionally, researchers tend to inflate sample sizes to make adequate allowance for drop-outs especially in studies with longer follow-up. Involvement of a statistician can help to mitigate these statistical issues. However, only 14% of orthodontic RCTs published between 2013 and 2017 involved a statistician [54].

7.2.2.4 Qualitative Research

The use of qualitative research in evidence-based medicine has become more established. The exploratory and explanatory nature of this type of research has prompted its use to complement quantitative studies, although qualitative research can also be conducted as a standalone approach. Qualitative research may also help to address concepts that cannot be measured, as well as to explore patient experiences and ideas from their perspective. This differs from quantitative methods which are based on clinicians' and researchers' preconceptions.

In the medical literature, qualitative research has been used in 22 ways to inform different aspects of RCTs, but mainly during the development of an intervention, and during study design conduct (e.g., exploring ways to improve participation) [73]. However, qualitative research involving orthodontic patients is relatively limited with, for example, only four qualitative studies published over a recent 18-month period (up to mid-2018) [74]. Therefore, researchers should be encouraged to undertake this type of research to enhance our understanding of unexplored topics, assist in refining interventions, and explain the findings from orthodontic trials.

7.2.2.5 Patient and Public Involvement

Patient and public involvement helps to make research more relevant and ensure it addresses unmet needs, therefore potentially reduces research waste [75, 76] [63]. Furthermore, such an involvement can also help researchers in understanding the area of research as well as patient needs, while also giving participants a sense of empowerment [77]. Patient and public involvement can also aid in directing and prioritizing research focus, refining research questions and selecting relevant outcomes, as well as during study design, conduct, and analysis of findings [75, 78]. Furthermore, feedback from participants on research information sheets and questionnaires can help improve their readability, layout, and content [75]. Additionally, patient and public involvement can be beneficial in dissemination of research findings [75]. The latter is particularly problematic in biomedical research, in which less than one-third of authors communicated their research findings with participants [79].

Patients perceive their condition differently compared to researchers, and therefore, they are likely to provide insightful feedback when involved in research [80]. The underrepresentation of patient-centered outcomes in orthodontic

RCTs has been highlighted in a previous systematic review [47]. Therefore, involvement of patients in orthodontic research might help address issues that might have been overlooked.

7.2.3 Quality of Reporting

7.2.3.1 Adherence to CONSORT

The quality of research can only readily be evaluated on the basis of explicit and transparent reporting of methods and findings. Inadequate reporting of trials limits their applicability, hampers their inclusion in synthesis of evidence, and therefore contributes to research waste [81]. Adherence to the Consolidated Standards of Reporting Trials (CONSORT) is incumbent on orthodontic researchers and has been endorsed by a number of journals [82]. However, the quality of reporting of 128 orthodontic RCTs published in four leading orthodontic journals was found to be suboptimal (using modified CONSORT checklist) with a mean percentage of reporting of 69%, with no description in relation to confidence intervals and allocation concealment in 71% and 64%, respectively [83]. As such, a bespoke CONSORT for orthodontics was developed to increase its accessibility to orthodontic researchers [82]. An orthodontic initiative geared at improving reporting of our RCTs by encouraging the use of subheadings to prompt adherence to the CONSORT checklist was subsequently developed [84]. This mandated use of subheadings in an orthodontic journal has shown promise and resulted in a 15% higher adherence to the CONSORT checklist [84].

7.2.3.2 The Effects of Patient Adherence

High levels of patient adherence tend to be associated with better treatment outcomes and experiences [50, 85]. In particular, interventions reliant on optimal compliance to achieve the best results include removable appliances and adjuncts. There is an acceptance, however, that patients within research studies tend to wear headgear and functional appliances by approximately a mean of 5 h daily less than that required, and also claim to wear these adjuncts more diligently than they actually do [86]. As such, the use of supplementary objective measures of adherence to advised protocols, harnessing newer technologies, is particularly important in trials involving removable components [12]. Other measures of overall adherence in orthodontic literature have encompassed oral hygiene levels, appliance wear and breakage, and appointment attendance [87].

7.2.3.3 Sharing Data Sets

The adoption of data set sharing allows the reuse of data and, therefore, optimizes the impact of the primary research [88]. Deposition of raw and deidentified orthodontic clinical trial data on online portals, such as institutional repositories, facilitates accessibility to the data. The individual-level data from different studies can be aggregated and transformed to homogenous data, which in turn facilitates data synthesis in systematic reviews [88, 89]. Additionally, raw data can be reused for secondary analysis and to answer different research questions, thus reducing duplication in studies and, therefore, mitigating against research waste [88–90]. However, data sharing is not mainstream in orthodontics and a clear protocol for data sharing practice is likely to facilitate this [73], before being uniformly encouraged by orthodontic journals, funders, and research ethics committees.

7.3 Conclusion

While significant progress has been made in relation to the publication, uptake, and application of evidence-based knowledge within orthodontics, concerns persist in relation to the focus of our research, with a failure to prioritize important areas, and continued use of inconsistent and less pertinent outcomes within randomized trials. This, in turn, has led to a limited yield from orthodontic systematic reviews relative to other biomedical areas. We highlighted numerous issues related to study design, bespoke methodology, and aspects concerning quality of reporting in orthodontic studies. Accounting for these issues can help to improve the relevance and utility of future orthodontic research.

7.4 Summary

Summary of key improvements required in relation to orthodontic research focus, design, conduct, and reporting.

- Prioritization of underexplored and clinically relevant topics.
- Selection of relevant outcomes by developing and adopting a core outcome set (COS).
- Undertaking more practice-based research.
- Follow-up of participants for longer periods.
- Involvement of statisticians in research design and analysis.
- Complementing RCTs with qualitative studies, where appropriate.
- Involvement of patients at different stages of research.
- Adherence to CONSORT statement in relation to trial reporting.
- Complete reporting of issues concerning patient compliance.
- Availability of trial data sets.

7.5 Case Scenario Exercise

7.5.1 Case Scenario

Box 7.2 Proposed Study Protocol

A comparative assessment of two methods of space closure: a randomized controlled trial.

Aim: To compare the efficacy of elastomeric chain and NiTi coil spring in terms of space closure.

Study setting: One University Hospital.

Methods: Eighty participants planned for space closure in the maxillary dental arch will be randomly assigned either to have spaces closed using elastic chain or NiTi coil spring. Randomization will be based on computer-generated random numbers and allocation concealment will involve the use of opaque, sealed envelopes. Maxillary study models will be taken at the start of space closure (T0) and 6 weeks later (T1).

Outcomes: The magnitude of spaces will be measured by one calibrated researcher using digital calipers. T-tests will be undertaken to compare the means between the groups at T1, as well as within the same group (T0–T1). The outcome data will be analyzed only for those who attended their follow-up appointment.

Questions

If you received the proposal for a trial comparing two methods of space closure (Box 7.2), based on the points discussed in this chapter:

1. How can you improve the following aspects:
   (a) Focus of the trial and outcomes.
   (b) Study setting.
   (c) Duration of the study.
   (d) Statistical analysis
2. How will the results be disseminated?

Answers:

1.
   (a) Consult a panel of prospective and former patients exploring their views on the relevance of the topic and, therefore, whether it should be prioritized. It would also be worth considering inclusion of aspects of space closure relevant to patients in the trial. Patients may point out that hindrance to oral hygiene, soft tissue trauma, esthetics, cost-effectiveness, and emergency appointments are more relevant to them than the rate of space closure.
   (b) Consider undertaking the study in more than one University Hospital as well as in a private practice setting. This approach will help to improve the generalizability of the findings, although it is important that calibration of researchers is undertaken with a clear research protocol in place.

(c) Follow-up of patients for the whole duration of treatment rather than the first 6 weeks of the space closure phase would assist in providing a more holistic assessment of the benefits and harms of the interventions.
(d) It is important to account for clustering effects related to measuring space closure in two sites per participant. Furthermore, it is important that the differential rate of space closure is assessed between groups only and avoiding within-group comparisons against the baseline. Consideration should be given to the use of intention-to-treat analysis by imputation of missing data and analysis of outcomes related to the entire sample.

2. In addition to publication of study findings, dissemination of the results to patients using lay language summaries through leaflets or online platforms such as websites is to be encouraged. Moreover, upload of the trial data set on an institutional repository is important to allow online access for secondary use and possible inclusion in meta-analyses.

References

1. Schulz KF, Chalmers I, Hayes RJ, Altman DG. Empirical evidence of bias. Dimensions of methodological quality associated with estimates of treatment effects in controlled trials. JAMA. 1995;273(5):408–12. https://doi.org/10.1001/jama.1995.03520290060030.
2. Moher D, Jones A, Cook DJ, Jadad AR, Moher M, Tugwell P, et al. Does quality of reports of randomised trials affect estimates of intervention efficacy reported in meta-analyses? Lancet. 1998;352(9128):609–13. https://doi.org/10.1016/S0140-6736(98)01085-X.
3. Buschang PH, Asiri SN. The present, past and future of orthodontic research. Semin Orthod. 2019;25(4):326–38. https://doi.org/10.1053/j.sodo.2019.10.008.
4. Shimada T, Takayama H, Nakamura Y. Quantity and quality assessment of randomized controlled trials on orthodontic practice in PubMed. Angle Orthod. 2010;80(4):713–8. https://doi.org/10.2319/090809-507.1.
5. Harrison JE. Clinical trials in orthodontics I: demographic details of clinical trials published in three orthodontic journals between 1989 and 1998. J Orthod. 2003;30(1):25–30. https://doi.org/10.1093/ortho/30.1.25.
6. Seehra J, Pandis N, Fleming PS. Clinical evaluation of marketed orthodontic products: are researchers behind the times? A meta-epidemiological study. Prog Orthod. 2017;18(1):14. https://doi.org/10.1186/s40510-017-0168-y.
7. Deane KH, Flaherty H, Daley DJ, Pascoe R, Penhale B, Clarke CE, et al. Priority setting partnership to identify the top 10 research priorities for the management of Parkinson's disease. BMJ Open. 2014;4(12):e006434. https://doi.org/10.1136/bmjopen-2014-006434.
8. Experts set top priorities for oral health research. Br Dent J. 2019;226:92. https://doi.org/10.1038/sj.bdj.2019.66.
9. Worthington H, Clarkson J, Weldon J. Priority oral health research identification for clinical decision-making. Evid Based Dent. 2015;16(3):69–71. https://doi.org/10.1038/sj.ebd.6401110.
10. Tulloch JF, Phillips C, Proffit WR. Benefit of early Class II treatment: progress report of a two-phase randomized clinical trial. Am J Orthod Dentofac Orthop. 1998;113(1):62–74.
11. O'Brien K, Wright J, Conboy F, Appelbe P, Davies L, Connolly I, et al. Early treatment for Class II Division 1 malocclusion with the Twin-block appliance: a multi-center, randomized, controlled trial. Am J Orthod Dentofac Orthop. 2009;135(5):573–9. https://doi.org/10.1016/j.ajodo.2007.10.042.
12. Parekh J, Counihan K, Fleming PS, Pandis N, Sharma PK. Effectiveness of part-time vs full-time wear protocols of Twin-block appliance on dental and skeletal changes: a randomized controlled trial. Am J Orthod Dentofac Orthop. 2019;155(2):165–72. https://doi.org/10.1016/j.ajodo.2018.07.016.
13. Mandall N, DiBiase A, Littlewood S, Nute S, Stivaros N, McDowall R, et al. Is early class III protraction facemask treatment effective? A multicentre, randomized, controlled trial: 15-month follow-up. J Orthod. 2010;37(3):149–61. https://doi.org/10.1179/14653121043056.
14. Mandall NA, Cousley R, DiBiase A, Dyer F, Littlewood S, Mattick R, et al. Is early class III protraction facemask treatment effective? A multicentre, randomized, controlled trial: 3-year follow-up. J Orthod. 2012;39(3):176–85. https://doi.org/10.1179/1465312512Z.00000000028.
15. Mandall N, Cousley R, DiBiase A, Dyer F, Littlewood S, Mattick R, et al. Early class III protraction facemask treatment reduces the need for orthognathic surgery: a multi-centre, two-arm parallel randomized, controlled trial. J Orthod. 2016;43(3):164–75. https://doi.org/10.1080/14653125.2016.1201302.
16. Dixon V, Read M, O'brien K, Worthington H, Mandall N. A randomized clinical trial to compare three methods of orthodontic space closure. J Orthod. 2002;29(1):31–6. https://doi.org/10.1093/ortho/29.1.31.
17. Mandall N, Lowe C, Worthington H, Sandler J, Derwent S, Abdi-Oskouei M, et al. Which orthodontic archwire sequence? A randomized clinical trial. Eur

J Orthod. 2006;28(6):561–6. https://doi.org/10.1093/ejo/cjl030.
18. Usmani T, O'Brien K, Worthington H, Derwent S, Fox D, Harrison S, et al. A randomized clinical trial to compare the effectiveness of canine lacebacks with reference to canine tip. J Orthod. 2002;29(4):281–6. https://doi.org/10.1093/ortho/29.4.281.
19. Irvine R, Power S, McDonald F. The effectiveness of laceback ligatures: a randomized controlled clinical trial. J Orthod. 2004;31(4):303–11. https://doi.org/10.1179/146531204225020606.
20. Fleming PS, DiBiase AT, Lee RT. Randomized clinical trial of orthodontic treatment efficiency with self-ligating and conventional fixed orthodontic appliances. Am J Orthod Dentofac Orthop. 2010;137(6):738–42. https://doi.org/10.1016/j.ajodo.2009.06.023.
21. Penning E, Peerlings R, Govers J, Rischen R, Zinad K, Bronkhorst E, et al. Orthodontics with customized versus noncustomized appliances: a randomized controlled clinical trial. J Dent Res. 2017;96(13):1498–504. https://doi.org/10.1177/0022034517720913.
22. Manning N, Chadwick S, Plunkett D, Macfarlane T. A randomized clinical trial comparing 'one-step'and 'two-step' orthodontic bonding systems. J Orthod. 2006;33(4):276–83. https://doi.org/10.1179/146531205225021825.
23. Banks P, Thiruvenkatachari B. Long-term clinical evaluation of bracket failure with a self-etching primer: a randomized controlled trial. J Orthod. 2007;34(4):243–51. https://doi.org/10.1179/146531207225022293.
24. Sandler J, Benson PE, Doyle P, Majumder A, O'Dwyer J, Speight P, et al. Palatal implants are a good alternative to headgear: a randomized trial. Am J Orthod Dentofac Orthop. 2008;133(1):51–7. https://doi.org/10.1016/j.ajodo.2007.04.032.
25. Stivaros N, Lowe C, Dandy N, Doherty B, Mandall N. A randomized clinical trial to compare the Goshgarian and Nance palatal arch. Eur J Orthod. 2010;32(2):171–6. https://doi.org/10.1093/ejo/cjp075.
26. Sandler J, Murray A, Thiruvenkatachari B, Gutierrez R, Speight P, O'Brien K. Effectiveness of 3 methods of anchorage reinforcement for maximum anchorage in adolescents: a 3-arm multicenter randomized clinical trial. Am J Orthod Dentofac Orthop. 2014;146(1):10–20. https://doi.org/10.1016/j.ajodo.2014.03.020.
27. Al-Moghrabi D, Pandis N, Fleming PS. The effects of fixed and removable orthodontic retainers: a systematic review. Prog Orthod. 2016;17(1):24. https://doi.org/10.1186/s40510-016-0137-x.
28. Forde K, Storey M, Littlewood SJ, Scott P, Luther F, Kang J. Bonded versus vacuum-formed retainers: a randomized controlled trial. Part 1: Stability, retainer survival, and patient satisfaction outcomes after 12 months. Eur J Orthod. 2018;40(4):387–98. https://doi.org/10.1093/ejo/cjx058.
29. Rowland H, Hichens L, Williams A, Hills D, Killingback N, Ewings P, et al. The effectiveness of Hawley and vacuum-formed retainers: a single-center randomized controlled trial. Am J Orthod Dentofac Orthop. 2007;132(6):730–7. https://doi.org/10.1016/j.ajodo.2006.06.019.
30. Gill DS, Naini FB, Jones A, Tredwin CJ. Part-time versus full-time retainer wear following fixed appliance therapy: a randomized prospective controlled trial. World J Orthod. 2007;8(3):300–6.
31. Shawesh M, Bhatti B, Usmani T, Mandall N. Hawley retainers full-or part-time? A randomized clinical trial. Eur J Orthod. 2010;32(2):165–70. https://doi.org/10.1093/ejo/cjp082.
32. Woodhouse N, DiBiase A, Johnson N, Slipper C, Grant J, Alsaleh M, et al. Supplemental vibrational force during orthodontic alignment: a randomized trial. J Dent Res. 2015;94(5):682–9. https://doi.org/10.1177/0022034515576195.
33. Robertson MA, Kau CH, English JD, Lee RP, Powers J, Nguyen JT. MI Paste Plus to prevent demineralization in orthodontic patients: a prospective randomized controlled trial. Am J Orthod Dentofac Orthop. 2011;140(5):660–8. https://doi.org/10.1016/j.ajodo.2010.10.025.
34. Huang GJ, Roloff-Chiang B, Mills BE, Shalchi S, Spiekerman C, Korpak AM, et al. Effectiveness of MI Paste Plus and PreviDent fluoride varnish for treatment of white spot lesions: a randomized controlled trial. Am J Orthod Dentofac Orthop. 2013;143(1):31–41. https://doi.org/10.1016/j.ajodo.2012.09.007.
35. Li X, Xu Z-R, Tang N, Ye C, Zhu X-L, Zhou T, et al. Effect of intervention using a messaging app on compliance and duration of treatment in orthodontic patients. Clin Oral Investig. 2016;20(8):1849–59.
36. Alkadhi OH, Zahid MN, Almanea RS, Althaqeb HK, Alharbi TH, Ajwa NM. The effect of using mobile applications for improving oral hygiene in patients with orthodontic fixed appliances: a randomised controlled trial. J Orthod. 2017;44(3):157–63. https://doi.org/10.1080/14653125.2017.1346746.
37. Al-Silwadi FM, Gill DS, Petrie A, Cunningham SJ. Effect of social media in improving knowledge among patients having fixed appliance orthodontic treatment: a single-center randomized controlled trial. Am J Orthod Dentofac Orthop. 2015;148(2):231–7.
38. Engleman HM, McDonald JP, Graham D, Lello GE, Kingshott RN, Coleman EL, et al. Randomized crossover trial of two treatments for sleep apnea/hypopnea syndrome: continuous positive airway pressure and mandibular repositioning splint. Am J Respir Crit Care Med. 2002;166(6):855–9. https://doi.org/10.1164/rccm.2109023.
39. Naoumova J, Kurol J, Kjellberg H. Extraction of the deciduous canine as an interceptive treatment in children with palatal displaced canines—part I: Shall we extract the deciduous canine or not? Eur J Orthod. 2015;37(2):209–18. https://doi.org/10.1093/ejo/cju040.
40. Parkin NA, Milner RS, Deery C, Tinsley D, Smith A-M, Germain P, et al. Periodontal health of palatally displaced canines treated with open or closed surgical technique: a multicenter, randomized controlled trial. Am J Orthod Dentofac Orthop. 2013;144(2):176–84. https://doi.org/10.1016/j.ajodo.2013.03.016.

41. Batista K, Thiruvenkatachari B, Harrison JE, O'Brien KD. Orthodontic treatment for prominent upper front teeth (Class II malocclusion) in children and adolescents. Cochrane Database Syst Rev. 2018;3:CD003452. https://doi.org/10.1002/14651858.CD003452.pub4.
42. Yassir YA, El-Angbawi AM, McIntyre GT, Revie GF, Bearn DR. A randomized clinical trial of the effectiveness of 0.018-inch and 0.022-inch slot orthodontic bracket systems: Part 1—duration of treatment. Eur J Orthod. 2019;41(2):133–42. https://doi.org/10.1093/ejo/cjy037.
43. Al-Moghrabi D, Johal A, O'Rourke N, Donos N, Pandis N, Gonzales-Marin C, et al. Effects of fixed vs removable orthodontic retainers on stability and periodontal health: 4-year follow-up of a randomized controlled trial. Am J Orthod Dentofac Orthop. 2018;154(2):167–74 e1. https://doi.org/10.1016/j.ajodo.2018.01.007.
44. Parkin NA, Deery C, Smith AM, Tinsley D, Sandler J, Benson PE. No difference in surgical outcomes between open and closed exposure of palatally displaced maxillary canines. J Oral Maxillofac Surg. 2012;70(9):2026–34. https://doi.org/10.1016/j.joms.2012.02.028.
45. Sackett DL, Rosenberg WMC, Gray JAM, Haynes RB, Richardson WS. Evidence based medicine: what it is and what it isn't. BMJ. 1996;312(7023):71–2. https://doi.org/10.1136/bmj.312.7023.71.
46. Fleming PS, Koletsi D, O'Brien K, Tsichlaki A, Pandis N. Are dental researchers asking patient-important questions? A scoping review. J Dent. 2016;49:9–13. https://doi.org/10.1016/j.jdent.2016.04.002.
47. Tsichlaki A, O'brien K. Do orthodontic research outcomes reflect patient values? A systematic review of randomized controlled trials involving children. Am J Orthod Dentofac Orthop. 2014;146(3):279–85.
48. Tsichlaki A, Chin SY, Pandis N, Fleming PS. How long does treatment with fixed orthodontic appliances last? A systematic review. Am J Orthod Dentofac Orthop. 2016;149(3):308–18. https://doi.org/10.1016/j.ajodo.2015.09.020.
49. Abed Al Jawad F, Cunningham SJ, Croft N, Johal A. A qualitative study of the early effects of fixed orthodontic treatment on dietary intake and behaviour in adolescent patients. Eur J Orthod. 2011;34(4):432–6. https://doi.org/10.1093/ejo/cjr032.
50. Al-Moghrabi D, Colonio Salazar FB, Johal A, Fleming PS. Factors influencing adherence to vacuum-formed retainer wear: a qualitative study. J Orthod. 2019;46(3):212–9.
51. El-Huni A, Salazar FBC, Sharma PK, Fleming PS. Understanding factors influencing compliance with removable functional appliances: a qualitative study. Am J Orthod Dentofac Orthop. 2019;155(2):173–81.
52. Koletsi D, Fleming PS, Eliades T, Pandis N. The evidence from systematic reviews and meta-analyses published in orthodontic literature. Where do we stand? Eur J Orthod. 2015;37(6):603–9. https://doi.org/10.1093/ejo/cju087.
53. Williamson P, Altman D, Blazeby J, Clarke M, Gargon E. Driving up the quality and relevance of research through the use of agreed core outcomes. J Health Serv Res Policy. 2012;17(1):1–2. https://doi.org/10.1258/jhsrp.2011.011131.
54. Al-Moghrabi D, Tsichlaki A, Pandis N, Fleming P. Collaboration in orthodontic clinical trials: prevalence and association with sample size and funding. Prog Orthod. 2018;19(1):1–7. https://doi.org/10.1186/s40510-018-0215-3.
55. Unverzagt S, Prondzinsky R, Peinemann F. Single-center trials tend to provide larger treatment effects than multicenter trials: a systematic review. J Clin Epidemiol. 2013;66(11):1271–80. https://doi.org/10.1016/j.jclinepi.2013.05.016.
56. Schäfer K, Ludwig B, Meyer-Gutknecht H, Schott TC. Quantifying patient adherence during active orthodontic treatment with removable appliances using microelectronic wear-time documentation. Eur J Orthod. 2015;37(1):73–80. https://doi.org/10.1093/ejo/cju012.
57. Read MJ, Deacon S, O'Brien K. A prospective cohort study of a clip-on fixed functional appliance. Am J Orthod Dentofac Orthop. 2004;125(4):444–9.
58. Kokich VG. Consider joining the orthodontic practice-based research network. Am J Orthod Dentofac Orthop. 2013;144(3):323. https://doi.org/10.1016/j.ajodo.2013.07.002.
59. Huang G, Baltuck C, Funkhouser E, Wang H-F, Todoki L, Finkleman S, et al. The National Dental Practice-Based Research Network Adult Anterior Open Bite Study: treatment recommendations and their association with patient and practitioner characteristics. Am J Orthod Dentofac Orthop. 2019;156(3):312–25. https://doi.org/10.1016/j.ajodo.2019.05.005.
60. Tsichlaki A, O'Brien K, Johal A, Fleming PS. Orthodontic trial outcomes: plentiful, inconsistent, and in need of uniformity? A scoping review. Am J Orthod Dentofac Orthop. 2018;153(6):797–807. https://doi.org/10.1016/j.ajodo.2017.10.022.
61. Edman Tynelius G, Petrén S, Bondemark L, Lilja-Karlander E. Five-year postretention outcomes of three retention methods—a randomized controlled trial. Eur J Orthod. 2014;37(4):345–53. https://doi.org/10.1093/ejo/cju063.
62. O'Rourke N, Albeedh H, Sharma P, Johal A. Effectiveness of bonded and vacuum-formed retainers: a prospective randomized controlled clinical trial. Am J Orthod Dentofac Orthop. 2016;150(3):406–15. https://doi.org/10.1016/j.ajodo.2016.03.020.
63. Koletsi D, Pandis N, Polychronopoulou A, Eliades T. Does published orthodontic research account for clustering effects during statistical data analysis? Eur J Orthod. 2012;34(3):287–92. https://doi.org/10.1093/ejo/cjr122.
64. Kerry SM, Bland JM. Statistics notes: sample size in cluster randomisation. BMJ. 1998;316(7130):549. https://doi.org/10.1136/bmj.316.7130.549.
65. Campbell MK, Elbourne DR, Altman DG. CONSORT statement: extension to cluster randomised trials. BMJ.

2004;328(7441):702–8. https://doi.org/10.1136/bmj.e5661.
66. Bland JM, Altman DG. Comparisons against baseline within randomised groups are often used and can be highly misleading. Trials. 2011;12(1):264. https://doi.org/10.1186/1745-6215-12-264.
67. Gratsia S, Koletsi D, Fleming PS, Pandis N. Statistical testing against baseline in orthodontic research: a meta-epidemiologic study. Eur J Orthod. 2019;41(2):165–71. https://doi.org/10.1093/ejo/cjy029.
68. Koletsi D, Pandis N, Fleming PS. Sample size in orthodontic randomized controlled trials: are numbers justified? Eur J Orthod. 2014;36(1):67–73. https://doi.org/10.1093/ejo/cjt005.
69. Clemmer EJ, Hayes EW. Patient cooperation in wearing orthodontic headgear. Am J Orthod. 1979;75(5):517–24. https://doi.org/10.1016/0002-9416(79)90070-8.
70. Bartsch A, Witt E, Sahm G, Schneider S. Correlates of objective patient compliance with removable appliance wear. Am J Orthod Dentofac Orthop. 1993;104(4):378–86. https://doi.org/10.1016/S0889-5406(05)81337-X.
71. Wertz RT. Intention to treat: once randomized, always analyzed. Clin Aphasiol. 1995;23:57–64.
72. Sterne JAC, White IR, Carlin JB, Spratt M, Royston P, Kenward MG, et al. Multiple imputation for missing data in epidemiological and clinical research: potential and pitfalls. BMJ. 2009;338:b2393. https://doi.org/10.1136/bmj.b2393.
73. O'Cathain A, Thomas K, Drabble S, Rudolph A, Hewison J. What can qualitative research do for randomised controlled trials? A systematic mapping review. BMJ Open. 2013;3(6):e002889.
74. Al-Moghrabi D, Tsichlaki A, Alkadi S, Fleming PS. How well are dental qualitative studies involving interviews and focus groups reported? J Dent. 2019;84:44–8. https://doi.org/10.1016/j.jdent.2019.03.001.
75. Brett J, Staniszewska S, Mockford C, Herron-Marx S, Hughes J, Tysall C, et al. Mapping the impact of patient and public involvement on health and social care research: a systematic review. Health Expect. 2014;17(5):637–50. https://doi.org/10.1111/j.1369-7625.2012.00795.x.
76. Sacristán JA, Aguarón A, Avendaño-Solá C, Garrido P, Carrión J, Gutiérrez A, et al. Patient involvement in clinical research: why, when, and how. Patient Prefer Adher. 2016;10:631. https://doi.org/10.2147/PPA.S104259.
77. Brett J, Staniszewska S, Mockford C, Herron-Marx S, Hughes J, Tysall C, et al. A systematic review of the impact of patient and public involvement on service users, researchers and communities. Patient. 2014;7(4):387–95. https://doi.org/10.1007/s40271-014-0065-0.
78. Trivedi P, Wykes T. From passive subjects to equal partners: qualitative review of user involvement in research. Br J Psychiatry. 2002;181(6):468–72. https://doi.org/10.1192/bjp.181.6.468.
79. Schroter S, Price A, Malički M, Richards T, Clarke M. Frequency and format of clinical trial results dissemination to patients: a survey of authors of trials indexed in PubMed. BMJ Open. 2019;9(10):e032701. https://doi.org/10.1136/bmjopen-2019-032701.
80. Boivin A, Richards T, Forsythe L, Grégoire A, L'Espérance A, Abelson J, et al. Evaluating patient and public involvement in research. BMJ. 2018;363:k5147. https://doi.org/10.1136/bmj.k5147.
81. Glasziou P, Altman DG, Bossuyt P, Boutron I, Clarke M, Julious S, et al. Reducing waste from incomplete or unusable reports of biomedical research. Lancet. 2014;383(9913):267–76. https://doi.org/10.1016/S0140-6736(13)62228-X.
82. Pandis N, Fleming PS, Hopewell S, Altman DG. The CONSORT statement: application within and adaptations for orthodontic trials. Am J Orthod Dentofac Orthop. 2015;147(6):663–79. https://doi.org/10.1016/j.ajodo.2015.03.014.
83. Lempesi E, Koletsi D, Fleming PS, Pandis N. The reporting quality of randomized controlled trials in orthodontics. J Evid Based Dental Pract. 2014;14(2):46–52. https://doi.org/10.1016/j.jebdp.2013.12.001.
84. Koletsi D, Fleming PS, Behrents RG, Lynch CD, Pandis N. The use of tailored subheadings was successful in enhancing compliance with CONSORT in a dental journal. J Dent. 2017;67:66–71. https://doi.org/10.1016/j.jdent.2017.09.009.
85. Al-Kurwi AS, Bos A, Kuitert RB. Overjet reduction in relation to wear time with the van Beek activator combined with a microsensor. Am J Orthod Dentofac Orthop. 2017;151(2):277–83. https://doi.org/10.1016/j.ajodo.2016.06.046.
86. Al-Moghrabi D, Salazar FC, Pandis N, Fleming PS. Compliance with removable orthodontic appliances and adjuncts: a systematic review and meta-analysis. Am J Orthod Dentofac Orthop. 2017;152(1):17–32. https://doi.org/10.1016/j.ajodo.2017.03.019.
87. Fleming PS, Scott P, DiBiase AT. Compliance: getting the most from your orthodontic patients. Dent Update. 2007;34(9):565–72.
88. Chan A-W, Song F, Vickers A, Jefferson T, Dickersin K, Gøtzsche PC, et al. Increasing value and reducing waste: addressing inaccessible research. Lancet. 2014;383(9913):257–66. https://doi.org/10.1016/S0140-6736(13)62296-5.
89. Naudet F, Sakarovitch C, Janiaud P, Cristea I, Fanelli D, Moher D, et al. Data sharing and reanalysis of randomized controlled trials in leading biomedical journals with a full data sharing policy: survey of studies published in the BMJ and PLOS medicine. BMJ. 2018;360:k400. https://doi.org/10.1136/bmj.k400.
90. Loder E, Groves T. The BMJ requires data sharing on request for all trials. BMJ. 2015;350:h2373. https://doi.org/10.1136/bmj.h2373.

Randomized Controlled Trials in Pediatric Dentistry

8

Chloe Meng Jiang, Gillian Hiu Man Lee, Chun Hung Chu, Edward Chin Man Lo, and May Chun Mei Wong

As approved and adopted by the National Commission on Recognition of Dental Specialties and Certifying Boards (NCRDSCB) of the American Dental Association, pediatric dentistry is one of dental specialties. It is recognized as "an age-defined specialty that provides both primary and comprehensive preventive and therapeutic oral health care for infants and children through adolescence, including those with special health care needs" [1].

Based on the findings of a bibliometric analysis of top-cited RCTs in pediatric dentistry, the majority of RCTs conducted in children and adolescents were in the discipline of cariology, followed by orthodontics, endodontics, behavior science and quality of life, oral and maxillofacial surgery, and oral hygiene [2]. In the discipline of cariology, fluoride agents used to prevent and/or arrest dental caries were the most frequently studied intervention in RCTs [3–5]. Dental restorations placed with different dental materials or techniques were compared in several RCTs [6–8]. There were several RCTs reporting on probiotic bacterium as food supplements [9, 10], and chewing gums with different ingredients to prevent dental caries [11, 12]. Besides, fissure sealant [13], toothpaste [14], motivational interviewing [15], and oral health education [16] were also investigated in RCTs in pediatric dentistry. In terms of orthodontics, most of the RCTs reported on the effect of using different appliances, for example, Bionator, Herbst, and Twin-block appliances, in orthodontic treatments [17, 18]. The effectiveness of adopting different pulpotomy techniques, such as using Er:YAG laser, calcium hydroxide, formocresol or mineral trioxide aggregate (MTA), to treat primary teeth was the most frequently studied research question in the discipline of endodontics [19]. In terms of behavior science and quality of life, RCTs were conducted to evaluate medicines (e.g., acetaminophen and ibuprofen) for pain control associated with dental procedures [20] and to compare the efficacy and safety of different drugs, like dexmedetomidine, midazolam, and ketamine in producing moderate sedation for uncooperative pediatric dental patients [21]. In addition, children's oral health-related quality of life

C. M. Jiang · E. C. M. Lo · M. C. M. Wong (✉)
Applied Oral Sciences and Community Dental Care, Faculty of Dentistry, The University of Hong Kong, Pokfulam, Hong Kong SAR, China
e-mail: cmjiang@hku.hk; hrdplcm@hku.hk; mcmwong@hku.hk

G. H. M. Lee
Paediatric Dentistry and Orthodontics, Faculty of Dentistry, The University of Hong Kong, Pokulam, Hong Kong SAR, China
e-mail: ghmlee@hku.hk

C. H. Chu
Restorative Dental Sciences, Faculty of Dentistry, The University of Hong Kong, Pokfulam, Hong Kong SAR, China
e-mail: chchu@hku.hk

R. Kohli et al. (eds.), *Randomized Controlled Trials in Evidence-Based Dentistry*,
https://doi.org/10.1007/978-3-031-47651-8_8

Table 8.1 Summary of the more commonly researched topics in the RCTs in pediatric dentistry and examples of the knowledge gaps

Thematic field	Intervention	Examples of knowledge gaps
Cariology	• Fluoride • Restoration • Probiotic bacterium • Chewing gum • Fissure sealant • Toothpaste • Motivational interviewing • Oral health education • Hall technique, nonrestorative • Casein phosphopeptide amorphous calcium phosphate (CPP-ACP)	• Clinical outcomes of treating primary molar teeth using preformed metal crowns (PMCs) vs. restorations with filling materials • Effectiveness of preventive and treatment methods in primary teeth of young children
Orthodontics	• Appliances • Force	• Efficacy of using clear aligners vs. fixed appliances
Endodontics	Pulpotomy	
Behavior science and quality of life	Use of medicine/drugs	• Effectiveness of sedation vs. general anesthesia for the provision of dental treatment for children
Oral and maxillofacial surgery	Surgery methods	
Oral hygiene	Oral health education	

(OHRQoL) and dental fear were also investigated in RCTs [22]. In the discipline of oral and maxillofacial surgery, most of the RCTs in pediatric patients focused on the orthopedics for children with cleft lip and palate [23, 24]. Apart from traditional oral health education methods which are mainly to provide lessons and to distribute brochures for participants to promote good oral hygiene practice, an innovative app-based approach which made participants actively involved in oral hygiene maintenance has also been evaluated in a recent RCT [25].

The interventions involved in RCTs in pediatric dentistry are frequently related to the prevention and control of dental diseases, such as dental caries prevention and oral health promotion. In addition to recruiting pediatric patients directly from dental clinic/hospitals, the pediatric population in the RCTs are commonly accessed from kindergartens, schools, and communities. Sometimes, various interventions, for example, fluoride application, fissure sealant, and milk containing probiotic bacterium, are delivered on a community basis. Dental public health is a specialty recognized by the NCRDSCB and is defined as "the science and art of preventing and controlling dental diseases and promoting dental health through organized community efforts on a community basis" [1]. It is difficult to completely separate RCTs in pediatric dentistry per se from dental public health. In fact, the RCTs investigating oral health-related issues of children and adolescents are frequently involved in both specialties where the crossover is inevitable.

It may be fair to say that a wide range of topics has been covered in RCTs in pediatric dentistry (Table 8.1). Nevertheless, a considerable number of knowledge gaps exist in various areas that are not well investigated, and well-conducted high-quality RCTs are insufficient in pediatric dentistry [26]. For example, the number of RCTs on the prevention and treatment of dental caries in the primary teeth is small and it is important to find out if the agents and methods that have been shown to be effective in the permanent teeth of school children are also effective in preschool children. It should be noted that the enamel of primary teeth is much thinner than that of permanent teeth, and it is much faster for the carious lesions in primary teeth to develop into cavities. On the one hand, due to the lack of RCTs in the literature, answers to many clinical questions remain unclear. For example, clinical outcomes of treating primary molar teeth using preformed metal crowns (PMCs) vs. restorations with filling materials, and effectiveness of sedation vs. gen-

Table 8.2 Important considerations in conducting and reporting RCTs

	Brief explanation
Intervention	Sufficient details of the study interventions as well as the control intervention should be described thoroughly
Sample size	Specified sample size calculation should be stated with sufficient details on all the essential elements
Randomization and allocation concealment	Generation of randomization allocation sequence should be provided together with how the randomization sequence is implemented with allocation concealment
Blinding	Adequate information on how the blinding is achieved in the trial should be stated comprehensively, even though no blinding or incomplete blinding is inevitable in some cases
Incomplete data	The amount and nature of the incomplete outcome data and how they are handled in the trial should be reported thoroughly
Statistical analysis	Proper statistical approach should be adopted. A general description of the data and the specified statistical method used should be clearly reported

eral anesthesia for the provision of dental treatment for pediatric patients, are some of the knowledge gaps that need to be filled based on reliable clinical evidence. On the other hand, sometimes the quality of existing RCTs in the literature is suboptimal, which weakens the reliability of the evidence provided by the trials.

There are important considerations in conducting and reporting RCTs (Table 8.2). A standardized reporting method, the Consolidated Standards for Reporting Trials (CONSORT), facilitates authors to completely and transparently report their RCTs and aids their critical appraisal and interpretation of the findings [26]. The CONSORT is widely endorsed by reputable medical/dental journals when evaluating submitted manuscripts on RCTs. Following the CONSORT, the published article provides comprehensive and detailed information of the RCT, so that readers can make their judgements about the reliability of the evidence provided by the trial. Even though authors claimed that they followed the CONSORT strictly, some major deviations from the CONSORT still exist in the published RCTs in pediatric dentistry.

8.1 Intervention

Sufficient details of interventions should be described thoroughly in the study so that other researchers who want to replicate the study can know exactly the way to deliver the intervention. For materials used in the trial, information including the name, brand (if commercial products), and usage should be provided. Similarly, for drug intervention, the name of the drug, dose, method of administration (such as oral and intravenous), timing, and duration of administration should be clearly described [26]. In terms of clinical procedures, implementation details such as specific step-by-step procedures and instruments used should be given. Besides, control interventions should be described thoroughly instead of using vague words like "usual care."

Two examples are illustrated below with the first example describing the step-by-step procedures of the interventions and the products used in each study group with sufficient information, for example, full name, brand, and instruction, for replication. The second example shows a lack of information on the products used (gray/white MTA and formocresol), makes it difficult for other researchers to replicate the study.

Example 1

Dilute formocresol (1:5 Buckley's solution), Erbium:Yttrium-Aluminum Garnet (Er:YAG) laser, calcium hydroxide, and ferric sulfate (15.5%) were used as parallel intervention methods. In all groups, after rubber dam isolation and caries removal, the pulp chamber was opened with a sterile high-speed diamond bur, and the coronal pulp was removed by a sterile slow-speed round bur (#830RL016, #H1SE.204021, Brasseler, Lemgo, Germany) under continuous water irrigation. Control of complete removal of the coronal pulp tissue down to the canal orifices was done by visual control and a sterile hand excavator in undercut areas. We controlled hemorrhage by placing sterile, saline wetted cotton wool pellets on the radicular pulp stumps under slight pressure (Thompson et al. 2001), waiting 5 min for primary hemostasis (Mielke et al. 1969), followed by removal of blood clot remnants and drying the cavity…Within the control group, formocresol-moistened pellets were placed on the pulp stumps for 5 min. Er:YAG laser radiation (wavelength, 2.94 μm) was delivered to the canal orifices with a special handpiece (KEY Laser 1242; handpiece 2051, KaVo, Biberach, Germany), with parameters set at 2 Hz and 180 mJ/pulse without water cooling (Keller and Hibst 1991). The mean number of laser pulses per tooth was 31.5 ± 5.9, equally distributed to each pulp stump. In the calcium hydroxide group, the canal orifices were dressed with aqueous calcium hydroxide (Calxyl®, OCO Präparate GmbH, Dirmstein, Germany), slightly dampened and covered with a calcium hydroxide cement (Kerr® Life, Kerr GmbH, Karlsruhe, Germany). Ferric-sulfate-wetted pellets (Astringedent®, Ultradent Products Inc., Salt Lake City, UT, USA) were placed on the pulp stumps for 15 s [19].

Example 2

…In test groups I and II, the pulp stumps were covered with gray or white MTA paste formed by mixing the MTA powder with sterile saline in a 3:1 powder/saline ratio, according to the manufacturer recommendations. In test group III, a cotton pellet moistened with formocresol was placed for 5 min on the pulp stumps and then the pulps were covered with zinc oxide and eugenol cement [27].

8.2 Sample Size Determination

The sample size of an RCT should be clearly stated and carefully estimated before the implementation of the trial for scientific and ethical reasons. On the one hand, an underpowered trial with insufficient sample size may fail to detect a clinical difference statistically. Thus, indeterminate results are generated and no reliable conclusion can be drawn. On the other hand, even though a trial with excess sample size has the power of detecting small difference statistically, it is perhaps unnecessary and a waste of resources. The essential elements to be considered when estimating sample size of an RCT are: (1) the effect size, which is determined by the "clinically important difference" to be tested in a study; (2) the α (type I) error level, usually set at 0.05 in a two-sided test; (3) the statistical power, namely the 1-β (type II) error level, usually set at 0.80 or 0.90 and (4) for continuous outcomes, an estimation of the standard deviation of the measurements [28]. Equal numbers in the two study groups (allocation ratio of 1:1) usually result in a given total sample size with maximum power; however, this is not always possible and practical. In some clinical trials, unequal group sizes may be adopted. If the number of study participants receiving one intervention is limited, then more participants will be needed in the other study group so as to achieve the statistical power to detect the anticipated difference [28].

In reporting sample size calculation, the primary outcome on which the calculation was based, and the values of the essential elements set in the calculation should be explicitly stated, and the resulting required sample size per study group should be reported [26]. Besides, possible attrition or non-compliance during the study should be considered in the sample size calculation as well [29].

Four examples are given below. The first example states clearly the primary outcome (caries arrested rate of 70%), and the determination of sample size is presented thoroughly with the essential elements: effect size (absolute difference of 10%), significance level ($\alpha = 5\%$), statistical power ($\beta = 80\%$), and an anticipated attrition rate of 10% annually. The second example illustrates apart from the essential elements in sample size calculation, namely effect size (0.7), significance level ($\alpha = 0.05$), statistical power ($\beta = 80\%$), an estimation of the standard deviation of the measurement (2), and an anticipated attrition rate (30–35%), the clustering effect of communities and an allocation ratio of 2:1 to include more communities in the experimental group than the control group had been taken into account to adjust the calculation. The third example states only the essential elements with ambiguous reporting for the adjustment of the clustering effect. In the last example, the effect size and other related details are not explicitly stated.

Example 1

The sample size was estimated based on a caries arrest rate of 70% (Chu et al., 2002), a 10% absolute difference in caries arrest rate being clinically significant, a statistical power of 80% ($\beta = 0.2$) and a statistical significance level of 5% ($\alpha = 0.05$). Calculation results showed that 360 carious tooth surfaces per group were required. Since the mean number of carious tooth surfaces in Hong Kong preschool children was four (Chu et al., 2012), approximately 90 children would be required in each group. With an anticipated 10% annual drop-out rate, over 300 children were recruited at baseline [5].

Example 2

The calculation of the sample size was based on a mean dmft increment in the children in the SLZ receiving standard care plus caregiver counseling of 3.5 (Lawerence et al., 2004), a common SD of 2 and a hypothesized minimum 20% treatment effect (0.7 difference). Assuming approximately (mean cluster size) 40 eligible children per community, the sample size was increased by a factor of 2 to adjust for the clustering effect (1 + #children in community or average size of each cluster of 40-1 × small intra cluster correlation coefficient (ICC) of 0.025) (Donner and Klar, 2000). Thus, the number of communities required for randomization to obtain 80% power at $\alpha = 0.05$ (two-sample t-test, two-sided) for detecting a mean difference in dmft of 0.7 was 6.4 (or 256 subjects per group). In practice, at least eight communities were randomly assigned per intervention group to adjust for the anticipated 30–35% attrition in 2 years (Lawerence et al., 2004). As a result of an increase in funding, we were able to further increase the number of communities to be enrolled in the FV group using the formula $k^2 = 1/2k(1 + Q)$, where k = 8 clusters per group under equal allocation (Q = 1) and we selected an allocation ratio of 2 (Q = 2) which yielded 12 communities in the experimental group and eight communities in the control group (Donner and Klar, 2000) [4].

Example 3

Sample size calculation was based on the findings of Farooq et al. (2000) and accounted for a 19% difference in success rates between the test and control groups using a significance level of 5% and power of 80%. The dependence of observations within each child was also taken into consideration. A sample size of 46 teeth per group was calculated. Given an expected attrition rate of 20%, we estimated that 55 teeth had to be included in each group [8].

Example 4

...The sample size was estimated from a power calculation ($\alpha = 0.05$ and $\beta = 0.20$) based on our previous findings using categorized bacterial scores. ... [30].

8.3 Randomization and Allocation Concealment

Sufficient information on the generation of the randomization allocation sequence should be provided so that readers can make their own judgements about the possible bias in the group allocation (selection bias). Using a computer-generated random number table, tossing a coin, throwing dice, and drawing lots are common methods to generate randomization sequence in RCTs. However, the term "random" is sometimes misused to report trials in the literature. It is improper to describe random sequence generated by using odd or even number alternatively to assign the study participants to the test and control groups. Similarly, the use of hospital or clinic record number and date of birth as "randomization sequence" is inappropriate. Instead of using a vague expression such as "random allocation," "randomization," or "randomly allocated," the method used for the randomization sequence generation needs to be explicitly described.

Furthermore, the randomization allocation sequence should be implemented with allocation concealment. This technique is used to prevent selection bias by shielding investigators who assign participants to intervention groups from being influenced by the allocation sequence before the assignment [31]. Central allocation (such as telephone and web-based randomization systems), sequentially numbered opaque-sealed envelopes or containers are desirable methods to achievement allocation concealment. However, in many cases, the description of the concealment method is neglected or inadequate.

Three examples are given. The first example clearly reports the generation of randomization sequence and allocation concealment of the study in details. The second example shows that the randomization has been achieved by tossing a coin, whereas whether the allocation concealment has been achieved remains unclear. The term "distributed randomly" is ambiguously used in the last example without information on the allocation concealment.

Example 1

> The study team's biostatisticians conducted the computer-generated random assignment of participants, stratified by center, using permuted blocks of various sizes unknown to the clinicians. Assignment was concealed in sealed, opaque, labeled envelopes, unopened until time for treatment by the clinician [3].

Example 2

> ...The split-mouth approach was employed for the allocation of the two restorative materials. Intraoral assignment of the material to the teeth was done by toss of coin... [7].

Example 3

> ...The selected teeth were randomly assigned and divided into 3 test groups according to the pulp dressings used. Group I included 24 teeth treated with gray MTA. Group II included 24 teeth treated with white MTA. Group III included 24 teeth treated with formocresol (control group). The treatments were distributed randomly to each of 3 teeth so that each child would receive 3 different treatments [27].

8.4 Blinding of Participants and Personnel

Blinding or masking is important in RCTs to avoid performance bias due to the disclosure of information on allocated interventions to people, such as participants and investigators, who are involved in the trial and may potentially be influenced by such information. In fact, different from allocation concealment, complete blinding may not be achieved in all cases. An RCT was conducted to compare failure rates of Hall technique crowns and control restorations, in which blinding is impossible due to the apparent differences between the two interventions [32]. Adequate information on how the blinding is achieved in the trial should be stated comprehensively, even though no blinding or incomplete blinding is inevitable in some cases. Thus, readers can judge whether or not and to what extent, the study outcomes are possibly influenced by the blinding.

With the use of identical milk containers, blinding for participants and investigators have been achieved successfully in the first example shown below. In the second example, even though the examiners were not informed about the group allocation, blinding for the examiners could not be achieved as they could distinguish the study groups according to the different appearances of the materials. The use of the term "double-blind" in the last example is confusing. It seems like only the examiner who evaluated the outcomes of restorations was blinded.

Example 1

> The children drank either LGG milk (Gefilus®, Valio Ltd., Riihimäki Dairy, Finland; pasteurized cow's milk containing 1% fat and live Lactobacillus rhamnosus GG, ATCC 53103, bacteria 5–10E105 CFU/ml) or control milk in the day-care centres 5 days a week for 7 months, from non-transparent colour-coded milk containers. The control milk came from the same dairy but contained no added lactobacilli. ... The day-care personnel, parents, children and investigators were unaware of which milk contained the LGG strain throughout the study... [9].

Example 2

> Children were followed up for oral health status at School Dental Service clinics of the WA Dental Health Services (6–12 months after group allocation) by the same examiners who conducted the baseline examination, and who were blinded to group allocation status. Although the examiners were blind to group allocation status, because of the distinct characteristics of the restorative materials used, such as stainless-steel crowns, composite resin or GIC, blind assessment of the material was not possible in all [33].

Example 3

> The double-blind evaluations were undertaken in a dental unit using the standard operating light, a mirror, an explorer and a WHO periodontal probe by an independent examiner experienced in the ART approach. Parameters for evaluating the qual-

ity of the restorations were retention, marginal integrity and wear according to the recommended codes used for evaluating ART restorations [34].

8.5 Incomplete Outcome Data

Attrition bias may arise due to incomplete (missing) data of RCTs. Authors should clarify the amount and nature of the incomplete outcome data and how they were handled in the trial so that the possible attrition bias can be assessed. Reasons for missing data in the study groups should be explained. As recommended by CONSORT, a diagram to describe the flow of participants through a trial is preferable [26]. With sufficient information, readers can evaluate whether the missing data are likely due to the intervention or dropouts due to other reasons, and also whether the missing data are balanced in numbers between the study groups in the trial. In fact, missing data may be imputed with various methods [35], and the details in data imputation should be reported.

In the first example shown below, the dropout rate of the trial is acceptable with less than 20% at the 30-month follow-up. The dropout rate of each study group is clearly reported and the missing data are balanced between the study groups. The amount of missing data is explicitly reported in the second example, together with the data imputation method adopted in the study described in detail. The last example shows a very high attrition rate (>50%) but the details of the missing data are not reported. Readers are not able to evaluate the attrition bias of this study based on the limited information provided.

Example 1

At the 30-month examination, 309 children remained in the study, giving an overall dropout rate of 17%. The subject dropout rates in Groups 1, 2 and 3 were 19%, 16% and 15%, respectively (χ^2 test, $p > 0.05$). There were no significant differences between the three groups of children regarding their demographic background, behaviors, clinical parameters and caries experience at the baseline and at the 30-month examinations… [5].

Example 2

Since 96 children had no follow-up examination, multiple imputation (Schafer, 1997) with the Markov Chain Monte Carlo estimation (20 imputations) used center, assigned group, number of actual fluoride varnish applications, factors related to loss-to-follow-up (mother's age, dental pain barrier, dental fear barrier, and fluoride toothpaste use), and salivary measures (log10MS and log10LB) to impute log (d2 + fs + 1) scores [3].

Example 3

…Using a parallel group design, 370 and 311 grade 2 children were randomly assigned to the ART and the TA group respectively…. A total of 108 children of the ART group and 84 children of the TA group were examined at evaluation year 6.3… [36].

8.6 Statistical Analysis

Data can be analyzed in various ways; thus, authors should specify the statistical approaches adopted in the study. Generally, a description of the data should be provided in detail. Accordingly, readers can have sufficient information on the characteristics of the data and make judgements about the validity of the further statistical approaches. To arrive at a conclusion supported by valid results, a proper statistical approach should be chosen according to the characteristics of the data. A common mistake in the data analysis of RCTs in pediatric dentistry is the neglect of the clustering effect, which indicates a potential correlation between observations. For many statistical analyses, the observations (unit of analysis) are required to be independent of each other. However, in many cases, observations are not independent, for example, multiple restorations placed in the same child. Appropriate statistical procedures should be employed to analyze the clustered observations. Ignoring the clustering effect and analyzing multiple correlated observations as an independent sample would lead to serious errors and invalid conclusions.

The intention-to-treat (ITT) approach is adopted in the first example shown below. Besides, the primary and further statistical analyses used in the study are reported with sufficient details. In the second example, fundamental statistical analyses methods are described, the clustering effect was taken into account by employing a multilevel logistic regression analysis and the formula to calculate the intracluster correlation coefficient (ICC) is clearly presented. In the last example, the statistical analysis unit (tooth) is not completely independent. As a child could have more than one tooth included in the trial, the clustering effect of the child should not be neglected. Fisher's exact test was inappropriately used without any further statistical analysis adjusting for the possible clustering effect.

Example 1

For primary analysis, we used the intention-to-treat (ITT) approach (Fisher et al., 1990). … Primary analysis tested two-year caries incidence among treatment groups, with a two-degree-of-freedom (d.f.) non-parametric extended Mantel-Haenszel (EMH) test stratifying on center (Koch and Edwards, 1988). A priori step-down comparisons (Koch and Gansky, 1996) of each varnish group vs. control were performed, each at $p \leq 0.05$: (1) 4FV vs. 0FV and (2) 2FV vs. 0FV; step (2) was performed only if step (1) was significant. A 1 d.f. EMH test, stratifying on center, tested trends across intended and actual number of applications. Logistic regression tested treatment group differences in incidence, with adjustment for covariates and treatment × center homogeneity. Supplemental analyses used linear regression to compare log (d2 + fs + 1) and log (d1 + fs + 1) among groups, adjusted for covariates (since dn+fs is skewed)... [3].

Example 2

Continuous data were analyzed by analysis of variance (ANOVA) and categorical data with 2 test, using the SPSS (version 16.0, SPSS, Inc., Chicago, Ill., USA). Bacterial counts were log-transformed before processing. Because of the clustered design, the outcomes in caries and general health were analyzed with age as covariate in a multilevel logistic regression using the software STATA (version 10.0, StataCorp, College Station, Tex., USA). The intra cluster correlation coefficient (ICC) (Killip et al., 2004), which reflects the homogeneity of the sample, was calculated using long one-way ANOVA with the software STATA. ICC is expressed as [(MSB − MSW)/(MSB + (m − 1) MSW)], MSB being the mean square between clusters, MSW the mean square within clusters and m the (average) size of the clusters. The level of significance was set at 5% ($p < 0.05$) [10].

Example 3

Sixteen children received only one restoration, while 17 children had two or more teeth restored. …The overall success rates (95% confidence interval [95% CI]) at the six-month follow- up for the GCP Glass Fill and Equia Fil were 69 percent (95% CI equals 51–83) and 83% (95% equals 66–93), respectively. No significant difference was detected between the study groups (Fisher's exact test, P = 0.20). However, at 12 months, the overall success rates of both materials were 56% (95% CI equals 37–73) for GCP Glass Fill and 86% (95% CI equals 69–94) for Equia Fil. This difference was statistically significant (Fisher's exact test, P = 0.03)... [37].

8.7 Other Considerations

8.7.1 Single-Center vs. Multiple-Center Trials

Many RCTs in the literature are single-center trials with small sample sizes, which may have insufficient statistical power in detecting the anticipated difference and lead to inconclusive results. Compared with single-center trials, multiple-center trials have several advantages [38, 39]. First, multiple-center trials have more heterogenous study participants which are recruited from more than one center/clinics located in different geographic regions. This strengthens the generalizability (external validity) of the research findings and augments the potential for subgroup analyses. Second, it is easier to achieve a sufficient sample size from multiple centers instead of a single one, especially for a RCT on a rare disease/condition. Third, multiple centers increase the rate of participant enrollment of the trial so that the attainment of the required sample size can be achieved in a relatively short period of time. However, it should be noted that multiple-center trials may be more complex and challenging to be conducted. Several considerations should be taken into account carefully, for example, to maintain the internal validity of the trial and to sustain commitment and collaboration with multiple centers. Besides, for research data obtained from multiple centers, proper statistical analysis approaches should be adopted to deal with the possible center effect within multiple-center trials [40].

8.7.2 Access to Pediatric Population

Participants for pediatric dental research are usually recruited from university-affiliated dental teaching hospitals, government dental clinics or hospitals, private dental clinics, schools or child daycare centers in the community. Schools and child daycare centers are the most common study sites for pediatric dental RCTs as many of them are public health related. Children go to school daily, and younger children may attend child daycare centers. Researchers can recruit children of the target age group for their study from the schools and daycare centers easily. Moreover, schools and daycare centers cover a population from a broad range of sociodemographic background. When participants are recruited from several schools with wide sociodemographic background, the recruited sample will provide good generalizability for RCTs that study the effects of public health interventions such as dental caries prevention measures [2, 4, 8] and oral health promotion [15].

RCTs that study the outcomes of dental treatments or materials usually recruit their participants from dental teaching hospitals or dental clinics [18, 31, 36]. Patients who attend the clinics usually present with a problem in oral health. The clinical settings provide good access to the population for the studies. Interventions can be provided in a proper clinical setting as well. It should be noted that the dental health care system of different geographic regions may influence how the recruitment centers are selected for research studies. For example, in Hong Kong, there is no dental insurance and government support for young children to visit dentists regularly. It is uncommon for children to attend a private dental clinic. Recruitment of children from private or government dental clinics are, therefore, impossible. However, RCTs conducted in Australia, UK, USA, or Europe often recruit child participants from different dental clinics [16, 17].

8.7.3 Equipoise

The key features of RCTs are the study participants randomly assigned either to the new intervention (test group, a novel but unproven treatment) or the control group. The controls can be concurrent controls in parallel studies or self-controls in crossover studies and the treatment received in the control group can be placebo or standard-of-care treatment [40]. The principle of equipoise comes into consideration to determine whether the control group should be placebo or standard-of-care. Even though the use of placebo control with no active treatment may be appealing, the rationale in adopting such control needs to be strongly justified. The (clinical) equipoise principle is an ethical requirement in conducting RCTs. There should be an equal uncertainty of the relative effectiveness of the study groups (either test or control treatment) before the start of the trial, and no study participants should receive a known inferior treatment [41, 42]. "The trial must be designed in a way that aims to resolve this uncertainty and bring consensus" [42]. In circumstances where a standard-of-care treatment exists, the control group should receive the standard-of-care instead of placebo.

8.7.4 Informed Consent and Assent

Obtaining informed consent is an important process in conducting a clinical trial. Participants should receive relevant and adequate information on the clinical trial in the form of an information sheet to allow them to make an informed decision about participation in the trial. In most cases, written consent should be obtained by asking the participants to sign on a consent form. According to the International Council for Harmonization of Technical Requirements for Pharmaceuticals for Human Use (ICH), child participants in a pediatric clinical trial are legally not able to provide informed consent. Therefore, informed consent from their parent(s) or guardian needs to be obtained to grant permission for their child to participate in the trial to protect the rights of the pediatric study participants (E11 ICH) [43].

In order to compensate the time and inconvenience that may have been occurred by the participation in research or simply to offer an incentive to encourage participation, monetary compensation may be given to parents for their children's participation in clinical trials [44]. Careful considerations about the amount and timing for providing such compensation are needed to avoid some parents being enticed to give consent for their children's participation against the children's best interest and the children are being coerced to participate [45]. Therefore, children should be approached whenever appropriate and have an opportunity to assess their willingness and give assent to participate in a trial to minimize the possible coercion in participation. However, such practice is not commonly reported in the literature on pediatric dentistry RCTs.

Assent has been defined as "a relational process whereby children's actions and adult responses taken together, reflect children's participation decisions" [44]. In order to seek the informed assent, age-appropriate and easy to understand information about the clinical trial should be given to the child participants to help them to decide if they want to take part in the trial [45]. It is not an easy process and researchers are encouraged to work together with the children to develop effective means of obtaining children's assent [44, 46–48]. Ford and coworkers involved children aged 6 and 12 years and collated the words that children can understand for the construction of information sheet and assent form [46]. Kumpunen and coworkers developed a storyboard and a word search approach for children aged 4–12 years [47].

8.7.5 Minimizing Distress and Non-cooperation

For daily oral health care, if children are uncooperative and refuse a necessary treatment, the dentists and their parents will try to find alternative treatment approaches, for example, a different form of drugs, non-surgical approaches, or non-invasive approaches. However, in RCTs, children who are randomly allocated to a particular study group cannot choose alternatives based on their own preferences. Despite this, it is not ethical to force the children to receive the intervention that they refuse. Thus, in most cases, non-cooperation is a criterion to exclude participant children from the trial. When children are unable to cooperate and complete the planned examination or intervention, they would be excluded from the trial. Investigators are encouraged to obtain good cooperation from participating children. Practical considerations should be exercised to ensure that the participants' experiences in the trial are positive, and efforts should be made to minimize discomfort and distress [43]. For example, in order to give a pleasant impression to the school children and encourage their participation in a clinical trial, Ly and coworkers have made use of a skit with an oral health message to be presented to the children during a school assembly to introduce the research team [49].

On the other hand, in gaining the children's cooperation during the clinical examination or sample collection for the research study, some common behavior management techniques such as tell-show-do, reinforcement, assimilation, and modelling can be practiced. Tell-show-do can help children understand what they will experience; reinforcement can encourage the children, build up trust, and rapport from them. For clinical trial under the school setting, modelling with schoolmates can set a good way for anxious children. Assimilation can help children adapt to the dental environment step-by-step. For example, instead of restoring caries cavities at the first dental visit, investigators of a trial used a two-stage approach to conducted interventions for the study children who were at a very young age [50]. In this RCT, only dental examinations and applications of fluoride agent were conducted at the first dental visit. These quick and painless procedures made the children feel less frightened about seeing a dentist and receiving dental treatments. This helped to gain trust from these young children, which made them less resistant to the restorative procedures at the second dental visit. This two-stage approach helped the children become more cooperative during the whole study. Therefore, when designing and conducting a trial, investigators should consider the most appropriate strategy and provide training to the research-related personnel to effectively implement such strategy to gain better cooperation from the participating children.

8.7.6 Arrangement for School-Based RCTs

As for RCTs conducted in kindergartens and schools, it is crucial to sustain a good collaboration with the involved kindergartens and schools. Implementing RCTs in kindergarten/schools may affect regular teaching schedules such as time conflicts between research activities and study courses, and involve entrance of unfamiliar people (research-related personnel who are not familiar to the kindergarten/school) into campus and occupation of classrooms or other school venues. Thus, efforts should be made to closely cooperate with the kindergarten/schools to balance research activities and regular teaching schedules. For example, in a RCT conducted in kindergartens which aimed to study the influence of prior application of silver diamine fluoride (SDF) solution on atraumatic restorative treatment, the investigators restored caries cavities 10 weeks after the application of SDF. Besides the scientific reason that a 10-week time period allows the active caries to become arrested after the application, another reason to adopt the 10-week interval is that the kindergartens could arrange the activities without interrupting their regular teaching schedules [50].

8.7.7 RCTs Testing Clinical Products

Newly invented treatments have to be substantially tested in human RCTs before they could be approved for wider use in the general population. In dentistry, the treatment could be dental materials, dental devices, or instruments. New treatments have to be studied in the laboratory first to determine the potential effect on people. Only treatments that are proved to have a promising effect and are at an acceptable safety level can be clinically investigated. Carefully designed RCTs, considered to be the gold standard, are usually conducted to test the new treatments. The rights and welfares of participants in the clinical trials of new treatments are always monitored by the institution sponsoring the trial. The study procedures have to be thoroughly reviewed by institutional review boards that are composed of experts and professionals from various healthcare disciplines, and lay people. Clinical trials testing new treatments are usually tested on adults first. The treatments may then be approved for the use in children even though the evidence of the safety and effectiveness in young age groups is limited. Inadequate trials for new treatments are problems in both medicine and dentistry. As the child population is relatively smaller, and not many new treatments are specifically developed for children, the incentive to conduct RCTs among children is usually low.

New products and treatments usually have to be approved by governmental authority before further clinical research can be conducted. A recent example would be the use of SDF in dental caries prevention. SDF has been approved and used in Japan for more than 80 years. It was cleared by the US Food and Drug Administration (FDA) in 2014 as an antihypersensitivity agent for dental use. Researchers can conduct study on SDF after it was approved by the authority.

8.8 Adverse Effects

When conducting an RCT to evaluate the benefits and efficacy of an intervention, information on harms, side, and unintended effects of the intervention should be provided for readers as well (consort). When deciding whether to accept or adopt the tested intervention in clinical practice, not only the benefits and efficacy, but also the adverse effects should be taken into account. In fact, not all trials have adverse events observed, and not all adverse events in a trial are the consequences of the intervention. So it is the authors' responsibility to provide sufficient information on whether there are harms or side effects, and if any, whether they are related to the intervention given. For example, in an RCT reporting on the atraumatic restorative treatment for primary teeth in preschool children, authors stated that "No obvious harms and adverse health outcomes due to the study interventions were observed" [50]. As for trials that may have various adverse events, details of the safety data should be collected and reported thoroughly. For instance, in an RCT applying SDF solution to treat dental caries among preschool children, a full report with details of the possible adverse effects of the intervention has been published [51]. However, it is found that the adverse effects are inadequately reported in the existing RCTs papers in pediatric dentistry. Majority of the papers did not define and list the adverse events during the trial, so readers did not have any clues to judge the possible adverse impacts of the intervention.

Regarding non-malfeasance, especially for a trial with a long follow-up time, an interim analysis can be performed with the intention "to compare treatment arms with respect to efficacy or safety at any time prior to formal completion of a trial" (E9 ICH) [52]. The interim analysis would help decide whether to stop early or to continue with the planned trial [26]. A trial can be stopped earlier than planned when the researchers find evidence showing more substantial benefits or harms than expected in the experimental intervention group. A trial can also be stopped earlier when no important difference between the test and control intervention groups are found as well. Interim analysis should be planned carefully and reported in detail because the number, methods, and consequences of these comparisons affect the interpretation of the trial [26, 52].

8.9 Dissemination

Conducting well-designed high-quality RCTs are crucial in evidence-based dentistry, as they provide reliable scientific evidence for practitioners to provide the best care for their patients. However, effective dissemination of research results is of paramount importance so that the new treatment will be adopted and implemented in clinical practice [53–55]. Without doubt, researchers presenting research findings at international conferences and writing up papers to be published in scientific journals are necessary for research results dissemination. Other stakeholders like the research and professional associations, research funders, and dental educators should also be proactive in disseminating the findings through clinical guidelines and dental education [53–55]. Besides, with the increasing emphasis of knowledge translation of research, researchers are also responsible for disseminating research findings to target audiences in the study communities especially when conducting community-based participatory research or research involving vulnerable populations [56, 57].

In summary, more well-designed high-quality randomized controlled trials (RCTs) are required to generate scientific evidence for use by clinical practitioners to provide the most appropriate care for their patients. In this chapter, published RCTs in pediatric dentistry are reviewed and knowledge gaps are identified. Important considerations and specific issues regarding the design, implementation, and dissemination of RCTs in pediatric dentistry are discussed.

8.10 Case Scenario Exercise

8.10.1 Case Scenario

> As a dental practitioner treating child patients, you would like to know the effective way to place preformed metal crowns (PMCs) in primary molars. Thus, a well-designed RCT is demanded to provide evidence on how to place PMCs in primary molars, and whether tooth preparation is necessary prior to the placement of PMCs. If you are the primary investigator, what would you do in designing and implementing this trial?

Questions

1. Who are the potential participants of the study and how to access the study population?
2. What is the primary outcome of the study? Is there any secondary outcome to be evaluated?
3. What are the potential interventions in the study?
4. How to determine the sample size of the study?
5. How to randomly allocate participants into different study groups? How to achieve allocation concealment?
6. How to achieve blinding in the study? Who should be blinded and by what methods?
7. What are the proposed statistical analyses of the study?
8. How to prevent attrition from the study? How to deal with missing outcome data?

Answers

1. Potential participants can be children with at least one primary molar tooth affected by decay recruited from different sources, for example, dental clinics, dental hospitals, kindergartens, primary schools, and communities.
2. The primary outcome can be the success of the PMCs (e.g., a composite outcome with no pain symptoms, no signs of infection, the restoration being intact, etc.) measured in the short term (less than 12 months) or long term (12 months or more). Apart from the primary outcome, various secondary outcomes can be evaluated, for example, the time used to place the PMCs, gingival conditions, and patient-reported outcome measures such as parental and child satisfaction.
3. Having tooth preparation prior to the placement of PMCs compared to no tooth preparation prior to the placement of PMCs.
4. Sample size calculation should be determined based on the study design (parallel or split-mouth design) and the primary outcome of the RCT (success or failure). As the primary outcome is dichotomous, risk ratio would be used to evaluate the difference in the success rates between PMCs with and without tooth preparation. The sample size can be determined based on the effect size, significance level, statistical power, allocation ratio, and the anticipated attrition rate. Intracluster correlation needs to be considered when multiple PMCs are placed in the same mouth so as to adjust for the clustering effect of the observations measured from the same child.
5. Computer-generated random number sequence and sequentially numbered opaque-sealed envelopes is a desirable method to achieve allocation concealment in this study.
6. In this study, the operator responsible for placing the PMCs cannot be blinded because the procedures in the study groups are different. However, the children, their parents, and the examiners responsible for assessing the study outcomes can be blinded by not informing them of the children's group allocation.
7. As the primary outcome is the success of the PMCs, survival analysis is a good option for analyzing the time-to-event variable. The clustering effect should not be neglected if multiple PMCs are placed in a child. As for the secondary outcomes, different statistical analysis methods may be chosen based on the measurement scales, such as comparing the means for continuous data and proportions for categorical data. Furthermore, appropriate statistical analysis should be used to compare the baseline characteristics between study groups in a parallel group design.
8. Several approaches can be adopted: (1) good communication with the participating parents and children during the recruitment process in explaining the project information and obtaining informed consent; (2) practical considerations to ensure positive experiences in the trial and make efforts to minimize discomfort and distress during the treatment; (3) providing incentives and (4) utilizing multiple strategies to follow up with the parents and maintaining their interests in the trial, such as making phone calls, sending reminders and emails. Depending on the amount and nature of the missing data, the missing data may be imputed and various methods can be adopted.

References

1. ADA. Specialty definitions. 2018. Available from: https://www.ada.org/en/ncrdscb/dental-specialties/specialty-definitions#.
2. Jiang CM, et al. Randomized controlled trials in dental journals on children and adolescents: a bibliometric analysis. J Evid Based Dent Pract. 2021;21(4):101621. https://doi.org/10.1016/j.jebdp.2021.101621.
3. Weintraub JA, et al. Fluoride varnish efficacy in preventing early childhood caries. J Dent Res. 2006;85(2):172–6.
4. Lawrence HP, et al. A 2-year community-randomized controlled trial of fluoride varnish to prevent early childhood caries in Aboriginal children. Community Dent Oral Epidemiol. 2008;36(6):503–16.
5. Duangthip D, et al. Caries arrest by topical fluorides in preschool children: 30-month results. J Dent. 2018;70:74–9.
6. Soncini JA, et al. The. longevity of amalgam versus compomer/composite restorations in posterior primary and permanent teeth—findings from the new England children's amalgam trial. J Am Dent Assoc. 2007;138(6):763–72.
7. Mandari GJ, Frencken JE, van't Hof MA. Six-year success rates of occlusal amalgam and glass-ionomer restorations placed using three minimal intervention approaches. Caries Res. 2003;37(4):246–53.
8. Franzon R, et al. Outcomes of one-step incomplete and complete excavation in primary teeth: a 24-month randomized controlled trial. Caries Res. 2014;48(5):376–83.
9. Nase L, et al. Effect of long-term consumption of a probiotic bacterium, Lactobacillus rhamnosus GG, in milk on dental caries and caries risk in children. Caries Res. 2001;35(6):412–20.
10. Stecksen-Blicks C, Sjostrom I, Twetman S. Effect of long-term consumption of milk supplemented with probiotic lactobacilli and fluoride on dental caries and general health in preschool children: a cluster-randomized study. Caries Res. 2009;43(5):374–81.
11. Thorild I, Lindau B, Twetman S. Caries in 4-year-old children after maternal chewing of gums containing combinations of xylitol, sorbitol, chlorhexidine and fluoride. Eur Arch Paediatr Dent. 2006;7(4):241–5.
12. Morgan MV, et al. The anticariogenic effect of sugar-free gum containing CPP-ACP nanocomplexes on approximal caries determined using digital bitewing radiography. Caries Res. 2008;42(3):171–84.
13. Poulsen S, Beiruti N, Sadat N. A comparison of retention and the effect on caries of fissure sealing with a glass-ionomer and a resin-based sealant. Community Dent Oral Epidemiol. 2001;29(4):298–301.
14. Nordstrom A, Birkhed D. Preventive effect of high-fluoride dentifrice (5000 ppm) in caries-active adolescents: a 2-year clinical trial. Caries Res. 2010;44(3):323–31.
15. Harrison R, et al. Effect of motivational interviewing on rates of early childhood caries: a randomized trial. Pediatr Dent. 2007;29(1):16–22.
16. Rong WS, et al. Effectiveness of an oral health education and caries prevention program in kindergartens in China. Community Dent Oral Epidemiol. 2003;31(6):412–6.
17. O'Brien K, et al. Effectiveness of early orthodontic treatment with the Twin-block appliance: a multicenter, randomized, controlled trial. Part 1: Dental and skeletal effects. Am J Orthod Dentofac Orthop. 2003;124(3):234–43.
18. O'Brien K, et al. Effectiveness of treatment for Class II malocclusion with the Herbst or Twin-block appliances: a randomized, controlled trial. Am J Orthod Dentofac Orthop. 2003;124(2):128–37.
19. Huth KC, et al. Effectiveness of 4 pulpotomy techniques—randomized controlled trial. J Dent Res. 2005;84(12):1144–8.
20. Bird SE, Williams K, Kula K. Preoperative acetaminophen vs ibuprofen for control of pain after orthodontic separator placement. Am J Orthod Dentofac Orthop. 2007;132(4):504–10.
21. Surendar MN, et al. A comparative evaluation of intrnasal dexmedetomidine, midazolam and ketamine for their sedative and analgesic properties: a triple blind randomized study. J Clin Pediatr Dent. 2014;38(3):255–61.
22. Klaassen MA, Veerkamp JSJ, Hoogstraten J. Young children's Oral Health-Related Quality of Life and dental fear after treatment under general anaesthesia: a randomized controlled trial. Eur J Oral Sci. 2009;117(3):273–8.
23. Prahl C, et al. A randomised prospective clinical trial into the effect of infant orthopaedics on maxillary arch dimensions in unilateral cleft lip and palate (Dutchcleft). Eur J Oral Sci. 2001;109(5):297–305.
24. Bongaarts CAM, et al. Infant orthopedics has no effect on maxillary arch dimensions in the deciduous dentition of children with complete unilateral cleft lip and palate (Dutchcleft). Cleft Palate Craniofac J. 2006;43(6):665–72.
25. Zotti F, et al. Usefulness of an app in improving oral hygiene compliance in adolescent orthodontic patients. Angle Orthod. 2016;86(1):101–7.
26. Mejàre IA, et al. A systematic map of systematic reviews in pediatric dentistry—what do we really know? PLoS One. 2015;10(2):e0117537.
27. Agamy HA, et al. Comparison of mineral trioxide aggregate and formocresol as pulp-capping agents in pulpotomized primary teeth. Pediatr Dent. 2004;26(4):302–9.
28. Campbell MJ, Julious SA, Altman DG. Estimating sample sizes for binary, ordered categorical, and continuous outcomes in two group comparisons. BMJ. 1995;311(7013):1145–8.
29. CONSORT. Explanation and Elaboration: updated guidelines for reporting parallel group randomised trials. BMJ. 2010;2011(343):d6131.
30. Çaglar E, et al. Short-term effect of ice-cream containing Bifidobacterium lactis Bb-12 on the number of salivary mutans streptococci and lactobacilli. Acta Odontol Scand. 2008;66(3):154–8.

31. Kim J, Shin W. How to do random allocation (randomization). Clin Orthop Surg. 2014;6(1):103–9.
32. Innes NPT, Evans DJP, Stirrups DR. Sealing caries in primary molars: randomized control trial, 5-year results. J Dent Res. 2011;90(12):1405–10.
33. Arrow P. Restorative outcomes of a minimally invasive restorative approach based on atraumatic restorative treatment to manage early childhood caries: a randomised controlled trial. Caries Res. 2016;50(1):1–8.
34. Ziraps A, Honkala E. Clinical trial of a new glass ionomer for an atraumatic restorative treatment technique in class I restorations placed in Latvian school children. Med Princ Pract. 2002;11(Suppl. 1): 44–7.
35. Carpenter JR, Kenward MG. Missing data in randomised controlled trials: a practical guide. Birmingham: Health Technology Assessment Methodology Programme; 2007. p. 199. https://researchonline.lshtm.ac.uk/id/eprint/4018500
36. Frencken JE, et al. Effectiveness of ART and traditional amalgam approach in restoring single-surface cavities in posterior teeth of permanent dentitions in school children after 6.3 years. Community Dent Oral Epidemiol. 2007;35(3):207–14.
37. de Franca Lopes CMC, et al. Randomized clinical trial of ART class II restorations using two glass ionomer cements: one-year follow-up. Pediatr Dent. 2018;40(2):98–104.
38. Chung KC, Song JW, WRIST Study Group. A guide to organizing a multicenter clinical trial. Plast Reconstr Surg. 2010;126(2):515–23.
39. Youssef N, Reinhart K, Sakr Y. The pros and cons of multicentre studies. Netherlands J Crit Care. 2008;12:120–2.
40. Zheng L, Zelen M. Multi-center clinical trials: randomization and ancillary statistics. Ann Appl Stat. 2008;2(2):582–600.
41. Garrocho-Rangel A, Cerda-Cristerna B, Pozos-Guillen A. Bioethical issues in conducting pediatric dentistry clinical research. J Clin Pediatr Dent. 2018;42(2):85–90.
42. Hoffer LJ. Understanding Equipoise. Nutr Clin Pract. 2020;35(3):495–8.
43. ICH Harmonised Guideline Addendum To ICH E11: Clinical Investigation of Medicinal Products in the Pediatric Population 2017. Available from: https://database.ich.org/sites/default/files/E11_R1_Addendum.pdf.
44. Dockett S, Perry B. Researching with young children: seeking assent. Child Indic Res. 2011;4:231–47.
45. Institute, N.C. Available from: https://www.cancer.gov/Common/PopUps/popDefinition.aspx?id=CDR0000688774&version=Patient&language=en.
46. Ford K, Sankey J, Crisp J. Development of children's assent documents using a child-centred approach. J Child Health Care. 2007;11(1):19–28.
47. Kumpunen S, et al. Practical approaches to seeking assent from children. Nurse Res. 2012;19(2):23–7.
48. Petten Consulting. 2020. Available from: http://www.pettenconsulting.com/obtaining-assent-from-children/.
49. Ly KA, et al. Xylitol gummy bear snacks: a school-based randomized clinical trial. BMC Oral Health. 2008;8:20.
50. Jiang M, et al. A 24-month randomized controlled trial on the success rates of restoring untreated and SDF-treated dentine caries lesions in primary teeth with the ART approach. J Dent. 2020;100:103435.
51. Duangthip D, et al. Adverse effects of silver diamine fluoride treatment among preschool children. J Dent Res. 2018;97(4):395–401.
52. ICH Harmonised Tripartite Guideline. Statistical Principles for Clinical Trial (E9). Available from: https://database.ich.org/sites/default/files/E9_Guideline.pdf.
53. Pitts N. Understanding the jigsaw of evidence-based dentistry: 1. Introduction, research and synthesis. Evid Based Dent. 2004;5(1):2–4.
54. Pitts N. Understanding the jigsaw of evidence-based dentistry. 2. Dissemination of research results. Evid Based Dent. 2004;5(2):33–5.
55. Pitts N. Understanding the jigsaw of evidence-based dentistry. 3. Implementation of research findings in clinical practice. Evid Based Dent. 2004;5(3): 60–4.
56. Bodison SC, et al. Engaging the community in the dissemination, implementation, and improvement of health-related research. Clin Transl Sci. 2015;8(6): 814–9.
57. McDavitt B, et al. Dissemination as dialogue: building trust and sharing research findings through community engagement. Prev Chronic Dis. 2016;13:E38.

9 Randomized Controlled Trials in Periodontology and Implantology

Harjit Singh Sehgal, Richie Kohli, and Joseph V. Califano

9.1 Introduction

Many research questions have been addressed in periodontal research, and more than 100 periodontology randomized controlled trials (RCTs) are published every year [1]. The RCTs address clinical issues in everyday decision-making. Often, however, poor study designs (inadequate sample size, inappropriate or absent controls, and poorly conceived statistical analysis) limit the quality of the data and thus the conclusions that can be derived. Moreover, there are other questions that have not been addressed by RCTs, leaving therapy based on clinical judgment alone.

The CONSORT (Consolidated Standards of Reporting Trials) statement, discussed throughout this textbook, was created to establish standards for the publication of drug studies with a 'standard' two-group parallel design [2]. In addition, a nonpharmacologic extension (CONSORT-NPE) was published [3] to aid and encourage full reporting of details of operative procedures [4]. This is particularly relevant to periodontal RCTs, many of which investigate operative or surgical interventions. Leow et al. (2016) assessed the quality of reporting in periodontology, changes from years 2013 to 2015, and adherence to CONSORT-NPE [3, 4]. In their review, the authors found that 84% of 173 studies included described randomization methods, 74% highlighted examiner blinding, 87% accounted for patients at the study conclusion, 50% addressed patient or clinician blinding, and 64% described allocation concealment. In addition, 62% contained detailed explanations of experimental treatments, but most (88%) lacked training and certification protocols to assure clinician fidelity to the intervention, and few (17%) described the clinician's expertise and experience. The review concluded that substantial improvements in reporting have occurred over time, but attention is required to all aspects of the CONSORT-NPE [4]. In particular, lack of blinding and statistical analysis that did not address participant attrition were some of the problems.

More recently, Meyer et al. (2023) assessed the inclusion of flow diagrams in RCTs published in periodontology and implantology from 2018 to 2022 [5]. The CONSORT checklist

H. S. Sehgal (✉)
Division of Periodontology, Department of Regenerative and Reconstructive Sciences, School of Dentistry, Oregon Health & Science University, Portland, OR, USA
e-mail: sehgal@ohsu.edu

R. Kohli
Division of Dental Public Health, School of Dentistry, Oregon Health & Science University, Portland, OR, USA
e-mail: kohli@ohsu.edu

J. V. Califano
Division of Periodontology, Regenerative and Reconstructive Sciences, School of Dentistry, Oregon Health & Science University, Portland, OR, USA
e-mail: califanj@ohsu.edu

R. Kohli et al. (eds.), *Randomized Controlled Trials in Evidence-Based Dentistry*,
https://doi.org/10.1007/978-3-031-47651-8_9

recommends the use of flow diagrams to help document and visualize the trial flow [2, 6]. Templates are available and help provide standardization. The authors included 544 eligible articles and reported that only 58% of the papers included a flow diagram, with reporting being more common in periodontology (73.1%) in contrast to implantology (51.5%). Only 56% of reports included a complete CONSORT flow diagram, with others having at least one point missing in their flow diagram from the CONSORT reporting template. The reasons for loss to follow-up were missing in a third of the flow diagrams (30.3%), and the RCT analysis type (intent-to-treat, per-protocol, or both) was not reported in the majority (84.6%) of the studies. Thus, the authors concluded that there is a need for greater author attention to the importance of complete flow diagrams.

CONSORT guidelines have also been developed for RCT abstracts to provide detail and clarity for readers to promptly assess a trial's validity and the applicability of its results [7]. Xie et al. (2020), assessed the quality of RCT abstracts on drug therapy for periodontal disease in the last 10 years [1]. Based on the assessment of 249 included studies, the authors found that reporting for CONSORT items on trial design, numbers analyzed, confidence intervals, intention-to-treat analysis or per-protocol analysis, harms, and registration was less than 30%. Blinding was reported by less than half of the abstracts, and very few of them accurately said who was blinded. Studies have shown that nonblinded assessors might overestimate the effect in the treatment groups and underestimate the effect in the control groups [8, 9]. Further, none of the abstracts reported funding. The literature points out that studies funded by pharmaceutical companies may selectively report funder favorable outcomes, leading to publication bias [10, 11]. So, one should be careful while interpreting drug RCTs to inform a particular drug use in clinical treatment. Future studies are needed to the CONSORT statement in this area of study.

9.2 Periodontology

9.2.1 Relative Effectiveness of Nonsurgical, Gingival Flap Procedures, and Resective Surgery Procedures

There are several RCTs that examine the relative effectiveness of nonsurgical, gingival flap procedures and resective surgery procedures [12–16]. In the review by Mailoa et al. [14], the authors searched peer-reviewed journals and selected RCTs that compared surgical to nonsurgical therapy in equal to or greater than ten patients diagnosed with periodontitis and studies were included if they measured clinical attachment level (CAL) and probing depth (PD) and had a follow-up equal to or greater than 2 years from the experimental clinical intervention.

The authors performed a meta-analysis to assess the outcome of therapy for shallow, moderate, and deep PDs at enrollment [14]. Eight trials met their criteria. The meta-analysis found that for shallow probing depths (1–3 mm), scaling and root planing (SRP), modified Widman flap (MWF), and osseous surgery (OS) resulted in a mean of 23.2%, 39.4%, and 61.39% CAL loss, respectively. For 4–6 mm probing depths, a mean of 8.4%, 6.5%, and 5.22% CAL gain, respectively, was found. In ≥7 mm probing depths, a 9.8%, 14.2%, and 9.38% CAL gain, respectively, were found. For probing depth, they found that for shallow probing depths (1–3 mm), scaling and root planing (SRP) and modified Widman flap (MWF) resulted in a mean increase in probing depth of 2.5% and 3.3%, respectively, while for osseous surgery (OS) probing depths were decreased by 6.3%. For 4–6 mm probing depths, a mean of 18.7%, 24.4%, and 30.8% probing depth reduction, respectively, was found. In ≥7 mm probing depths, there was a 21.6%, 33.1%, and 42.8% probing depth reduction, respectively. The relative changes in CAL and PD from baseline indicated that OS resulted in a greater PD reduction than either SRP or MWF in initially shallow probing sites. However, SRP resulted in less CAL loss than either surgical approach. For initial probing depths of 4–6 mm, MWF resulted in more PD reduction than either SRP or OS, which were not statistically different from each other. However, SRP resulted in more CAL gain than either MWF or OS. For an initial probing of ≥7 mm, OS resulted in a significantly greater PD reduction than either SRP or MWF, which were not different from each other. Regarding CAL for an initial probing of ≥7 mm, SRP had a more favorable effect for CAL than either MWF or OS. Four other systematic reviews/meta-analyses found similar results [12, 13, 15, 16].

Mailoa et al. [14] noted that all of the studies included in the meta-analysis had a high risk of bias. For example, only one study provided details on the randomization method, and none provided methods used to conceal the allocation sequence and blind the participants and outcome assessment. Three studies reported incomplete outcome data. Similarly, in their meta-analysis on flap procedures compared to subgingival treatment of periodontitis, Sanz-Sánchez, 2020 [16] also found serious methodological inadequacies associated with bias. The most common risk of bias was incomplete reporting of the randomization process (sequence and allocation concealment) and examiner blinding. Thus, future studies need to address these deficiencies.

9.2.2 Scaling and Root Planing Alone and with Adjunctive Agents

Three recent systematic reviews/meta-analyses compared manual and ultrasonic instrumentation in nonsurgical periodontal therapy. Two of the analyses found no difference in PD reduction or CAL gain from baseline for either therapy [17, 18]. One of the reviews [19] found that manual instrumentation was significantly better for initial probing depths of 4–6 mm than ultrasonic scaling for PD reduction at 6 months post-treatment, with no difference for CAL gain. When the probing depth was >6 mm, both PD reduction and CAL gain were significantly better for manual SRP [19]. However, the authors pointed out that the data on the outcome of treatment on initially shallow pockets was generally of low quality as sample sizes were small. The review also pointed to publication bias, with some studies with no significant findings not being published. The published work came primarily from highly developed countries: there was only a single study from a developing country; hence, more research is needed in developing countries.

The studies discussed above did not include smoking as a variable. Since smoking has a highly significant effect on periodontal health and the response to periodontal therapy, failure to consider this variable may have resulted in reported differences in outcomes that were due to a failure to balance the test and control groups for this variable. Future studies of therapies need to include and document the smoking history of the study participants as well.

New RCTs may yield greater findings if, in addition to CAL and PD, the studies include other measures such as bleeding on probing, Periodontal Index, Gingival Index, and microflora changes. Results of experimental therapies for single and multi-rooted teeth should be reported separately, as they may respond differently to treatment [20].

Two recent systematic reviews/meta-analyses compared full-mouth disinfection FMD (SRP full mouth within 24 h, with 2 weeks of chlorhexidine rinses after SRP), FMSRP (SRP full mouth within 24 h only), and conventional SRP (CSD). One found a small but significant difference in PD reduction (0.2 mm) and CAL gain (0.2–0.4 mm) for FMD and FMSRP as compared to CSD, but the differences were not deemed clinically significant [21]. The other review did not find a significant difference between the three approaches [22]. Two reviews compared FMD with FMSRP. They both found a significant difference between the approaches for PD at 40–60 days and 180 days of 0.24 mm and 0.33 mm, respectively, with no difference in

CAL. The differences were not considered clinically significant [23, 24].

Eberhard et al. (2015) discuss the design limitations and considerations for future studies assessing the clinical outcomes of full-mouth disinfection and full-mouth scaling [22]. They found that there is low-quality existing evidence and that special attention should be paid to allocation concealment, complete outcome data reporting, and blinding of outcome assessors. The blinding of outcome assessment can be compromised by participant awareness of differences between interventions and visible signs of differences in intervention groups, for example, debridement completion differences between the groups or stains on the teeth from pharmaceuticals [22]. Objective outcomes like tooth loss may be less amenable to bias, but the duration of follow-up needed would increase to 3–5 years [22]. Future studies should address economic costs and patient burden, and the authors should follow the CONSORT guidelines [22].

The addition of local delivery antibiotics to scaling and root planing was also assessed in two systematic reviews/meta-analyses. The meta-analyses indicated a significant improvement in PD reduction (0.36–0.65) but not for CAL [25, 26]. A third review examined the use of locally applied antibiotics during surgery and found a significant improvement in PD reduction (0.41 mm) and CAL (0.61 mm) [27]. Future RCTs should also include other periodontal endpoints such as tooth survival and oral health outcomes in addition to PD and CAL, identify the ideal antibiotic agent, its dosage, delivery methods (e.g., into membranes or bone grafts), release kinetics, antimicrobial spectrum, and effects on periodontal healing [27].

Adjunctive systemic antibiotics were examined in a systematic review by Khattri et al. [28]. SRP plus amoxicillin and metronidazole, metronidazole alone, azithromycin, doxycycline, tetracycline, and clindamycin were compared to SRP alone. Each of the antibiotic regimens was also compared to each other. This was done in both chronic periodontitis and aggressive periodontitis patients. The outcome measures included PD, CAL, pocket closure, and bleeding on probing (BOP). Among all the comparisons made for different adjunctive antibiotics, the differences in the outcome measures were either not significant or the differences were small. Even when a significant difference was found, the analysis indicated that differences were small and of very low certainty. Most trials testing amoxicillin, metronidazole, and azithromycin reported adverse events such as nausea, vomiting, diarrhea, mild gastrointestinal disturbances, and metallic taste. No serious adverse events were reported.

The authors concluded that there was very low-certainty evidence to inform clinicians and patients as to whether adjunctive systemic antimicrobials are of any benefit in the nonsurgical treatment of periodontitis. There is insufficient evidence to decide whether some antibiotics are better than others when used with SRP. The authors also suggested some important considerations for future studies. These include standardizing dosage and duration of antibiotic administration and control treatment, assessment of antibiotic resistance, consistent reporting of adverse events, results stratified by periodontitis severity and age, and a priori defining the 'minimally important clinical difference for the outcomes percentage of closed pockets, CAL, pocket depth, and percentage of BOP'.

There are five other systematic reviews/meta-analyses of adjunctive treatment with systemic antibiotics. These reviews found a limited PD reduction (0.44 mm) and CAL gain (0.21 mm); however, significant improvements were noted in PD reduction for moderate (0.88 mm) and deep (1.26 mm) pockets and CAL gain for moderate (0.83 mm) and deep (1 mm) pockets at 12 months in patients with untreated aggressive periodontitis [29–33]. One review examined whether assessing the presence/absence of a periodontal pathogen before treatment resulted in a better outcome, but no evidence was found to suggest that baseline detection of periodontopathogenic bacteria should be used as a criterion for prescribing adjunctive antibiotics [31].

The adjunctive use of subantimicrobial-dose doxycycline (SDD) was also examined. The meta-analysis, conducted by Reddy et al. indicated a significant effect of SDD for PD decrease (0.442 mm for initial probing depth of 4–6 mm, and 0.452 mm for initial probing depth of ≥7 mm) and CAL gain (0.448 mm for initial probing depth of 4–6 mm, and 0.481 mm for initial probing depth of ≥7 mm) when added to SRP [34]. A second review also found similar differences for CAL and PD [32].

Five systematic reviews/meta-analyses compared SRP with adjunctive probiotics (orally administered *Lactobacillus reuteri*) compared to SRP alone. One review found a significant effect on PD reduction and CAL gain at 3 and 12 months but not at 6 and 9 months [35]. A similar early small but significant effect for PD reduction and CAL gain that could not be confirmed at 6 months was found by Hu et al. [36]. Three other reviews found a significant decrease in PD and CAL. However, all of these short-term studies found inconsistent effects, therefore, they do not support the use of probiotics as an adjunct to periodontal therapy [37–39].

Four systematic reviews/meta-analyses compared SRP with locally delivered statins to SRP alone. The authors hypothesize that statins may support the production of growth factors that enhance bone deposition. All of these reviews found a significant effect on PD reduction (1–1.76 mm) and CAL gain (1–1.84 mm). But, three of the reviews found a high level of heterogeneity among the studies and stated that the results should be viewed with caution [40–43].

One systematic review, including four studies, examined SRP with adjunctive locally delivered metformin gel. The authors indicate that there is evidence that metformin increases the osteogenic activity of osteoblasts and decreases the number of osteoclasts. All the studies were conducted in the same research center. They found a significant difference in a decrease in PD (2.12 mm) and CAL gain (2.29 mm). While this result is of interest, especially because of the magnitude of the difference, the findings should be confirmed by other investigators/centers [44] to increase generalizability as well as confidence in the results.

9.2.3 Regenerative Surgical Procedures

A recent comprehensive review of regenerative surgical procedures by Tsai et al. [45] included 60 RCTs. The meta-analysis allowed comparisons of several regenerative procedures including all combinations of regenerative approaches and gingival flap procedure alone. The regenerative procedures included guided tissue regeneration (GTR), enamel matrix derivative (EMD), bone graft, and platelet-rich plasma (PRP). Differences between the regenerative therapies were small, with GTR resulting in the greatest PD reduction (1.33 mm greater than a gingival flap alone) and EMD + BG and EMD + GTR gaining the most attachment (1.5 mm greater than a gingival flap alone). For PD reduction and CAL gain, the gingival flap procedure was the least effective [45]. The results of two other systematic reviews/meta-analyses that focused on EMD were different: they did not find a significant effect of EMD when combined with a bone graft, compared to a bone graft alone [46, 47].

Several systematic reviews/meta-analyses examined regenerative techniques and found the same results as Tsai et al. [31, 48–51]. The paucity of data, the risk of methodological and the potential publication bias suggested caution in interpreting these results and indicated the need for multicenter studies for this specific application. The authors highlighted that although publication biases could not be detected with funnel plots analysis in their study, the small size of the included trials may underpower such analyses. Publication bias is also possible, particularly in emerging fields of research.

One systematic review/meta-analysis examined RCTs that studied the use of EMD as an adjunct to scaling and root planing. They found that EMD did not have a significant effect [52]. Another meta-analysis examined the use of EMD as part of a gingival flap procedure where there were supra bony pockets. This analysis indicated there was no significant effect of EMD in sites without vertical defects [53]. The authors reported that although no differences were found in tooth survival, EMD application resulted in clinical and radiographic additional benefits compared to Open Flap Debridement (OFD) alone.

Three systematic reviews/meta-analyses examined the effect of the growth factors rhPDGF-BB (recombinant human platelet-derived growth factor) and rhFGF-2 (recombinant human fibroblast growth factor) in the surgical treatment of intrabony defects. The results were in agreement: the analyses found a significant increase of 20–40% more bone gain and 1 mm more linear bone fill for rhPDGF-BB. One study found an additional 1 mm of CAL gain. Two of the reviews also looked at rhFGF-2 and reported similar enhancement of bone fill and linear bone gain [54–56].

A systematic review/meta-analysis of the adjunctive effect of autologous platelet concentrates (APCs) – [platelet-rich plasma (PRP), plasma rich in growth factors (PRGF), and platelet-rich fibrin (PRF)] to a gingival flap procedure with or without a bone graft, gingival flap procedure with GTR, or gingival flap procedure with EMG [57]. They found there was very low-quality evidence that the adjunct of APC to OFD or OFD + bone graft when treating infrabony defects improves PD, CAL, and radiographic bone defect fill. For GTR or EMD, there was insufficient evidence of a significant enhancement of PD decrease or CAL gain for the addition of autologous platelet concentrates. Two other reviews yielded similar results and conclusions [58, 59]. One review found that platelet-rich plasma had a significant effect on PD decrease (0.55 mm), CAL gain (0.58 mm), and linear bone gain (0.76 mm increase) [60]. A review by Miron, et al. found a significant effect of PRF when used in conjunction with a gingival flap procedure. However, when combined with a variety of regenerative procedures, there was no additional benefit of adding PRF [61].

Several systematic reviews/meta-analyses examined regenerative procedures in furcation defects. The consensus among these studies was that a significant increase in attachment gain was found for GTR in class II furcation defects. The amount of improvement was consistent with the reviews of regeneration in intrabony defects. The authors also indicated that GTR does not have a significant positive effect on class III furcation defects. Finally, while these procedures may be helpful for class I defects, the authors noted that nonregenerative therapy may also be similarly effective [62–64].

Several reviews examined cell-based regenerative therapies (periodontal ligament stem cells, pulp stem cells, periosteum derived stem cells, gingival fibroblasts, and their associated stem cells) and concluded that while there are promising results, the number and quality of the studies do not allow conclusions as to efficacy [65–67].

9.2.4 Use of Lasers in Periodontal Therapy

Lasers of varying wavelengths in devices manufactured by several companies have been used as an adjunct to scaling and root planing. The laser has been used in two ways in studies. First, the laser can be used to debride the root surfaces and tissues and aid in the degranulation of periodontitis lesions. Or, the laser can be used to serve in an antimicrobial fashion with photosensitizers in the presence of oxygen. When the photosensitizers are exposed to the laser energy, reactive oxygen species are produced that can be bactericidal and are described as antimicrobial photodynamic therapy (aPDT).

A recent multicenter RCT examined the Erbium, chromium-doped yttrium, scandium, gallium, and garnet, the Er,Cr:YSGG laser (Biolase™), as an adjunct to scaling and root planing where the comparator was a minimally invasive surgical procedure. The investigators reported decreases in PD and CAL gain in both study arms, but they were not different [68]. Several systematic reviews/meta-analyses examined the use of lasers in nonsurgical and surgical protocols. They concluded that the data available did not indicate a significant effect on the outcome of periodontal therapy over conventional periodontal therapy alone [69–72].

Several RCTs examined the adjunctive effect of lasers in a photodynamic effect protocol as compared to SRP alone or SRP with systemic antibiotics. Most of the meta-analyses indicated that there was no significant benefit of this laser therapy and did not support its use in this fashion for periodontal therapy [73–77]. One study found a statistically significant benefit for PD decrease and CAL gain but indicated that the differences were modest and may not be clinically significant [78]. A meta-analysis by Souza *et al* found a significant adjunctive effect of the laser-induced photodynamic effect in conjunction with SRP that resulted in clinical improvements similar to that obtained when amoxicillin and metronidazole were used as an adjunct for SRP [79].

There are some important methodological considerations while designing RCTs examining the adjunctive effect of lasers. Significant heterogeneity has been noted in terms of laser type, tip diameter, wavelength, photosensitizer, model of periodontal treatment, number of treated sites, etc. [75]. There is no consensus on the parameters of the laser and the photosensitizers used, and these were often inadequately reported. There is a need for the scientific community to establish and require minimum parameters of information in order to replicate or compare studies with different models of lasers and different protocols [79].

9.2.5 Root Coverage Procedures

RCTs concerned with surgical procedures for root coverage have examined and compared a number of different surgical procedures and diverse materials. Surgical procedures include the coronally advanced flap (CAF) and tunneling. Materials utilized with these surgeries include subepithelial connective tissue grafts (SCTG), GTR with resorbable membranes (GTRrm), acellular dermal matrix grafts (ADMG), enamel matrix derivative (EMD), xenogenic collagen, and root conditioning with ethylenediaminetetraacetic acid (EDTA).

A 2018 Cochrane systematic review paper by Chambone et al. [80] examined 48 RCTs. Most were found to have an uncertain risk of bias: one had a low risk of bias, 12 had a high risk of bias, and 35 had an unclear risk of bias. These trials compared a CAF alone, CAF with EMD, GTRrm and CAF, and SCTG and CAF. The results of their meta-analysis indicated that a greater reduction in gingival recession for SCTG) + CAF compared to GTRrm + CAF (mean difference = −0.37 mm, $p = 0.002$; 3 studies; 98 participants; low-quality evidence). There was insufficient evidence of a difference in gingival recession reduction between ADMG + CAF and SCTG + CAF, or EMD + CAF and SCTG + CAF. Regarding CAL changes, GTRrm + CAF promoted additional gains compared to SCTG + CAF (mean difference = 0.35, $p = 0.02$; 3 studies; 98 participants; low-quality evidence), but there was insufficient evidence of a difference between ADMG + CAF and SCTG + CAF or between EMD + CAF and SCTG + CAF. Greater gains in the keratinized tissue were found for SCTG + CAF when compared to EMD + CAF (mean difference − 1.06 mm $p < 0.00001$; 2 studies; 62 participants; low-quality evidence), and SCTG + CAF when compared to GTR rm. + CAF (mean difference = −1.77 mm, $p < 0.0001$; 3 studies; 98 participants; very low-quality evidence). There was insufficient evidence of a difference in keratinized tissue gain between ADMG + CAF and SCTG + CAF. Few data exist on aesthetic condition change related to patients' opinions and patients' preferences for a specific procedure. The authors concluded that subepithelial connective tissue grafts with CAF, CAF alone or associated with other biomaterial, and guided tissue regeneration may be used as root coverage procedures for treating localized or multiple recession-type defects. The available evidence base indicates that in cases where both root coverage and gain in the width of keratinized tissue are desired, the use of subepithelial connective tissue grafts shows a slight improvement in outcome. There is also some weak evidence suggesting that acellular dermal matrix grafts appear as the soft tissue substitute that may provide the most similar outcomes to those achieved by subepithelial connective tissue grafts [80].

For future studies, split-mouth trials should include patient preferences for a specific periodontal plastic surgery procedure, precise and objective aesthetic evaluations, use of the visual analog scale (VAS) for more precise evaluations of patient-based outcomes, the inclusion of baseline and final individual defect measurements with subgroup evaluations in patients presenting similar defects [80]. The outcome measures should include gingival recession depth and width, clinical attachment level, width and thickness of keratinized tissue, and root surface conditions (i.e., presence of caries, abrasions, or restorations) [80]. Other considerations are to provide relevant training and certification of the operators in following the protocol, multicenter studies for the inclusion and evaluation of appropriate sample sizes of patients, and more long-term RCTs. Further, considering limited data availability for lateral positioned flaps and for free gingival grafts and platelet-rich fibrin, these procedures should be evaluated by future research. The authors should also make their data available for other researchers to reuse and analyze to overcome this issue and advance medical knowledge and developing improved treatments as has been proposed as a policy for medical journals [81].

An earlier meta-analysis of 22 RCTs by the same first author compared SCTG plus CAF, Xenogenic collagen graft plus CAF, EMD plus CAF to CAF alone and found the CAF alone was less effective in achieving complete root coverage than the other procedures [82].

A systematic review by Hwang *et al* compared several soft tissue coverage procedures and also assessed the effect of CAF thickness on the outcome. The analysis showed there was a critical threshold of >1.1 mm for flap thickness for complete root coverage ($p < 0.02$) [83].

Three meta-analyses compared SCTG plus CAF to xenogenic collagen graft plus CAF. Two found that the two procedures were not significantly different in their ability to achieve complete root coverage [84, 85] while the third found that SCTG exhibited significantly higher mean root coverage as compared to the xenogenic graft (91.79% vs 80.10%) that was not significantly different at 12 months ($p = 0.06$). The SCTG also achieved significantly greater gingival thickness when compared to the xenogenic collagen graft ($p < 0.05$) [86].

An RCT compared Xenogenic collagen matrix (CM) plus CAF plus EMD, CM plus CAF, CAF plus EMD, and CAF alone and found the obtained root coverage was 68.04% – 24.11% for CAF; 87.20% – 15.01% for CAF plus CM; 88.77% – 20.66% for CAF plus EMD; and 91.59% – 11.08% for CAF + CM + EMD after 6 months. Groups that received biomaterials showed greater complete root coverage ($p < 0.05$). Complete root coverage was 70.59% for CAF + EMD, which was significantly superior to CAF alone (23.53%), CAF + CM (52.94%), and CAF + CM + EMD (51.47%) ($p < 0.05$). Keratinized tissue thickness gain was significant only in CM-treated groups ($p < 0.05$) [87].

A meta-analysis by Cortellini *et al* compared an SCTG plus CAF with CAF alone and found that both procedures were effective with similar outcomes; however, the SCTG plus CAF combination treatment had a significantly better outcome with respect to complete root coverage ($p = 0.0016$), reduction in recession ($p < 0.0001$), and increase in keratinized tissue ($p < 0.0001$), especially if the gingival flap was thin (≤0.8 mm). This finding was in agreement with that of an earlier review by the same author [88, 89].

A meta-analysis by Carvelli *et al* compared the SCTG plus CAF with EMD with the SCTG plus CAF alone. The results indicated that the amount of root coverage was significantly better with the addition of EMD (mean difference = 0.3 mm, $p = 0.04$), although the difference is probably not clinically meaningful [90]. This is in agreement with the results of a meta-analysis by Mauricio et al. [91] and an RCT by Mercado *et al* [92]. Mercado *et al* also found a significant increase in keratinized tissue width with the addition of EMD ($p < 0.01$) [92]. One multicenter RCT found equivalence in the result with and without EMD [93].

A systematic review and meta-analysis comparing a CAF with tunneling using either SCTG or ADMG considered 20 articles and utilized six in the meta-analysis. They found that the CAF and tunneling were both effective when used with either an SCTG or ADMG with comparable mean root coverage. When comparing the CAF plus SCTG and Tunneling plus SCTG or CAF plus ADMG and Tunneling plus ADMG, the CAF achieved significantly better complete root coverage ($p < 0.003$ for SCTG and $p < 0.0007$ for ADMG). There was no difference in keratinized tissue gain for any of the procedures [94].

Gingival margin stability after periodontal plastic surgery for root coverage was examined in an RCT where a manual versus an oscillating-rotating powered toothbrush was compared. There were no significant differences in PD or CAL for the two groups. Complete root coverage was significantly higher in subjects that used the oscillating-rotating powered toothbrush at 6 months (manual, 66.67%; powered, 96.67%; $p = 0.002$) [95].

Finally, two other RCTs examined the use of EDTA root conditioning and autologous platelet concentrate as adjuncts to root coverage procedures. Both were found to have no effect on the outcome of root coverage procedures [59, 96].

9.2.6 Smoking and Periodontitis

Three systematic reviews and meta-analyses examined smoking and periodontitis and the effect of smoking on the success of periodontal therapy. All agreed that the findings of studies reviewed confirmed that smoking decreased the PD reduction (mean of 0.2–0.39 mm less reduction) and attachment gain (0.32–0.35 mm less) as compared to nonsmokers and former smokers, with both nonsurgical and surgical periodontal therapy. Smokers were also found to have an 80% higher risk of periodontitis as compared to nonsmokers and former smokers [97–99]. Future RCTs should include smokers and analyze them as a distinct subgroup population.

9.2.7 Periodontitis and Preterm/Low Birth Weight

In the systematic review and meta-analysis by Iheozor-Ejiofor *et al* examined RCTs assessing the effect of periodontal therapy on preterm birth/low birth weight (PTB/LBW). Fifteen RCTs met the inclusion criteria and were studied. Eleven compared periodontal treatment with no treatment during pregnancy. The meta-analysis showed no clear difference in preterm birth <37 weeks between periodontal treatment and no treatment (11 studies; low-quality evidence). There is low-quality evidence that periodontal treatment may reduce low birth weight < 2500 g (9.70% with periodontal treatment versus 12.60% without treatment; seven studies) [100].

A meta-analysis by Fogacci et al. similarly found that in all meta-analyses, the effect of periodontal treatment on preterm birth and LBW was not statistically significant [101].

9.2.8 Periodontitis, Diabetes, and Obesity

Several RCTs have examined the effect of periodontal therapy on glycemic control in type 2 diabetics. The periodontal therapy was either scaling and root planing (SRP) or SRP and systemic antibiotics. The results of the systematic reviews and meta-analyses are similar, although the conclusions the authors have drawn are somewhat different. The meta-analysis by Baeza et al. found that the mean decrease in HbA1c was 0.56 ($p < 0.01$) and for the serum level of C-reactive protein 1.89 ($p < 0.01$) [102]. Simpson et al. also found a similar result with a mean percentage reduction in HbA1c of 0.29% at 4 months [103]. In contrast, a meta-analysis by Wang et al. found no significant difference in the HbA1c for patients receiving no periodontal treatment, SRP, SRP plus doxycycline, or SRP plus placebo [104]. The meta-analysis was hampered by the small number of studies available to be analyzed and the small number of participants. Engebretson et al. found in a multicenter RCT that the HbA1c was not significantly different in patients receiving periodontal therapy versus those without periodontal therapy [105]. These studies are too short and too small to reach definitive conclusions about the impact of various periodontal treatments on diabetic health. Often, the results of the studies are confounded because other risk factors for diabetes are either not assessed at all or inadequately [90]. In a systematic review and meta-analysis examining the effect of obesity on the response to periodontal therapy, 15 studies were assessed. The results of the analysis found no difference in clinical periodontal parameters when comparing otherwise healthy overweight/obese patients to normal-weight patients [106]. Box 9.1 provides summary of the main findings from the key RCTs, systematic reviews, Cochrane reviews and meta-analyses in Periodontology.

Box 9.1 Summary of the Main Findings from the Key RCTs, Systematic Reviews, Cochrane Reviews, and Meta-Analyses in Periodontology

- Scaling and Root Planing (SRP), Modified Widman Flap (MWF) and Osseous Surgery (OS) result in loss of attachment in shallow pockets (1–3 mm) and all of these result in attachment gain for deeper pockets. While MWF results in better pocket depth (PD) reduction than SRP and OS in 4–6 mm deep pockets and OS results in better PD reduction in >7 mm deep pockets, SRP results in better attachment gain in both these scenarios.
- Adjunctive use of local delivery antibiotic to scaling and root planing provide improvement in periodontal parameters however their clinical significance appears to be limited.
- Adjunctive use of systemic antimicrobials found small but significant differences in PD reduction and CAL (Clinical Attachment Level) gain. There is insufficient evidence to decide whether some antibiotics are better than others when used with SRP. There is no evidence to suggest that baseline detection of periodontopathogenic bacteria should be used as a criterion for prescribing adjunctive antibiotics.
- Adjunctive use of Subantimicrobial-Dose Doxycycline (SDD) with SRP results in additional PD decrease (0.442 mm for initial probing depth of 4–6 mm, and 0.452 mm for initial probing depth of ≥7 mm) and CAL gain.
- Adjunctive use of probiotics (orally administered *Lactobacillus reuteri*) with SRP provides a significant effect on PD reduction and CAL gain at 3 and 12 months but not at 6 and 9 months.
- Adjunctive use of lasers in the treatment of periodontitis does not provide any additional benefit over conventional periodontal therapy alone.
- Differences between the regenerative therapies for intrabony defects were small with GTR (Guided Tissue Regeneration) resulting in the greatest PD reduction (1.33 mm greater than a gingival flap alone) and EMD (Enamel Matrix Derivative) + BG (Bone Graft) and EMD + GTR gaining the most attachment.
- GTR also results in a significant increase in attachment gain in class II furcation defects. The amount of improvement was consistent with that reported above for intrabony defects.
- Growth factors rhPDGF-BB (recombinant human platelet derived growth factor) and rhFGF-2 (recombinant human fibroblast growth factor) when used in the surgical treatment of intrabony defects result in a significant increase of 20–40% more bone gain and 1 mm more linear bone fill for rhPDGF-BB while no difference in CAL.
- Adjunctive use of Autologous platelet concentrates (APCs) - [platelet rich plasma (PRP), plasma rich in growth factors (PRGF), platelet rich fibrin (PRF)] to Open Flap Debridement (OFD) or OFD + bone graft does not provide any additional significant benefit when treating infrabony defects.
- Subepithelial connective tissue grafts SCTG plus Coronally Advanced Flap (CAF) had a significantly better outcome as far as complete root coverage ($p = 0.0016$), reduction in recession ($p < 0.0001$), and increase in keratinized tissue ($p < 0.0001$), especially if the gingival flap was thin (≤0.8 mm).
- Adjunctive use of EMD with SCTG and CAF resulted in significantly better root coverage (mean difference = 0.3 mm,

$p = 0.04$) and increase in keratinized tissue width ($p < 0.01$).

- Adjunctive use of EDTA root conditioning and autologous platelet concentrate with root coverage procedure have no significant effect on the outcome of root coverage procedures.
- Smokers have an 80% higher risk of periodontitis as compared to non-smokers and former smokers. Smoking decreases the PD reduction (mean of 0.2–0.39 mm less reduction) and attachment gain (0.32–0.35 mm less) with periodontal therapy as compared to non-smokers and former smokers.
- Periodontal therapy does not have an effect on adverse pregnancy outcomes of preterm birth and low birth weight however may result in a mean decrease in HbA1c of 0.56 and in serum level of C-reactive protein of 1.89 in diabetics.

9.3 Implantology

Tooth loss from dental caries, periodontal disease, or trauma sadly occurs, and among tooth replacement options, dental implants are key options. In this section, we review the current evidence from RCTs, systematic reviews, and meta-analysis of RCTs and their quality and identify gaps in current research as well as future directions on Implant-site development, short vs long dental implants, timing of implant placement, guided vs nonguided implant placement, management of peri-implant diseases and implant maintenance. Because modern implantology is a relatively new area of dentistry, there is much opportunity for research.

9.3.1 Implant-site Development

Several RCTs have examined the effects of different materials and techniques for Implant-site development. In a systematic review of RCTs [107], alveolar ridge preservation was shown to prevent horizontal, vertical mid-buccal, and vertical mid-lingual bone resorption compared to tooth extraction alone. Various ridge preservation modalities including using bovine bone particles, bovine bone with porcine collagen, cortico-cancellous porcine bone particles, allograft particles, alloplastic particles, autologous blood-derived products, cell therapy, recombinant bone morphogenic protein or socket sealing alone have compared. While no one technique was deemed superior, particulate xenogenic or allogenic materials covered with an absorbable collagen membrane or rapidly absorbable collagen sponge provided the most favorable outcome for horizontal ridge preservation. Only 2 of 22 RCTs included patient-related outcome measures (PROM) and found no difference in reported discomfort, perceived benefit, and quality of life scores between the test and control groups. Future studies should be designed to include PROM and local, systemic, and surgical procedure-related variables as well [107]. In addition, the US Food and Drug Administration (FDA), which regulates regenerative medicine products, also has a high priority that patient-related measures are included in studies submitted for review.

Dam et al. (2022) [108] reviewed the recent advances in bone augmentation for dental implants and concluded that no single biomaterial or clinical technique is ideal and that each graft procedure has advantages and disadvantages in each clinical application. The clinician needs to choose the graft material with a high success rate and less morbidity. Autogenous bone is considered as the gold standard because of its biocompatibility, osteoconductive, osteoinductive, and osteogenic properties. The use of different scaffold material types, growth factors, and stem cells shows promise in regenerative treatment interventions for maxillofacial defects. There is, however, limited evidence to support the use of biological mediators such as growth factors as an adjunct to regeneration of alveolar ridge preservation and ridge augmentation procedures; hence, clinicians should determine if the additional effort and expense will significantly enhance clinical outcomes [109]. The authors suggest that growth factors may provide the greatest benefit for enhanced wound healing in a compromised patient or in sites with severe hard and soft tissue defects, or during retreatment. Another narrative review [110] acknowledges the great heterogeneity of the available studies for the use of bioactive factors and the limited number of RCTs; hence, no robust conclusions can be drawn. Future studies should investigate the optimal carriers for bioactive agents, dosage, and timing of administration as well as the possibility of combining different agents to promote synergistic.

Atieh et al. [111] in 2021 also assessed the clinical effects of various materials and techniques for alveolar ridge preservation (ARP) after tooth extraction compared with extraction alone or other methods of ARP, or both, in patients requiring dental implant placement following healing of extraction sockets. The comparisons were assessed for xenograft or alloplast vs. extraction alone; allograft or alloplast vs. xenograft, alloplast with and without membrane, synthetic cell-binding peptide P-15 as an adjunct to allograft, and alloplasts with different particle sizes. The authors found that there was very low-certainty evidence for the reduction in loss of alveolar ridge width and height in favor of ARP techniques. In addition, there was a lack of evidence if ARP techniques lead to any differences in the need for additional augmentation at the time of implant placement, implant failure, aesthetic outcomes, or prosthodontic outcomes due to a lack of information or long-term data. Evidence is also lacking for any clinically significant difference between different grafting materials and barriers used for ARP.

In their Cochrane Review, Esposito *et al* concluded that although various techniques can augment bone horizontally and vertically, it is unclear which are the most efficient [112]. They reported that short implants appear to be a better alternative to vertical bone grafting of resorbed mandibles and complications, especially for vertical augmentation. Bone substitutes (Bio-Oss or Cerasorb) may replace autogenous bone for sinus lift procedures of atrophic maxillary sinuses, but more studies are needed to confirm that. They also reported that distraction osteogenesis allows for more vertical bone augmentation than other techniques, which, on the other hand, can allow for horizontal augmentation at the same time. Titanium screws may be preferred as compared to resorbable screws to fixate onlay bone grafts. The authors pointed out that these conclusions are based on a few trials including few patients, who sometimes had short follow-ups, often with a high risk of bias. Answers to many of these questions require proper RCTs. The authors suggested that it is difficult to provide clear indications with respect to which augmentation procedures should be tested first. Clinical situations that would benefit from augmentation procedures need to be determined as well. Priority should be given to those interventions that look simpler, less invasive, involve less risk of complications, and reach their goals within the shortest timeframe. It is also important to further evaluate the potential ability of bone morphogenetic proteins (rhBMP-2) to favor bone growth in conjunction with bone substitutes, autogenous bone, and a combination of the two. Future research is needed to confirm which autogenous graft donor sites provide a sufficient amount of bone with less risk of complications and patient discomfort. It is also imperative to evaluate the objective aesthetic outcomes assessed by blind outcome assessors and the patient's own perception of aesthetics.

In a more recent systematic review and meta-analysis [113], horizontal bone augmentation was seen to successfully increase bone width prior to implant placement. Sites with initially smaller bone dimensions presented with larger bone width gains, demonstrating effective horizontal bone augmentation [113]. In another systematic review and meta-analysis [114], horizontal bone augmentation was also seen to be a successful treatment modality when performed simultaneously with dental implant placement. The most common type of intervention was using a xenogenic particulate graft with a resorbable collagen membrane [114]. Vertical ridge augmentation is also a feasible and effective treatment modality for the reconstruction of vertical ridge defects; however, complications with these procedures are more common. In a systematic review and meta-analysis [115], distraction osteogenesis was shown to provide the most vertical bone gain; however, it also had the most complication rate. Guided bone regeneration (GBR) procedures and the use of bone blocks were the other successful treatment options, with bone blocks also presenting with significant complication rates [115]; hence, no clear evidence is present for the superiority of a particular augmentation technique. The authors advise caution while interpreting these results due to high heterogeneity between studies, conflicting inter-study outcomes, uncontrolled confounders inherent in each study design, and the multiple sub-types of interventions. In addition, the long-term outcome of the augmented bone and implant outcomes in the augmented bone are unclear.

Pneumatized maxillary sinuses and resorbed alveolar ridges present novel challenges for implant therapy in the posterior maxilla and require specialized maxillary sinus floor augmentation (MSFA) techniques. In a systematic review and meta-analysis [116], MSFA was shown to be a reliable treatment modality in the long-term for patients with partially and fully edentulous maxillae. There were no significant differences in implant loss between edentulous or dentate patients, between implants placed simultaneously with or delayed after MSFA, and between MSFA performed using solely autogenous bone or with bone substitutes.

9.3.2 Short vs. Long Dental Implants

While there are many predictable bone augmentation techniques and graft materials with high success rates, severe ridge deficiencies require extensive ridge augmentation, which requires additional time and expense and results in greater morbidity. Systematic reviews and meta-analyses have examined the clinical outcomes of short dental implants (≤8 mm) and extra-short dental implants (≤6 mm) as an alternative to standard-length implants (>8 mm) as a less invasive approach.

Iezzi et al. conducted a systematic review and meta-analysis of RCTs and found that short dental implants (<7 mm) placed in native bone can be equally effective as standard-length implants placed in augmented bone for rehabilitation of partially edentulous and posterior atrophic jaws in the medium term up to 5 years [117]. There was a trend for significantly lower marginal bone loss and lower incidence of complications with short implants and no difference in implant survival rates. Most of the studies were randomized. However, the majority were judged to have a moderate to high risk of bias, primarily due to unclear blinding of outcome assessment (detection bias) and incomplete outcome data (attrition bias). Another recent meta-analysis compared clinical outcomes of extra-short (δ6 mm) implants to long (ε 8 mm) implants with or without bone augmentation [118] and found comparable 1- and 3-year implant survival rates with a significantly higher survival rate in the longer implant group at 5-years post-treatment. The significantly improved survival rate seen in the longer implant group was found only in implants placed in the native bone; the rates were not different in the reconstructed bone group. Similarly, mandibular longer implants with vertical augmentation displayed slightly poorer survival than extra-short implants at 1 year. Also, the marginal bone loss and biological complications rate, e.g., paresthesia, graft infection, graft resorption, and perforation of the sinus membrane, favored extra-short implants while the prosthetic complications rate was not different among the groups. Oral health study designs frequently collect information from multiple sites within the same subject, hence introducing a generally positive correlation among responses within subjects. This may lead to an overestimation of the performance of implants. Future RCTs should adjust for within-patient correlations to help draw appropriate conclusions. In addition, only 20 out of 31 studies conformed to the CONSORT statement, and only 8 out of 30 RCTs were registered in a public database. Dental researchers should adhere to the CONSORT statement and register their trials in public databases, as has been required by many medical journals as well, to improve the quality of the RCTs and, consequently, improve patient care [118].

9.3.3 Timing of Implant Placement

Speakers at the sixth European Association for Osseointegration (EAO) Consensus Conference 2021 [119] assessed four systematic reviews evaluating the impact of dental implant placement timing and loading, and the EAO released consensus statements for implant timing:

- The heterogeneity and quality of the data did not allow for drawing any conclusions on immediate placement in conjunction with different timings of loading and marginal bone changes following different timings of implant placement/loading for implant-supported multiple-unit fixed dental prosthesis;
- The limited amount of data on the effect of implant surface and design on implant survival following different timings of implant placement/loading did not allow us to draw any robust conclusion;
- Based on the studies assessed in relation to aesthetic outcomes (mid-facial mucosa changes, papilla height, and aesthetic indexes), no recommendation could be made in favor of a specific timing for implant placement;
- There are no differences in aesthetic outcomes between IP + IL (Immediate implant placement with immediate provisionalization/ loading), EP + IL (Early implant placement with immediate provisionalization/ loading), and DP + DL (Late implant placement with immediate provisionalization/loading). There is a trend that the mid-facial mucosa and PES (Pink Esthetic Score) changes observed in the first 12 months of healing are not maintained/observed in the long term for up to 5 years;
- There is no strong evidence that the timing for implant placement or loading of implant-supported single crowns influences patients´ comfort or satisfaction. There is some evidence that patients rehabilitated with full-arch fixed dental prosthesis demonstrate higher patient satisfaction with immediate than with early or delayed loaded implant reconstructions for a period of up to 3 months, but the difference is not frequently found 1 year after baseline registration.

Troiano et al. (2018) [46], analyzed the current evidence regarding differences in early and late implant failure as well as in marginal bone level (MBL) changes between submerged and nonsubmerged healed dental implants. They reported a small higher rate (2%) of early implant failure when a nonsubmerged healing approach is performed. The authors found that late implant failure does not appear to be different in submerged or nonsubmerged healing, but the power of evidence, as determined by trial sequential analysis, was not high. With regards to marginal bone level changes at 1 year from implant load, they found that nonsubmerged healing may better preserve marginal bone, although with a small effect size (0.13 mm). Thus, more studies are needed in this area.

9.3.4 Guided vs Nonguided Implant Placement

Implants may be placed with a flap or a flapless approach, free-handed without the use of a surgical guide, partially-guided with the use of a nonrestrictive or restrictive surgical guide or fully guided with the use of a static computer-aided surgical guide or with a dynamic computer-aided guided approach. Interactive CT studies containing anatomic and prosthetic information can be used to plan partially- (i.e., no depth or vertical control) and fully guided (i.e., mesio-distal and buccolingual positions, vertical depth, and hex timing are controlled) implant surgery [120].

A multicenter clinical trial evaluated the accuracy and precision of CAD/CAM (computer-aided design/computer-assisted manufacture) surgical guides [121]. Implants placed using bone- and mucosa- supported guides were more precise than guides supported by teeth or a combination of teeth and mucosa; however, the differences were not statistically significant. The authors advised maintaining a safe distance of 2 mm between implants and anatomical structures, considering the mean positional discrepancies between the planned and actual implant outcomes [121].

A recent systematic review of the RCTs [122] found that a flapless static computer-guided implant placement showed improved outcomes than a flapped freehanded implant placement and a cast-based partially guided implant placement in terms of less depth deviation, less angular deviation, less 3D bodily deviation (moderate/high certainty evidence) besides significantly reducing the surgery time and less intra- and post-operative morbidity (very low/low-certainty evidence). The authors point out that the long-term efficacy outcomes of these approaches, especially on implant survival, success, and incidence of peri-implant diseases, are yet to be determined [122]. A combined static and dynamic computer-guided implant surgery was shown to have better accuracy of 3D positioning at the platform and the apex and less angular deviation than either approach alone and also freehand surgery for single implant placement [123]. It must be emphasized that the flapless and guided surgical approaches have a learning curve and require additional preoperative and intraoperative planning; hence, the clinician should become familiar with these techniques.

9.3.5 Peri-implant Diseases and Treatment

Despite high implant survival rates of 92.8%–97.1% over a follow-up period of 10 years for partially and fully edentulous patients [124, 125], dental implants are prone to complications like peri-implantitis [126]. Peri-implantitis can be asymptomatic, with only signs of bleeding on probing, attachment loss, and bone loss. It can also have clinical signs of increasing probing depths, suppuration, draining sinus, and peri-implant mucosal swelling or recession. If not detected and treated earlier, the bony destruction could extend the whole length of the implant, resulting in loss of implant stability [127].

Ting et al. (2018) performed a comprehensive overview of systematic reviews and meta-analyses pertaining to peri-implantitis in humans, including the prevalence and incidence, the diagnostic findings, microbial findings, effects of systemic diseases, and treatment of peri-implantitis [128]. They concluded that the occurrence of peri-implantitis was higher in patients with periodontitis, in patients who smoke, and after 5 years of implant function. The microbial profile of peri-implantitis was different from periodontitis. In addition to the prevalent periodontal pathogens, peri-implantitis sites can also have opportunistic bacteria like *Staphylococcus aureus*, *Staphylococcus intermedius*, *Streptococcus mitis,* and *Hemophilus influenzae*. The risk for peri-implantitis was higher in patients with uncontrolled diabetes and cardiovascular disease. Surgical treatment of peri-implantitis can reduce probing depths, and guided bone regeneration can be unpredictable in peri-implantitis treatment. Different combinations of adjunctive treatments for surgical and nonsurgical interventions can produce successful peri-implantitis treatment outcomes. There was no strong evidence to suggest the most effective treatment intervention for peri-implantitis; however, any other single or combined interventions were better in peri-implantitis treatment than debridement alone. Finally, postimplant maintenance may be crucial in patients with a high risk of peri-implantitis. The authors cautioned that the included studies have various degrees of heterogeneity in study design, case selection, and treatment. And since there is no accepted standard protocol for treating peri-implantitis, the majority of studies were designed as a comparison between two completely different types of intervention rather than between a recognized control. Future RCTs are also needed using standardized definitions for peri-implantitis for all forms of peri-implantitis treatment interventions.

9.3.6 Implant Maintenance

Peri-implantitis occurs with a frequency from 1% to 47% at implant level [129]. To date, there is no evidence-based guideline or protocol for the prevention of peri-implant diseases. Monje et al. [130] assessed the impact of peri-implant maintenance therapy (PIMT) on the prevention of peri-implant diseases. The authors found that there is a positive impact of PIMT on peri-implant tissue health as well as implant survival rate (ISR) and that a reasonable interval of PIMT might be 5–6 months because of the positive significant impact on the incidence of peri-implantitis. The authors concluded that PIMT as supportive periodontal therapy must be customized according to patients' risk profiling. It is also important to assess patient-, clinical-, and implant-related factors. As pointed out by these authors, there are many design considerations and limitations for studies on implant maintenance. Because of ethical principles, peri-implantitis cannot be studied by restricting the patient from conducting oral hygiene to observe the appearance and development of the disease. Therefore, the existing studies may not reflect the state of the art on PIMT. Box 9.2 provides summary of the main findings from the key RCTs, systematic reviews, Cochrane reviews and meta-analyses in Implantology.

Box 9.2 Summary of the Main Findings from the Key RCTs, Systematic Reviews, Cochrane Reviews, and Meta-Analyses in Implantology

- Alveolar ridge preservation may prevent horizontal, vertical mid-buccal and vertical mid-lingual bone resorption as compared to tooth extraction alone. Particulate xenogenic or allogenic materials covered with an absorbable collagen membrane or rapidly absorbable collagen sponge provided the most favorable outcome for horizontal ridge preservation.
- Horizontal bone augmentation successfully increases bone width when performed simultaneously or prior to dental implant placement.
- Vertical ridge augmentation is a feasible and effective treatment modality for reconstruction of vertical ridge defects however complications with these procedures are more common.
- Maxillary sinus floor augmentation is a reliable treatment modality in the long-term for patients with partially and fully edentulous maxillae.
- There is limited evidence to support the use of biologic mediators such as growth factors as adjunct to regeneration of alveolar ridge preservation and ridge augmentation procedures.
- Short dental implants (<7 mm) placed in native bone can be equally effective as standard-length implants placed in augmented bone for rehabilitation of partially edentulous and posterior atrophic jaws in the medium term up to 5 years. Extra-short implants (6 mm) can also be an acceptable alternative to longer implants in the atrophic posterior arches.
- There are no differences in marginal bone level changes, implant survival, aesthetic outcomes or patient comfort or satisfaction with different timing of implant placement (immediate or delayed) or loading (immediate provisionalization or loading or delayed loading).
- Flapless static computer-guided implant placement showed improved outcomes than a flapped free-handed implant placement and a cast-based partially-guided implant placement in terms of less depth deviation, less angular deviation, less 3D bodily deviation (moderate/high certainty evidence) besides significantly reducing the surgery time and less intra- and post-operative morbidity (very low/low certainty evidence).
- Prevalence of peri-implantitis is higher in patients with periodontitis, in patients who smoke, and after 5 years of implant function. The microbial profile of peri-implantitis is different from periodontitis. The risk for peri-implantitis is higher

in patients with uncontrolled diabetes and cardiovascular disease.
- Surgical treatment of peri-implantitis can reduce probing depths and guided bone regeneration can be unpredictable in peri-implantitis treatment. Different combination of adjunctive treatments for surgical and non-surgical interventions can produce successful peri-implantitis treatment outcomes.
- 0Peri-implant maintenance therapy (PIMT) has a positive impact on peri-implant tissue health as well as implant survival rate.

9.4 Conclusions

A significant increase in the number of randomized clinical trials over the last 20 years in Periodontology and Implantology attests to the interest in high-level evidence for existing and constantly evolving materials and treatment modalities. There are numerous methodological and quality control issues in the existing body of work that prevent definitive conclusions. These limitations cause many trials to be excluded from systematic reviews and meta-analyses or convey low certainty to the generated evidence, both of which further reduce the value of the research to the practice community. We have underscored many such issues noted in various studies and have identified areas for future research. There are many knowledge gaps and important topics for further investigation. Examples are:

- There is a need for greater author and journal editor awareness of the importance of complete CONSORT flow diagrams in periodontology and implantology RCTs.
- Risk of bias must be minimized. The randomization process (sequence and allocation concealment) and examiner blinding should be described. Outcome data should be reported completely.
- Future studies should utilize the new 2018 classification for periodontitis and peri-implant diseases. In addition to PD and CAL changes, studies should also consider other indicators such as bleeding on probing, periodontal Index, and gingival Index, bacterial changes, when comparing different periodontal pocket depths.
- Single and multi-rooted teeth should be measured separately because they may respond differently to treatment due to local anatomical conditions and complex morphology in the furcation area.
- Objective outcomes like tooth loss should be studied as these may be less amenable to bias.
- Economic costs and patient burden should also be addressed for different treatment modalities.
- Standardized dosage and duration for antibiotic administration, assessment of antibiotic resistance, and consistent reporting of adverse events should be done.
- The authors should also plan to make their data available for other researchers to reuse and analyze to overcome the issue of limited data availability and to advance medical knowledge and develop improved treatments.
- Optimal carriers for bioactive agents, dose, and timing of administration as well as the possibility of combining different agents to promote synergistic effects should be investigated.
- Long-term outcomes of the augmented bone and implant outcomes in the augmented bone need to be studied.
- Future studies should be designed to include patient-related outcome measures (PROM) and local, systemic, and surgical procedure-related variables as well.

The information in this chapter should aid clinical researchers in their development of sound clinical trials to generate more meaningful and robust scientific data of value to clinical practice.

9.5 Case Scenario Exercise

9.5.1 Case Scenario (Based on Koromantzos et al. 2011) [131]

The proposed randomized, controlled clinical trial study aims to assess the effect of nonsurgical periodontal therapy on glycemic control of type 2 diabetes patients with moderate-to-severe periodontitis.

Questions

1. What outcome would you use to assess the glycemic control of type 2 diabetes patients?
2. Provide an example of your detailed protocol for providing periodontal treatment for the experimental and control group.

Answers

1. Glycemic control in type 2 diabetes patients can be evaluated using three parameters: glycosylated hemoglobin (HbA1c), fasting blood glucose (FBG), and postprandial glucose (P PG). Glycosylated hemoglobin is the gold standard for glycemic control estimation. Thus, we will use that as the outcome. We will use a cutoff of glycated hemoglobin (Hb1Ac) of 7%, as defined by the American Diabetes Association (ADA) as good diabetic control.
2. All participants will receive oral hygiene instructions at baseline. The intervention group will receive nonurgical periodontal therapy in the form of full-mouth scaling and root planing (SRP) in two sessions, 1 week apart, with the use of a specific ultrasonic scaler and hand instruments, under local anesthesia. Patients in the control group will receive periodontal prophylaxis at baseline in the form of supragingival removal of plaque and calculus with the same type of ultrasonic scaler. SRP will be performed in the control group after the completion of the study (after the 6-month visit). Teeth with hopeless teeth will be extracted at SRP visits. All patients will receive oral hygiene instructions after each visit, while the intervention group will receive additional supportive SRP at each visit if judged necessary (with the presence of sites with bleeding on probing and/or increased periodontal pocket depth). Periodontal treatment will be administered by the same trained periodontist.

References

1. Xie L, Qin W, Yu T, Pathak JL, Zeng S, Du M. Quality assessment of randomized controlled trial abstracts on drug therapy of periodontal disease from the abstracts published in dental science citation indexed journals in the last ten years. Med Oral Patol Oral Cir Bucal. 2020;25(5):e626–e33.
2. Begg C, Cho M, Eastwood S, Horton R, Moher D, Olkin I, et al. Improving the quality of reporting of randomized controlled trials—the CONSORT statement. JAMA. 1996;276(8):637–9.
3. Boutron I, Moher D, Altman DG, Schulz KF, Ravaud P. Extending the CONSORT statement to randomized trials of nonpharmacologic treatment: explanation and elaboration. Ann Intern Med. 2008;148:295–309.
4. Leow NM, Hussain Z, Petrie A, Donos N, Needleman IG. Has the quality of reporting in periodontology changed in 14 years? A systematic review J Clin Periodontol. 2016;43:833–8.
5. Meyer HJ, Pandis N, Seehra J, et al. Reporting of flow diagrams in randomised controlled trials published in periodontology and implantology: a survey. BMC Med Res Methodol. 2023;23(1):105.
6. Schulz KF, Altman DG, Moher D. CONSORT 2010 statement: updated guidelines for reporting parallel group randomized trials. Ann Intern Med. 2010;152:726–32.
7. Hopewell S, Clarke M, Moher D, Wager E, Middleton P, Altman DG, Schulz KF, CONSORT Group. CONSORT for reporting randomized controlled trials in journal and conference abstracts: explanation and elaboration. PLoS Med. 2008;5(1):e20.
8. Hrobjartsson A, Emanuelsson F, Skou TA, Hilden J, Brorson S. Bias due to lack of patient blinding in clinical trials. A systematic review of trials randomizing patients to blind and nonblind sub-studies. Int J Epidemiol. 2014;43:1272–83.
9. Hrobjartsson A, Thomsen AS, Emanuelsson F, Tendal B, Hilden J, Boutron I, et al. Observer bias in randomised clinical trials with binary outcomes: systematic review of trials with both blinded and nonblinded outcome assessors. BMJ. 2012;344:1–11.
10. Lexchin J, Bero LA, Djulbegovic B, Clark O. Pharmaceutical industry sponsorship and research outcome and quality: systematic review. BMJ. 2003;326(7400):1167–70.
11. Bero L, Oostvogel F, Bacchetti P, Lee K. Factors associated with findings of published trials of drug-

drug comparisons: why some statins appear more efficacious than others. PLoS Med. 2007;4(6): e184.
12. Ferrarotti F, Giraudi M, Citterio F, Fratini A, Gualini G, Piccoli GM, et al. Pocket elimination after osseous resective surgery: a systematic review and meta-analysis. J Clin Periodontol. 2020;47(6):756–67.
13. Kaldahl WB, Kalkwarf KL, Patil KD. A review of longitudinal studies that compared periodontal therapies. J Periodontol. 1993;64(4):243–53.
14. Mailoa J, Lin GH, Khoshkam V, MacEachern M, Chan HL, Wang HL. Long-term effect of four surgical periodontal therapies and one non-surgical therapy: a systematic review and meta-analysis. J Periodontol. 2015;86(10):1150–8.
15. Polak D, Wilensky A, Antonoglou GN, Shapira L, Goldstein M, Martin C. The efficacy of pocket elimination/reduction compared to access flap surgery: a systematic review and meta-analysis. J Clin Periodontol. 2020;47(Suppl. 22):303–19.
16. Sanz-Sanchez I, Montero E, Citterio F, Romano F, Molina A, Aimetti M. Efficacy of access flap procedures compared to subgingival debridement in the treatment of periodontitis. A systematic review and meta-analysis. J Clin Periodontol. 2020;47(Suppl 22):282–302.
17. Muniz F, Langa GPJ, Pimentel RP, Martins JR, Pereira DH, Rosing CK. Comparison between hand and sonic/ultrasonic instruments for periodontal treatment: systematic review with meta-analysis. J Int Acad Periodontol. 2020;22(4):187–204.
18. Suvan J, Leira Y, Moreno Sancho FM, Graziani F, Derks J, Tomasi C. Subgingival instrumentation for treatment of periodontitis. A systematic review. J Clin Periodontol. 2020;47(Suppl. 22): 155–75.
19. Zhang X, Hu Z, Zhu X, Li W, Chen J. Treating periodontitis-a systematic review and meta-analysis comparing ultrasonic and manual subgingival scaling at different probing pocket depths. BMC Oral Health. 2020;20(1):176.
20. Van der Weijden GA, Dekkers GJ, Slot DE. Success of non-surgical periodontal therapy in adult periodontitis patients: a retrospective analysis. Int J Dent Hyg. 2019;17:309–17.
21. Lang NP, Tan WC, Krahenmann MA, Zwahlen M. A systematic review of the effects of full-mouth debridement with and without antiseptics in patients with chronic periodontitis. J Clin Periodontol. 2008;35(Suppl. 8):8–21.
22. Eberhard J, Jepsen S, Jervoe-Storm PM, Needleman I, Worthington HV. Full-mouth treatment modalities (within 24 hours) for chronic periodontitis in adults. Cochrane Database Syst Rev. 2015;(4):CD004622.
23. da Costa L, Amaral C, Barbirato DDS, Leao ATT, Fogacci MF. Chlorhexidine mouthwash as an adjunct to mechanical therapy in chronic periodontitis: a meta-analysis. J Am Dent Assoc. 2017;148(5):308–18.
24. Oh TJ. Adjunctive use of chlorhexidine mouthwash to nonsurgical periodontal therapy may enhance periodontal pocket depth reduction. J Evid Based Dent Pract. 2018;18(4):358–9.
25. Herrera D, Matesanz P, Martin C, Oud V, Feres M, Teughels W. Adjunctive effect of locally delivered antimicrobials in periodontitis therapy: a systematic review and meta-analysis. J Clin Periodontol. 2020;47(Suppl. 22):239–56.
26. Wang CY, Yang YH, Li H, Lin PY, Su YT, Kuo MY, et al. Adjunctive local treatments for patients with residual pockets during supportive periodontal care: a systematic review and network meta-analysis. J Clin Periodontol. 2020;47(12):1496–510.
27. Yusri S, Elfana A, Elbattawy W, Fawzy El-Sayed KM. Effect of locally delivered adjunctive antibiotics during surgical periodontal therapy: a systematic review and meta-analysis. Clin Oral Investig. 2021;25(9):5127–38.
28. Khattri S, Kumbargere Nagraj S, Arora A, Eachempati P, Kusum CK, Bhat KG, et al. Adjunctive systemic antimicrobials for the non-surgical treatment of periodontitis. Cochrane Database Syst Rev. 2020;11:CD012568.
29. Haffajee AD, Socransky SS, Gunsolley JC. Systemic anti-infective periodontal therapy. A systematic review. Ann Periodontol. 2003;8(1):115–81.
30. Keestra JA, Grosjean I, Coucke W, Quirynen M, Teughels W. Non-surgical periodontal therapy with systemic antibiotics in patients with untreated aggressive periodontitis: a systematic review and meta-analysis. J Periodontal Res. 2015;50(6):689–706.
31. Nibali L, Koidou VP, Hamborg T, Donos N. Empirical or microbiologically guided systemic antimicrobials as adjuncts to non-surgical periodontal therapy? A systematic review. J Clin Periodontol. 2019;46(10):999–1012.
32. Sgolastra F, Petrucci A, Gatto R, Giannoni M, Monaco A. Long-term efficacy of subantimicrobial-dose doxycycline as an adjunctive treatment to scaling and root planing: a systematic review and meta-analysis. J Periodontol. 2011;82(11):1570–81.
33. Teughels W, Feres M, Oud V, Martin C, Matesanz P, Herrera D. Adjunctive effect of systemic antimicrobials in periodontitis therapy: a systematic review and meta-analysis. J Clin Periodontol. 2020;47(Suppl 22):257–81.
34. Reddy MS, Geurs NC, Gunsolley JC. Periodontal host modulation with antiproteinase, anti-inflammatory, and bone-sparing agents. A systematic review. Ann Periodontol. 2003;8(1):12–37.
35. Ho SN, Acharya A, Sidharthan S, Li KY, Leung WK, McGrath C, et al. A systematic review and meta-analysis of clinical, immunological, and microbiological shift in periodontitis after nonsurgical periodontal therapy with adjunctive use of probiotics. J Evid Based Dent Pract. 2020;20(1):101397.
36. Hu D, Zhong T, Dai Q. Clinical efficacy of probiotics as an adjunctive therapy to scaling and root planning in the management of periodontitis: a systematic review and meta-analysis of randomized controlled trails. J Evid Based Dent Pract. 2021;21(2):101547.

37. Gheisary Z, Mahmood R, Harri Shivanantham A, Liu J, Lieffers JRL, Papagerakis P, et al. The Clinical, microbiological, and immunological effects of probiotic supplementation on prevention and treatment of periodontal diseases: a systematic review and meta-analysis. Nutrients. 2022;14(5):1036.
38. Martin-Cabezas R, Davideau JL, Tenenbaum H, Huck O. Clinical efficacy of probiotics as an adjunctive therapy to non-surgical periodontal treatment of chronic periodontitis: a systematic review and meta-analysis. J Clin Periodontol. 2016;43(6):520–30.
39. Song D, Liu XR. Role of probiotics containing Lactobacillus reuteri in adjunct to scaling and root planing for management of patients with chronic periodontitis: a meta-analysis. Eur Rev Med Pharmacol Sci. 2020;24(8):4495–505.
40. Ambrosio LMB, Rovai ES, Sendyk DI, Holzhausen M, Pannuti CM. Does the adjunctive use of statins provide additional benefits to nonsurgical periodontal treatment? A systematic review and meta-analysis. J Periodontal Res. 2018;53(1):12–21.
41. Cecoro G, Piccirillo A, Martuscelli G, Del Fabbro M, Annunziata M, Guida L. Efficacy of locally delivered statins as an adjunct to scaling and root planning in the treatment of periodontitis: a systematic review and meta-analysis. Eur Rev Med Pharmacol Sci. 2021;25(18):5737–54.
42. Meza-Mauricio J, Soto-Penaloza D, Penarrocha-Oltra D, Montiel-Company JM, Peruzzo DC. Locally applied statins as adjuvants to non-surgical periodontal treatment for chronic periodontitis: a systematic review and meta-analysis. Clin Oral Investig. 2018;22(7):2413–30.
43. Sinjab K, Zimmo N, Lin GH, Chung MP, Shaikh L, Wang HL. The effect of locally delivered statins on treating periodontal intrabony defects: a systematic review and meta-analysis. J Periodontol. 2017;88(4):357–67.
44. Nicolini AC, Grisa TA, Muniz F, Rosing CK, Cavagni J. Effect of adjuvant use of metformin on periodontal treatment: a systematic review and meta-analysis. Clin Oral Investig. 2019;23(6):2659–66.
45. Tsai SJ, Ding YW, Shih MC, Tu YK. Systematic review and sequential network meta-analysis on the efficacy of periodontal regenerative therapies. J Clin Periodontol. 2020;47(9):1108–20.
46. Troiano G, Laino L, Zhurakivska K, Cicciu M, Lo Muzio L, Lo Russo L. Addition of enamel matrix derivatives to bone substitutes for the tréatment of intrabony defects: a systematic review, meta-analysis and trial sequential analysis. J Clin Periodontol. 2017;44(7):729–38.
47. Zhou S, Sun C, Huang S, Wu X, Zhao Y, Pan C, et al. Efficacy of adjunctive bioactive materials in the treatment of periodontal intrabony defects: a systematic review and meta-analysis. Biomed Res Int. 2018;2018:8670832.
48. Aimetti M, Fratini A, Manavella V, Giraudi M, Citterio F, Ferrarotti F, et al. Pocket resolution in regenerative treatment of intrabony defects with papilla preservation techniques: a systematic review and meta-analysis of randomized clinical trials. J Clin Periodontol. 2021;48(6):843–58.
49. Diaz-Faes L, Fernandez-Somoano A, Magan-Fernandez A, Mesa F. Efficacy of regenerative therapy in aggressive periodontitis: a systematic review and meta-analysis of randomised controlled clinical trials. Clin Oral Investig. 2020;24(4):1369–78.
50. Esposito M, Grusovin MG, Papanikolaou N, Coulthard P, Worthington HV. Enamel matrix derivative (Emdogain) for periodontal tissue regeneration in intrabony defects. A Cochrane systematic review. Eur J Oral Implantol. 2009;2(4):247–66.
51. Matarasso M, Iorio-Siciliano V, Blasi A, Ramaglia L, Salvi GE, Sculean A. Enamel matrix derivative and bone grafts for periodontal regeneration of intrabony defects. A systematic review and meta-analysis. Clin Oral Investig. 2015;19(7):1581–93.
52. Roccuzzo A, Imber JC, Stahli A, Kloukos D, Salvi GE, Sculean A. Enamel matrix derivative as adjunctive to non-surgical periodontal therapy: a systematic review and meta-analysis of randomized controlled trials. Clin Oral Investig. 2022;26(6):4263–80.
53. Graziani F, Gennai S, Cei S, Ducci F, Discepoli N, Carmignani A, et al. Does enamel matrix derivative application provide additional clinical benefits in residual periodontal pockets associated with suprabony defects? A systematic review and meta-analysis of randomized clinical trials. J Clin Periodontol. 2014;41(4):377–86.
54. Darby IB, Morris KH. A systematic review of the use of growth factors in human periodontal regeneration. J Periodontol. 2013;84(4):465–76.
55. Khoshkam V, Chan HL, Lin GH, Mailoa J, Giannobile WV, Wang HL, et al. Outcomes of regenerative treatment with rhPDGF-BB and rhFGF-2 for periodontal intra-bony defects: a systematic review and meta-analysis. J Clin Periodontol. 2015;42(3):272–80.
56. Li F, Yu F, Xu X, Li C, Huang D, Zhou X, et al. Evaluation of recombinant human FGF-2 and PDGF-BB in periodontal regeneration: a systematic review and meta-analysis. Sci Rep. 2017;7(1):65.
57. Del Fabbro M, Karanxha L, Panda S, Bucchi C, Nadathur Doraiswamy J, Sankari M, et al. Autologous platelet concentrates for treating periodontal infrabony defects. Cochrane Database Syst Rev. 2018;11:CD011423.
58. Hou X, Yuan J, Aisaiti A, Liu Y, Zhao J. The effect of platelet-rich plasma on clinical outcomes of the surgical treatment of periodontal intrabony defects: a systematic review and meta-analysis. BMC Oral Health. 2016;16(1):71.
59. Li R, Liu Y, Xu T, Zhao H, Hou J, Wu Y, et al. The additional effect of autologous platelet concentrates to coronally advanced flap in the treatment of gingival recessions: a systematic review and meta-analysis. Biomed Res Int. 2019;2019:2587245.
60. Rosello-Camps A, Monje A, Lin GH, Khoshkam V, Chavez-Gatty M, Wang HL, et al. Platelet-rich plasma for periodontal regeneration in the treatment of intrabony defects: a meta-analysis on prospective

clinical trials. Oral Surg Oral Med Oral Pathol Oral Radiol. 2015;120(5):562–74.
61. Miron RJ, Moraschini V, Fujioka-Kobayashi M, Zhang Y, Kawase T, Cosgarea R, et al. Use of platelet-rich fibrin for the treatment of periodontal intrabony defects: a systematic review and meta-analysis. Clin Oral Investig. 2021;25(5):2461–78.
62. Avila-Ortiz G, De Buitrago JG, Reddy MS. Periodontal regeneration—furcation defects: a systematic review from the AAP Regeneration Workshop. J Periodontol. 2015;86(Suppl. 2):S108–30.
63. Graziani F, Gennai S, Karapetsa D, Rosini S, Filice N, Gabriele M, et al. Clinical performance of access flap in the treatment of class II furcation defects. A systematic review and meta-analysis of randomized clinical trials. J Clin Periodontol. 2015;42(2):169–81.
64. Oliveira HFE, Verri F, Lemos CA, Cruz R, Batista VES, Pellizzer E, et al. Clinical evidence for treatment of class II periodontal furcation defects. Systematic review and meta-analysis. J Int Acad Periodontol. 2020;22(3):117–28.
65. Cecoro G, Guida L, Iuorio A, Nucci L, Pesce P, Annunziata M. Cell-based therapies for the surgical treatment of periodontal intrabony defects: a systematic review. Eur Rev Med Pharmacol Sci. 2021;25(21):6592–602.
66. Novello S, Debouche A, Philippe M, Naudet F, Jeanne S. Clinical application of mesenchymal stem cells in periodontal regeneration: a systematic review and meta-analysis. J Periodontal Res. 2020;55(1):1–12.
67. Zhang Y, Zhao W, Jia L, Xu N, Xiao Y, Li Q. The application of stem cells in tissue engineering for the regeneration of periodontal defects in randomized controlled trial: a systematic review and meta-analysis. J Evid Based Dent Pract. 2022;22(2):101713.
68. Clem D, Heard R, McGuire M, Scheyer ET, Richardson C, Toback G, et al. Comparison of Er, Cr:YSGG laser to minimally invasive surgical technique in the treatment of intrabony defects: six-month results of a multicenter, randomized, controlled study. J Periodontol. 2021;92(4):496–506.
69. Behdin S, Monje A, Lin GH, Edwards B, Othman A, Wang HL. Effectiveness of laser application for periodontal surgical therapy: systematic review and meta-analysis. J Periodontol. 2015;86(12):1352–63.
70. Ma L, Zhang X, Ma Z, Shi H, Zhang Y, Wu M, et al. Clinical Effectiveness of Er: YAG lasers adjunct to scaling and root planing in non-surgical treatment of chronic periodontitis: a meta-analysis of randomized controlled trials. Med Sci Monit. 2018;24:7090–9.
71. Mailoa J, Lin GH, Chan HL, MacEachern M, Wang HL. Clinical outcomes of using lasers for peri-implantitis surface detoxification: a systematic review and meta-analysis. J Periodontol. 2014;85(9):1194–202.
72. Schwarz F, Aoki A, Becker J, Sculean A. Laser application in non-surgical periodontal therapy: a systematic review. J Clin Periodontol. 2008;35(8 Suppl):29–44.
73. Akram Z, Hyder T, Al-Hamoudi N, Binshabaib MS, Alharthi SS, Hanif A. Efficacy of photodynamic therapy versus antibiotics as an adjunct to scaling and root planing in the treatment of periodontitis: a systematic review and meta-analysis. Photodiagn Photodyn Ther. 2017;19:86–92.
74. Azarpazhooh A, Shah PS, Tenenbaum HC, Goldberg MB. The effect of photodynamic therapy for periodontitis: a systematic review and meta-analysis. J Periodontol. 2010;81(1):4–14.
75. Salvi GE, Stahli A, Schmidt JC, Ramseier CA, Sculean A, Walter C. Adjunctive laser or antimicrobial photodynamic therapy to non-surgical mechanical instrumentation in patients with untreated periodontitis: a systematic review and meta-analysis. J Clin Periodontol. 2020;47(Suppl. 22):176–98.
76. Xue D, Tang L, Bai Y, Ding Q, Wang P, Zhao Y. Clinical efficacy of photodynamic therapy adjunctive to scaling and root planing in the treatment of chronic periodontitis: a systematic review and meta-analysis. Photodiagn Photodyn Ther. 2017;18:119–27.
77. Zhao Y, Pu R, Qian Y, Shi J, Si M. Antimicrobial photodynamic therapy versus antibiotics as an adjunct in the treatment of periodontitis and peri-implantitis: a systematic review and meta-analysis. Photodiagn Photodyn Ther. 2021;34:102231.
78. Chambrone L, Wang HL, Romanos GE. Antimicrobial photodynamic therapy for the treatment of periodontitis and peri-implantitis: an American Academy of Periodontology best evidence review. J Periodontol. 2018;89(7):783–803.
79. Souza EQM, da Rocha TE, Toro LF, Guiati IZ, Ervolino E, Garcia VG, et al. Antimicrobial photodynamic therapy compared to systemic antibiotic therapy in non-surgical treatment of periodontitis: systematic review and meta-analysis. Photodiagn Photodyn Ther. 2020;31:101808.
80. Chambrone L, Salinas Ortega MA, Sukekava F, Rotundo R, Kalemaj Z, Buti J, et al. Root coverage procedures for treating localised and multiple recession-type defects. Cochrane Database Syst Rev. 2018;10:CD007161.
81. Naudet F, Siebert M, Pellen C, Gaba J, Axfors C, Cristea I, Danchev V, Mansmann U, Ohmann C, Wallach JD, Moher D, Ioannidis JPA. Medical journal requirements for clinical trial data sharing: ripe for improvement. PLoS Med. 2021;18(10):e1003844. https://doi.org/10.1371/journal.pmed.1003844.
82. Chambrone L, Pannuti CM, Tu YK, Chambrone LA. Evidence-based periodontal plastic surgery. II. An individual data meta-analysis for evaluating factors in achieving complete root coverage. J Periodontol. 2012;83(4):477–90.
83. Hwang D, Wang HL. Flap thickness as a predictor of root coverage: a systematic review. J Periodontol. 2006;77(10):1625–34.
84. AlSarhan MA, Al Jasser R, Tarish MA, AlHuzaimi AI, Alzoman H. Xenogeneic collagen matrix versus connective tissue graft for the treatment of

multiple gingival recessions: a systematic review and meta-analysis. Clin Exp Dent Res. 2019;5(5):566–79.
85. Tonetti MS, Cortellini P, Bonaccini D, Deng K, Cairo F, Allegri M, et al. Autologous connective tissue graft or xenogenic collagen matrix with coronally advanced flaps for coverage of multiple adjacent gingival recession. 36-month follow-up of a randomized multicentre trial. J Clin Periodontol. 2021;48(7):962–9.
86. Meza-Mauricio J, Cortez-Gianezzi J, Duarte PM, Tavelli L, Rasperini G, de Faveri M. Comparison between a xenogeneic dermal matrix and connective tissue graft for the treatment of multiple adjacent gingival recessions: a randomized controlled clinical trial. Clin Oral Investig. 2021;25(12):6919–29.
87. Sangiorgio JPM, Neves F, Rocha Dos Santos M, Franca-Grohmann IL, Casarin RCV, Casati MZ, et al. Xenogenous collagen matrix and/or enamel matrix derivative for treatment of localized gingival recessions: a randomized clinical trial. Part I: Clinical outcomes. J Periodontol. 2017;88(12):1309–18.
88. Cairo F, Cortellini P, Pilloni A, Nieri M, Cincinelli S, Amunni F, et al. Clinical efficacy of coronally advanced flap with or without connective tissue graft for the treatment of multiple adjacent gingival recessions in the aesthetic area: a randomized controlled clinical trial. J Clin Periodontol. 2016;43(10):849–56.
89. Cortellini P, Tonetti M, Baldi C, Francetti L, Rasperini G, Rotundo R, et al. Does placement of a connective tissue graft improve the outcomes of coronally advanced flap for coverage of single gingival recessions in upper anterior teeth? A multi-centre, randomized, double-blind, clinical trial. J Clin Periodontol. 2009;36(1):68–79.
90. Carvelli G, Caton JG, Barmak AB, Tsigarida A. Comparison of coronally advanced flap and connective tissue graft with or without enamel matrix derivative for gingival recession treatment: a systematic review and meta-analysis of randomized clinical trials. Int J Periodontics Restorative Dent. 2022;42(5):e121–e31.
91. Meza Mauricio J, Furquim CP, Bustillos-Torrez W, Soto-Penaloza D, Penarrocha-Oltra D, Retamal-Valdes B, et al. Does enamel matrix derivative application provide additional clinical benefits in the treatment of maxillary Miller class I and II gingival recession? A systematic review and meta-analysis. Clin Oral Investig. 2021;25(4):1613–26.
92. Mercado F, Hamlet S, Ivanovski S. Subepithelial connective tissue graft with or without enamel matrix derivative for the treatment of multiple Class III-IV recessions in lower anterior teeth: a 3-year randomized clinical trial. J Periodontol. 2020;91(4):473–83.
93. Rasperini G, Roccuzzo M, Francetti L, Acunzo R, Consonni D, Silvestri M. Subepithelial connective tissue graft for treatment of gingival recessions with and without enamel matrix derivative: a multicenter, randomized controlled clinical trial. Int J Periodontics Restorative Dent. 2011;31(2):133–9.
94. Tavelli L, Barootchi S, Nguyen TVN, Tattan M, Ravida A, Wang HL. Efficacy of tunnel technique in the treatment of localized and multiple gingival recessions: a systematic review and meta-analysis. J Periodontol. 2018;89(9):1075–90.
95. Acunzo R, Limiroli E, Pagni G, Dudaite A, Consonni D, Rasperini G. Gingival margin stability after mucogingival plastic surgery. The effect of manual versus powered toothbrushing: a randomized clinical trial. J Periodontol. 2016;87(10):1186–94.
96. Barootchi S, Tavelli L, Ravida A, Wang CW, Wang HL. Effect of EDTA root conditioning on the outcome of coronally advanced flap with connective tissue graft: a systematic review and meta-analysis. Clin Oral Investig. 2018;22(8):2727–41.
97. Chambrone L, Preshaw PM, Rosa EF, Heasman PA, Romito GA, Pannuti CM, et al. Effects of smoking cessation on the outcomes of non-surgical periodontal therapy: a systematic review and individual patient data meta-analysis. J Clin Periodontol. 2013;40(6):607–15.
98. Kotsakis GA, Javed F, Hinrichs JE, Karoussis IK, Romanos GE. Impact of cigarette smoking on clinical outcomes of periodontal flap surgical procedures: a systematic review and meta-analysis. J Periodontol. 2015;86(2):254–63.
99. Leite FRM, Nascimento GG, Baake S, Pedersen LD, Scheutz F, Lopez R. Impact of smoking cessation on periodontitis: a systematic review and meta-analysis of prospective longitudinal observational and interventional studies. Nicotine Tob Res. 2019;21(12):1600–8.
100. Iheozor-Ejiofor Z, Middleton P, Esposito M, Glenny AM. Treating periodontal disease for preventing adverse birth outcomes in pregnant women. Cochrane Database Syst Rev. 2017;6:CD005297.
101. Fogacci MF, Vettore MV, Thome Leao AT. The effect of periodontal therapy on preterm low birth weight: a meta-analysis. Obstet Gynecol. 2011;117(1):153–65.
102. Baeza M, Morales A, Cisterna C, Cavalla F, Jara G, Isamitt Y, et al. Effect of periodontal treatment in patients with periodontitis and diabetes: systematic review and meta-analysis. J Appl Oral Sci. 2020;28:e20190248.
103. Simpson TC, Weldon JC, Worthington HV, Needleman I, Wild SH, Moles DR, et al. Treatment of periodontal disease for glycaemic control in people with diabetes mellitus. Cochrane Database Syst Rev. 2015;(11):CD004714.
104. Wang TF, Jen IA, Chou C, Lei YP. Effects of periodontal therapy on metabolic control in patients with type 2 diabetes mellitus and periodontal disease: a meta-analysis. Medicine (Baltimore). 2014;93(28):e292.
105. Engebretson SP, Hyman LG, Michalowicz BS, Schoenfeld ER, Gelato MC, Hou W, et al. The effect of nonsurgical periodontal therapy on hemoglobin A1c levels in persons with type 2 diabetes and chronic periodontitis: a randomized clinical trial. JAMA. 2013;310(23):2523–32.

106. Papageorgiou SN, Reichert C, Jager A, Deschner J. Effect of overweight/obesity on response to periodontal treatment: systematic review and a meta-analysis. J Clin Periodontol. 2015;42(3):247–61.
107. Avila-Ortiz G, Chambrone L, Vignoletti F. Effect of alveolar ridge preservation interventions following tooth extraction: a systematic review and meta-analysis. J Clin Periodontol. 2019;46:195–223.
108. Dam VV, Trinh HA, Rokaya D, Trinh DH. Bone Augmentation for Implant Placement: Recent Advances. Int J Dent. 2022;2022:8900940. https://doi.org/10.1155/2022/8900940. PMID: 35386549; PMCID: PMC8977324.
109. Sehgal H, Hokett SD, Katancik JA. The use of growth factors for guided bone regeneration in clinical periodontics. Curr Oral Health Rep. 2019;6:244–9.
110. Donos N, Dereka X, Calciolari E. The use of bioactive factors to enhance bone regeneration: a narrative review. J Clin Periodontol. 2019;46:124–61.
111. Atieh MA, Alsabeeha NH, Payne AG, Ali S, Faggion CM Jr, Esposito M. Interventions for replacing missing teeth: alveolar ridge preservation techniques for dental implant site development. Cochrane Database Syst Rev. 2021;4(4):CD010176.
112. Esposito M, Grusovin M, Felice P, Karatzopoulos G, Worthington HV, Coulthard P. Interventions for replacing missing teeth: horizontal and vertical bone augmentation techniques for dental implant treatment. Cochrane Database Syst Rev. 2009;(4):CD003607.
113. Naenni N, Hyun-Chang L, Papageorgiou SN, et al. Efficacy of lateral bone augmentation prior to implant placement: a systematic review and meta-analysis. J Clin Periodontol. 2019;46:287–306.
114. Thoma DS, Bienz SP, Figuero E, Jung RE, Sanz-Martín I. Efficacy of lateral bone augmentation performed simultaneously with dental implant placement: a systematic review and meta-analysis. J Clin Periodontol. 2019;46:257–76.
115. Urban IA, Montero E, Monje A, Sanz-Sánchez I. Effectiveness of vertical ridge augmentation interventions: a systematic review and meta-analysis. J Clin Periodontol. 2019;46:319–39.
116. Raghoebar GM, Onclin P, Boven GC, et al. Long-term effectiveness of maxillary sinus floor augmentation: a systematic review and meta-analysis. J Clin Periodontol. 2019;46:307–18.
117. Iezzi G, Perrotti V, Felice P, Barausse C, Piattelli A, Del Fabbro M. Are <7-mm long implants in native bone as effective as longer implants in augmented bone for the rehabilitation of posterior atrophic jaws? A systematic review and meta-analysis. Clin Implant Dent Relat Res. 2020;22:552–66.
118. Yu X, Xu X, Zhang Z, Yang Y, Deng F. A meta-analysis indicating extra-short implants (≤ 6 mm) as an alternative to longer implants (≥ 8 mm) with bone augmentation. Nat Portfolio Sci Rep. 2021;11(1):8152.
119. Donos N, Asche NV, Akbar AN, Francisco H, Gonzales O, Gotfredsen K, Haas R, Happe A, Leow N, Navarro JM, Ornekol T, Payer M, Renouard F, Schliephake H. Impact of timing of dental implant placement and loading: summary and consensus statements of group 1-The 6th EAO Consensus Conference 2021. Clin Oral Implants Res. 2021;32:85–92.
120. Califano JV, Rosenfeld A, Mandelaris G. A logical and progressive approach to computed tomography-guided implantology. Clin Adv Periodont. 2012;2(4):264–73.
121. Testori T, Robiony M, Parenti A, Luongo G, Rosenfeld AL, Ganz SD, Mandelaris GA, Del Fabbro M. Evaluation of accuracy and precision of a new guided surgery system: a multicenter clinical study. Int J Periodontics Restorative Dent. 2014;34:s59–69.
122. Romandini M, Ruales-Carrera E, Sadilina S, Hämmerle CHF, Sanz M. Minimal invasiveness at dental implant placement: a systematic review with meta-analyses on flapless fully guided surgery. Periodontol. 2000;2023(91):89–112.
123. Yotpibulwong T, Arunjaroensuk S, Kaboosaya B, Sinpitaksakul P, Arksornnukit M, Mattheos N, Pimkhaokham A. Accuracy of implant placement with a combined use of static and dynamic computer-assisted implant surgery in single tooth space: a randomized controlled trial. Clin Oral Implants Res. 2023;34:330–41.
124. Albrektsson T, Donos N, Working G. Implant survival and complications. The Third EAO consensus conference 2012. Clin Oral Implants Res. 2012;23:63–5.
125. Srinivasan M, Vazquez L, Rieder P, et al. Survival rates of short (6 mm) micro-rough surface implants: a review of literature and meta-analysis. Clin Oral Implants Res. 2014;25:539–45.
126. Klinge B, Meyle J, Working Group 2. Peri-implant tissue destruction. The third EAO consensus conference. Clin Oral Implants Res. 2012;23:108–10.
127. Klinge B, Hultin M, Berglundh T. Peri-implantitis. Dent Clin N Am. 2005;49:661–76.
128. Ting M, Craig J, Balkin BE, Suzuki JB. Peri-implantitis: a comprehensive overview of systematic reviews. J Oral Implantol. 2018;44:225–47.
129. Derks J, Tomasi C. Peri-implant health and disease. A systematic review of current epidemiology. J Clin Periodontol. 2015;42:S158–71.
130. Monje A, Aranda L, Diaz KT, Alarcón MA, Bagramian RA, Wang HL, Catena A. Impact of maintenance therapy for the prevention of peri-implant diseases: a systematic review and meta-analysis. J Dent Res. 2016;95:372–9.
131. Koromantzos PA, Makrilakis K, Dereka X, Katsilambros N, Vrotsos IA, Madianos PN. A randomized, controlled trial on the effect of non-surgical periodontal therapy in patients with type 2 diabetes. Part I: Effect on periodontal status and glycaemic control. J Clin Periodontol. 2011;38:142–7.

10 Randomized Controlled Trials in Restorative Dentistry and Prosthodontics

Yasuhiko Kawai, Raphael de Souza, and Jocelyne Feine

10.1 Introduction

The randomized clinical trial (RCT) is a well-established, powerful research tool in healthcare. The continuous use of RCTs has improved clinical practice in all fields of health over the decades, from pioneering trials in the 1950s [1] to ongoing efforts to mitigate the SARS-CoV-2 pandemic [2]. In brief, the contribution of RCTs is a result of asking straightforward clinical questions with relatively simple designs and strong control of confounding factors.

RCTs are particularly applicable in restorative dentistry and prosthodontics. Dental researchers should be aware of some peculiarities that might impact on optimal results, however. As an example, several well-established methodological approaches used in RCTs refer to pharmaceutical testing, whereas our specialty of interest is solely operative. This may raise important challenges regarding blinding and operator experience, which would be inconsequential with pharmaceutical interventions. Thus, while the clinicians and participants may not be blinded to the specific intervention, blinding can be successfully handled for individuals who measure and enter the data, as well as those who carry out the statistical analyses. In that way, bias can be minimized.

A simple conceptual explanation of what an RCT can be: an (i) experimental study carried out with (ii) human participants assigned to receive (iii) healthcare interventions (iv) randomly. Taken into our specialty context:

(i) *In experimental studies*, the participants receive dental restorations or prostheses as part of the study protocol or maintenance methods for those treatment modalities. This means that an operator or care provider will apply those assigned interventions to each participant, instead of observing results of interventions applied outside a study protocol.

(ii) *Human participants* refer to the need for real human beings as research individuals, instead of animal models, computer simulations, in vitro specimens or extracted human cells, teeth, or other organs. For example, a trial would test different restorative materials in human participants instead of extracted human teeth.

(iii) *Healthcare interventions* refer to any treatment or approach intended to prevent health

Y. Kawai (✉)
Nihon University School of Dentistry at Matsudo, Chiba, Japan
e-mail: kawai.yasuhiko@nihon-u.ac.jp

R. de Souza · J. Feine
McGill University Faculty of Dental Medicine and Oral Health Sciences, Montreal, Canada
e-mail: raphael.desouza@mcgill.ca; jocelyne.feine@mcgill.ca

R. Kohli et al. (eds.), *Randomized Controlled Trials in Evidence-Based Dentistry*, https://doi.org/10.1007/978-3-031-47651-8_10

conditions or other health outcomes. More specifically, these include interventions of interest (experimental), active comparators/controls (well-known healthcare interventions, e.g., traditional complete dentures), placebo/sham procedures, or no intervention (the shortened dental arch could be listed in this latter category in a study about restoring molars with implants or removable denture, for example). Normally, participants are allocated to different groups to receive one of the interventions or no intervention.

(iv) The term "*randomly*" implies that participants receive any of the interventions by chance only; in other words, a sample of participants is divided into groups that are practically similar, except for the interventions controlled by the study. Any between-group difference is assumed to be caused by the tested interventions instead of unknown confounders, which is different from observational studies. For example, the decision about providing conventional instead of implant-retained prostheses to a participant should be totally by chance, not because the edentulous ridge has unfavorable conditions.

10.1.1 Before Starting an RCT of Prosthetic and Restorative Dentistry

A protocol must be prepared and registered before the clinical trial begins. Registering a protocol requires a protocol that includes clear information, the number and type of potential participants and referring professionals, as well as avoidance of duplication of efforts by different researcher groups. Trial registration is considered an ethical requirement in many fields, including prosthetic and restorative dentistry. Most dental journals require a protocol registration number before accepting submissions of a manuscript reporting a clinical trial. This benefits the scientific community in many ways, including the future allocation of funds and minimization of publication bias (i.e., when researchers choose to publish just part of their trial results, depending on what they find) [3].

A PubMed search using the keyword "clinical trial registry" and filtering by RCT showed 7187 results. The articles per year were 100 articles in 2008 and 922 in 2019, showing a significant increase in the last decade. Presently, registration of RCTs before their initiation has become mandatory, and the trend is particularly significant for high-quality journals. In North America, ClinicalTrials.gov (https://clinicaltrials.gov/), a privately and publicly funded clinical trial database, is common. In Japan and Brazil, the UMIN Clinical Trials Registry (https://www.umin.ac.jp/ctr/index.htm) and ReBEC (https://ensaiosclinicos.gov.br), respectively, are widely known among local researchers.

Before a study begins, researchers should be reminded that even studies with negative results must be published in the same manner as studies with positive results. The bias created when studies with negative results are not published is called publication bias. When appropriate sample sizes are used, negative results should be published, as these are important in guiding clinical practice. Issues with publication bias have been widely described in the medical field and seem to be the same in dentistry [4]. Another potential issue is the partial publication of the outcomes considered for a trial, i.e., published manuscripts do not report those outcomes showing unfavorable results for an intervention. Trial protocol registries require outcomes to be specified a priori, and results are promptly and properly reported.

RCTs require rigorous planning, meticulous management, and generous funding for success. In a nutshell, the purpose of conducting an RCT is to generate reliable evidence to support evidence-based decision-making by patients and clinicians. The type of prosthesis, techniques, materials, and outcome variables specific to restorative dentistry and prosthodontics should be carefully considered when developing the study protocol. Jokstad et al. [5] concluded two decades ago in "The Reporting of Randomized Controlled Trials in Prosthodontics," that few RCTs in prosthodontics are reported in accordance with contemporary guidelines for adequate reporting of trials. While reports have improved somewhat from those days, there are still issues that are often overlooked at the planning stage of the trial.

10.1.2 Specific Issues in Restorative Dentistry and Prosthodontics

There are specific issues to consider when studying restorative dentistry and prosthodontics; these may be different than in pharmaceutical studies. First, many technologies exist for a single treatment. For example, several manufacturing companies produce different impression materials for the same purpose. Second, there are differences among clinicians in operative techniques and skills. Third, blinding of the clinician and/or study participant may not be possible. For studies in which it is impossible to keep the treatment provider and patient blind to treatment assignment, it is important to blind others who deal with the data (e.g., biostatisticians).

Many prosthodontic and restorative RCTs have been conducted. However, meta-analyses using these reports have been shown to have a low degree of homogeneity due to the factors already mentioned, including differences in outcome variables, methods, and materials. This reduces our ability to combine the results of many studies to produce robust evidence-based clinical recommendations.

10.1.3 Issues of Baseline Data and Trial Validity

A key problem in many studies is the lack of a baseline measure that can be compared to the outcome. If the intention of the investigators is to demonstrate a change in one or more clinical parameters, the baseline measures should be the same as those used for the study outcomes, which should be validated, appropriate, and comparable to those used in other studies. For example, a trial measuring the chewing ability (outcome) of edentulous patients after receiving implants should measure the same variable before the surgery (chewing ability on baseline). Using established measures from the literature and not creating new, unvalidated measures is essential to quality trials. Such practices enhance the generalizability of the trial results and allow more precise estimates of prognosis for specific patient groups. As an example, different implant treatments may reveal different effects depending on chewing ability at baseline (i.e., baseline chewing ability acts as a moderator of treatment outcomes). Moreover, including the same measure at baseline and at all appropriate follow-up sessions will enable the observation of changes (e.g., pre- and post-intervention improvement of chewing performance with implants and its evolution through the follow-up appointments). Of course, some clinical trial designs do not use pre/post or change measures, which are also discussed in this chapter.

Trial results must be generalizable beyond a given setting, patient, and care provider in order to be useful. Moreover, the application of evidence to the patient in any clinical setting can only be assured when the dentist is confident in the individual patient's prognosis. Thus, an RCT must include a thorough data collection plan at baseline to ensure that participants and the care they receive are comparable to true clinical situations. This includes a precise list of sociodemographic and clinical characteristics of participants. Age and sex/gender are intuitive requirements in that list, given their general influence on healthcare outcomes (please refer to Sect. 10.4.1 for more details). Baseline data can also lead to subgroup analyses, preferably if decided a priori to minimize bias. There are situations when one treatment is better than another for one subgroup of patients but not for a different subgroup. For example, Kawai et al. divided a sample of edentulous participants according to their mandibular ridge heights into "high" and "low" sub-groups at baseline, compared the occlusal scheme of different complete dentures and showed that lingualized occlusion was effective in improving overall satisfaction only in the low group [6]. Studies need to be designed and adequate samples recruited to answer the specific questions posed. Failure to do results in underpowered analyses. A lack of power to detect treatment effects in subgroups is due to lack of an adequate sample size. Differences in treatment effects based on the sizes of outcomes observed within the subgroups may lead to erroneous conclusions unless the uncertainty of the estimates is taken into account. Ideally, an RCT must be planned to detect differences when subgroups are compared, in a well-defined sample size and analyses plan. Another point is that subgroup analyses often are done to allow for planning better targeted future studies.

10.1.4 Dental Biomaterials

The extensive use of biomaterials in restorative dentistry and prosthodontics raises significant challenges for the external validity of RCTs. Researchers must be transparent regarding devices and biomaterials used. For example, a trial in which dental implants are compared must provide details on the fixtures and abutments used, including size, shape, and composition. Proprietary names must be provided in such a way as to ensure that the RCT is reproducible, including batch numbers. Sponsors must also be mentioned to disclose potential conflicts of interest (e.g., RCTs funded by manufacturers of dental materials), and strategies to mitigate such conflicts must be discussed when applicable. It is also important to make sure that donated in-kind materials correspond to those used in real clinical practice—ideally, they should come from same commercially available batches and used in comparable conditions (e.g., same technique, similar time before expiry date). An exception for the latter aspect would reside in studies about novel biomaterials/devices that are being tested before commercialization. With the materials that are in production, industrial partners may not be willing to completely describe the materials that are tested. This is problematic, because without that information, the study can never be replicated.

10.2 Overview of RCTs in Restorative Dentistry and Prosthodontics

10.2.1 Existing Evidence

10.2.1.1 Restoration and Materials

Research on composite resins is a major subject in restorative dentistry. During the preparation of this text, the authors identified 150 reports of RCTs on dental composite restorations in PubMed (last update: March 2021). These papers were further narrowed down to 29 papers by using the keywords "RCTs" and "differences in materials of composite resin" or "differences in adhesion between composite resin and dentin" [7–35]. Composite resin restoration usually targets different cavity classifications. Among the 29 selected articles, 16 involved class II [7, 11, 13, 15, 16, 19–21, 23, 24, 27–29, 33–35], 3 class I [9, 17, 21–23, 25, 31, 34], and 3 cervical cavities [8, 10, 12]. Focused research questions include comparisons of different composite materials [9, 10, 15, 16, 20, 21, 23–25, 27–29, 31], different surface treatments, different adhesives [8, 12, 14, 17, 19] and different techniques [7, 9, 11, 13, 14, 18, 22, 26, 30, 32–35].

Most of the articles examined restorations in molars or cervical filling procedures (cavity classes I, II, and V), but few examined anterior teeth (classes III and IV). Frequently measured outcomes referred to the clinical performance of the restorations (occurrence of fractures, retention, marginal adaptation, recurrent caries, and post-operative sensitivity), as well as patient satisfaction. However, there are few studies on treatment time and material costs. The toxicity of the material itself (e.g., adverse effects on soft tissues, the oral cavity, and the whole body) has not been thoroughly investigated. The changes in bisphenol A levels in saliva and urine after placing lingual bonded retainers were the subject of a study in the field of Orthodontics [36].

The next common search is "various treatment methods/materials": 20 RCTs on glass ionomer sealants [37–43] and cements [41,

44–47]. There are also 20 articles on "caries removal methods": laser [48, 49], incomplete [26, 50–53], and complete excavation before restoration [48–65]. Many studies have compared complete or incomplete caries removal in terms of clinician-assessed success rates. Also, pulp vitality, recurrent caries, pain and discomfort, and the retention of restorations have been examined. However, these studies did not consider the baseline status (including different cavity depths or distance to the pulp) in relation to the observed outcomes and, thus, the effect of baseline status on prognosis. It would aid clinical decision-making if any indication for incomplete removal could be predicted from the baseline examination. Furthermore, there is no gold standard that might indicate the effectiveness of incomplete caries removal on outcomes.

A distinctive feature in restorative research is the use of a split-mouth design [7, 10, 16, 22, 25, 28, 30, 66, 67] that cannot be used in many other dental procedures. In those studies, participants receive restorations on both sides of the mouth, with each side randomly assigned to receive one of the trial interventions. A major advantage of this design is that it tests different restorative materials under the same intraoral conditions, although there may be some drawbacks. Another advantage includes smaller sample sizes and the possibility of applying more than one intervention at the same time. Specific comments on split-mouth studies can be found in Sect. 10.5.1 (Table 10.1).

Table 10.1 Key randomized controlled trials in the restorative dentistry literature

Topic	Subtopic (number of studies)	Studies
Composite resin restorations (29)	Materials (13)	Balkaya et al. [16], Colak et al. [20], Correia et al. [10], Efes et al. [31], Fatma Dilsad et al. [9], Kupietzky et al. [15], Lawson et al. [25], Rocha Gomes Torres et al. [28], van Dijken and Lindberg [24], van Dijken and Pallesen [21, 23, 27, 29]
	Adhesives (5)	Kemaloğlu et al. [8], Loguercio et al. [14], Marques et al. [17], Oz et al. [12], van Dijken and Pallesen [19]
	Cavity Class I (8)	dos Santos et al. [34], Efes et al. [31], Fatma Dilsad et al. [9], Lawson et al. [25], Marques et al. [17], Olegário et al. [22], van Dijken and Pallesen [21, 23]
	Cavity Class II (16)	Balkaya et al. [16], Coelho-de-Souza et al. [33], Colak et al. [20], dos Santos et al. [34], Kuijs et al. [35], Kupietzky et al. [15], Menezes-Silva et al. [13], Rocha Gomes Torres et al. [28], Torres et al. [7], Tunac et al. [11], van Dijken and Lindberg [24], van Dijken and Pallesen [19, 21, 23, 27, 29]
	Cervical cavity (3)	Correia et al. [10], Kemaloğlu et al. [8], Oz et al. [12]
	Techniques (13)	Banomyong et al. [32], Coelho-de-Souza et al. [33], Dias et al. [18], dos Santos et al. [34], Fatma Dilsad et al. [9], Franzon et al. [26], Fron Chabouis et al. [30], Kuijs et al. [35], Loguercio et al. [14], Menezes-Silva et al. [13], Olegário et al. [22], Torres et al. [7], Tunac et al. [11]
Restorative materials	Resin and Glass ionomer sealants (7)	Baseggio et al. [41], Chen et al. [40], Chen et al. [39], Kervanto-Seppälä et al. [42], Liu et al. [38], Muñoz-Sandoval et al. [37], Poulsen et al. [43]
	Resin and Cements (5)	Amaral et al. [45], Baseggio et al. [41], Donly and Segura [46], Ferreira et al. [44], ten Cate and van Duinen [47]
Caries removal	Laser (2)	([49], [48]
	Incomplete excavation (5)	Bressani et al. [51], Franzon et al. [50], Franzon et al. [26], Hevinga et al. [52], Yildiz et al. [53]
	Complete excavation (17)	Bjørndal et al. [61], Bressani et al. [51], Dalpian et al. [58], Franzon et al. [50], Hadley et al. [49], Hesse et al. [54], Hevinga et al. [52], Kirzioglu et al. [64], Lula et al. [63], Maltz et al. [56], Orhan et al. [60], Peric et al. [62], Peters et al. [65], Shabzendedar et al. [59], Sirin Karaarslan et al. [57], Valério et al. [48], Viral et al. [55], Yildiz et al. [53]

Table 10.2 Key randomized controlled trials in the prosthodontic literature

Topic	Subtopic (number of studies)	Studies
Complete dentures	Conventional and simplified methods (10)	Ceruti et al. [69], Cunha et al. [71], de Villa Camargos et al. 2019; Heydecke et al. [73], Kawai et al. [76], Kawai et al. [74], Kawai et al. [72], Lira-Oetiker et al. [68], Mengatto et al. [75], [70])
	Different impression materials (5)	Hyde et al. [82], Hyde et al. [81], Jo et al. [80], Komagamine et al. [78], Miyayasu et al. [79]
	Different occlusal scheme (4)	Brandt et al. [83], Farias Neto et al. [84], Heydecke et al. [85], Kawai et al. [6]
	Different denture cleaning (12)	Aoun et al. [94], Arruda et al. [90], de Andrade et al. [97], Duyck et al. [96], Moffa et al. [92], Nishi et al. [95], Paranhos et al. [98], Peracini et al. [91], Ramage et al. [89], Ribeiro et al. [88], Salles et al. [93], Valentini-Mioso et al. [87]

10.2.1.2 Prosthodontics

A total of 29 complete denture studies were identified. Among them, 10 compared conventional and simplified fabrication methods [68–77]. This comparison of techniques includes different impression materials [78–82], occlusal schemes [6, 83–85], dietary advice after insertion [86], and denture cleaning [87–98]. The studies in which simplified and traditional methods were compared involved a broad age range of participants. As no significant difference was detected between both treatments on various outcomes, complete dentures fabricated by simplified methods are considered more cost-effective. However, it is unclear whether simplified approaches are helpful for all patients. In this regard, it would be desirable to develop criteria to determine which treatment method is more beneficial for individual patients based on baseline indicators such as radiographic examination, oral status, and patient characteristics, as well as patient-reported outcomes of their satisfaction and quality of life. These outcome variables should be gathered throughout the study. Also, the participants in the study were patients who were physically able to travel to the dental clinic. Future research should focus on examining the usefulness of simplified fabrication in patients with limited access to dentists, such as in nursing homes (Table 10.2).

10.2.2 Knowledge Gaps

10.2.2.1 Restoration and Materials

The research questions on lining materials [99–106], remineralization [107, 108], and root caries [109–113] are scarce. Among them, root surface caries is undoubtedly an important issue in our increasingly aging society. Silver diamine fluoride (SDF) is a conventional treatment method, but it is expected to have a preservation effect on root caries in the elderly. Compared with composite resin, SDF is assumed to have a lower cost and shorter treatment time, but evidence on its cost-effectiveness is needed and compared with other restorative materials. The same could be mentioned about whether the use of SDF can reduce the risk of recurrent caries.

Furthermore, there are very few RCTs in which crowns and direct restorations for endodontically treated teeth are compared [114, 115]. A single RCT, conducted in the 90 s, compared direct and indirect veneers [116–119]—newer materials and different patient groups demand testing through the use of RCTs.

10.2.2.2 Prosthodontics

Clinicians want to know the prognosis of endodontically treated teeth. In addition, clinicians prefer to choose the method and materials to support endodontically treated teeth according to the condition of the teeth. However, focusing on the causal factor of prognosis of fixed prostheses is rare [120–123]. There is no strong evidence to support decisions on which material should be selected, as well as the most appropriate treatment method, based on the baseline condition of endodontically treated teeth (remaining tooth structure, ferrule effect, root condition, etc.); at this time, there is inadequate evidence on this topic to support clinical decision-making.

The RCTs on partially edentate patients varied in the research questions: modified resin denture

[124], shortened dental arch [125–128], laser-sintered dentures [129], preparation of rest seats [130], and double-crown-retained removable partial dentures [131]. Based on the difficulty of the case, it is desirable to narrow down the target, for example, the number of molar supports (Eichner index) or Kennedy classification class 1. Furthermore, the effect of wearing the appliance should be evaluated through clinician- and patient-based measures, as well as the costs assessed.

RCTs with nutritional outcomes are few but have been increasing in the recent decade [86, 132–138]. Prosthodontics and nutrition are important issues. However, there is evidence that prosthetic quality is not necessarily related to nutritional intake. In the future, it would be desirable to conduct RCTs to examine the evidence of the effect of interventions that can cause behavioral changes in an individuals' nutritional intake, perhaps with simple advice before or after appliance insertion.

10.3 Funding for Your RCT

Securing research funds can be one of the most challenging tasks in conducting any proposal (along with participant recruitment). Resources for trials in restorative dentistry and prosthodontics can come from two sources: (1) funding agencies and (2) industry.

10.3.1 Funding Agencies

Probably the most reputable sponsors for research in restorative and prosthetic dentistry are government funding agencies. Most of these agencies support broad areas of research and accept investigator-initiated proposals. Government agencies are often flexible in terms of the aims of a proposal and milestones, but lengthy, rigorous peer-review processes with relatively low success rates can be daunting to investigators. Examples of funding sources for oral health include: (i) the

Box 10.1 Summary of Important Essential Research Areas in Restorative and Prosthetic Dentistry

New Technologies

Restorative Dentistry

1. Development and testing are essential for new biocompatible restorative materials without mercury or other toxic materials in both developed and developing countries, especially for use in low-resource settings.
2. Sealants and glass ionomers should be tested, as well as silver diamine fluoride (SDF), for their longevity and cost effectiveness.
3. Development and testing are needed for new technologies to produce less costly restorative materials for all types of lesions and loss of tooth structure.
4. The short- and long-term clinical performance of different cavity liners and pulp capping agents, from traditional calcium hydroxide-based materials to novel alternatives, should be assessed.
5. Alternatives to traditional dental handpieces and burs should be tested, as well as chemo-mechanical agents and lasers, as a way to promote patient comfort and reduce aerosols. The latter aspect is critical to maintain dental care during crises such as the current COVID-19 pandemic.

Prosthetic Dentistry

6. More evidence is needed on minimally invasive implant technologies, including small-sized (short and/or narrow) implants, minimal numbers and guided surgery.
7. The development and testing of implant abutment connection types are warranted.
8. Studies on implant coating materials to reduce corrosion and biofilm accumulation are essential.

9. We need to better understand how different implant designs are or are not associated with success/survival.
10. Removable denture studies should focus on fabrication protocols and technologies that are aimed to improve performance (including fit) and to reduce costs and operative complexity.
11. Studies are needed on any new technology already on the market with little or no supporting evidence of efficacy/effectiveness; this includes digital workflows, intraoral scanning and computer-assisted manufacturing for fixed and removable prostheses.
12. Newer adhesive methods (zirconia and other novel ceramic-based materials) should be assessed.
13. We need long-term evidence on the success and survival of zirconia, PEEK and other materials used in dental implants.
14. Better maintenance methods should be confirmed for prosthetic appliances, including oral and denture hygiene methods (e.g., soft tissue hygiene), antimicrobial materials to compensate non-ideal compliance (e.g., dependent seniors or inpatient care receivers).

Box 10.2 Summary of Essential Research Methodologies Lacking in Restorative and Prosthetic Dentistry

Methodologies

1. Pairing traditional data analysis (quantitative) with qualitative appraisal via mixed methods approaches may be desirable.
2. Long-term studies are needed on dental implants involving participant groups with important systemic health conditions, e.g. diabetes, osteoporosis, H&N radiotherapy, etc.
3. The toxicity of composite and other restorative materials must be established, following up on the plethora of in vitro and preclinical studies on this subject.

Box 10.3 Summary of Essential Research Outcomes Lacking in Restorative and Prosthetic Dentistry

Outcomes

1. Patient-reported outcomes should be applied in appropriate prosthodontic research studies; these include patient perceptions of and satisfaction with treatment, oral health-related quality of life, preferences for a particular treatment (cross-over RCTs) and esthetic appraisal.
2. Appropriate, validated measurement tools should be developed when unavailable.
3. Appropriate cost analyses should be included as an outcome in all prosthodontic and restorative studies.
4. The effect of medications that alter bone metabolism on implant success, e.g. SSRIs, beta-blockers, etc., are essential.
5. Outcomes associated with different amounts of caries removal (e.g., incomplete vs complete) should be measured.
6. Clarification of the clinical relevance of old concepts is needed; old concepts can include the amount of ferrule for a crown, indication for posts and core (including recommended type), need for indirect restorations instead of direct fillings (e.g., cusp protection, anterior veneers), different designs and fabrication methods for removable dentures, etc.

Note: Please keep in mind that the highest quality evidence is derived from meta-analyses of numerous RCTs in a topic area. Thus, replication studies are highly valuable and required for evidence-based clinical recommendations.

Canadian Institutes of Health Research (CIHR), which has a specific committee for RCTs; (ii) the National Institutes of Health (NIH), one of the main funding sources for dental research worldwide, specifically the National Institute of Dental and Craniofacial Research (NIDCR); (iii) in Japan, ministerial Grants-in-Aid Programs (Japan Society for the Promotion of Science, and Ministry of Health, Labor and Welfare); (iv) in Brazil, federal and state research funding agencies (e.g., CNPq, CAPES, and FAPESP); (v) in Hong Kong, Health and Medical Research Fund (HMRF, Research Fund Secretariat); (vi) in EU (European Research Council grant), etc. The authors strongly encourage early career researchers to attend seminars and other events promoted by funding agencies and universities, which explain how to apply for specific funding competition announcements. Those events provide strong guidelines on how to structure ideas before submitting a grant, thus increasing success rates. Some agencies provide "reviewer in training"/observer programs that can help young applicants to succeed. Another advice for young clinical researchers in our field is to seek mentoring from senior researchers in allied fields, including biostatistics, engineering, epidemiology, and materials sciences. Besides adding an interdisciplinary component to grant applications, those researchers have more exposure to the challenges of grantsmanship than clinician-scientists.

Diverse foundations are important sources of funding in our specialty. Many organizations launch calls for research proposals that can be used for RCTs in oral health. Depending on the specific goals of the foundations, these calls tend to be rather specific. One of the best examples in our specialty is the International Team for Implantology (ITI), a non-profit organization that focuses on education and research in implant dentistry. The ITI accepts research proposals twice a year and can accommodate the budget of RCTs to test dental implants and prostheses. Professional organizations also may provide research funding directly or by means of research organisms such as research networks or universities.

10.3.2 Industry

The direct applicability of research in restorative and prosthetic dentistry opens a strong potential for industrial funding. Most manufacturers of dental biomaterials have an interest in carrying out studies in collaboration with external researchers as a way to further clarify the properties of their products as well as to gain credibility. This includes materials used for direct restorations (e.g., composites, adhesive systems), dental implants, and prostheses. In the latter example, both the type of biomaterial (e.g., different ceramic materials for crowns and bridges) and the manufacturing methods (e.g., CAD/CAM vs conventional) may be highly relevant to companies.

An application for industrial funds follows a different workflow. Whereas government agencies and foundations launch calls and follow strict timelines, direct involvement with industries often demands networking and preliminary discussions on the research question and protocol. Often based on an executive summary, discussion involves some meetings to define what would be relevant for the company and the researchers. After that, a full proposal is prepared for further discussion. Some companies have well-defined investigator-initiated grant programs but may still reach out for discussion of potentially interesting proposals. Finally, any acceptance of industry funding must undergo a formal agreement (contract), in which the rights and duties of each partner are well-established—for example, research universities often have strict guidelines to ensure impartiality in research conduct and dissemination of the results.

10.4 Study Design and Methodology

10.4.1 Selection of Baseline Data

Obtaining baseline information has the following objectives: first, to ascertain the homogeneity of both randomly assigned groups when conducting RCTs in a parallel design. For this purpose, the data to be collected are generally on typical confounding factors, such as gender and age. Furthermore, if the pre-procedure examination separates the groups into subgroups and if the outcome is divided into successful and unsuccessful cases between the subgroups, then the researcher may be able to determine effective modifiers or important markers that predict and affect the outcome. For example, the presence or absence of edentulous mandibular ridge resorption is believed to be the influencing factor in complete denture intervention outcome. This factor will be assured and proven by choosing a reasonable pretest item, recording the participants' ridge conditions at baseline, and then analyzing the relationship between the outcomes. If they are related, the baseline examination will prove to be a useful preoperative marker. Such validated testing methods have been developed in recent years, and their use may allow for more evidence-based treatment and prognosis predictions. However, careful selection of baseline items is essential. Otherwise, this will lead to costly and labor-intensive research.

Examples of useful baseline data collection tools include the three Prosthodontic Diagnostic Index (PDI) versions by the American College of Prosthodontics [139–141]. Each version of the PDI classifies the case complexity of patients and trial participants who would receive restorative interventions and deal with complete edentulism, partial edentulism, and dentate individuals separately. Partial tooth loss can be classified by functional systems as the Eichner classification [142], which categorizes cases according to the number and distribution of antagonist occlusal units. Different classification systems can be used for edentulous ridges, depending on the research question—for example, the Kapur classification seems more interesting if the focus of an RCT is masticatory function [143], whereas the Cawood and Howell classification may be more relevant to determine surgical challenges when placing implants [144].

10.4.2 Outcomes

Since tooth loss cannot be cured, i.e., we cannot provide people with a new natural tooth, it is a chronic condition that requires prosthetic therapeutic approaches. The primary purpose of prosthetic devices is to restore or improve aesthetics, function, and quality of life. It is logical, therefore, that the best judge of a prosthetic device is the person who is wearing or using the device. Thus, the choice of outcome for a prosthetic device (removable or fixed restoration) should be based on the perceptions of the patient. For this purpose, patient-reported outcome measures have been developed and validated, e.g., Oral Health Impact Profile (OHIP) [145] and Geriatric/General Oral Health Assessment Index (GOHAI) for oral health-related quality of life/self-perception of oral health [146], McGill Denture Satisfaction Questionnaire (MDSQ) [147, 148] and Patient's Denture Assessment (PDA) [149] for patient satisfaction. Conversely, studies that examine materials, tissues, etc., may require outcomes that focus on clinical or laboratory variables.

10.4.3 Patient Recruitment Strategy and Who Conducts the Interventions?

Efficacy or effectiveness: The first question to consider is whether the RCT is primarily concerned with efficacy or effectiveness. In general, RCTs often identify efficacy under strict protocols involving specialist clinicians, frequent follow-ups, careful patient selection, and "ideal" provision of care. In other words, RCTs aim to determine whether, under ideal circumstances, one intervention is better than another. On the other hand, effectiveness research, which should be carried out following RCTs, is carried out to understand whether or not the findings from rigorous RCTs are similar in "real world" circumstances.

It may be difficult or impossible to blind participants to treatment allocation in many prosthodontic RCTs. Thus, it is important to recruit "unbiased" participants. For example, imagine that you are planning to measure patient-reported outcomes in a study in which participants will be randomized into groups, such that one group would receive implants and the other would not. Ideally, one wants an "equipoise" (the understanding that there is no convincing evidence that one approach is better than another) in the minds of both the investigators and participants [150]. If you advertise that you are seeking participants for an implant study, then those who are already interested in getting implants will respond; if they are then allocated to the non-implant group, they may decide not to participate, which would bias the sample. On the other hand, if you advertise a complete denture study, those who prefer implants may not respond. It is important to consider these issues when preparing study recruitment advertisements. The authors' research group has advertised our implant studies seeking people who wished to replace their conventional dentures [151]. Thus, they were able to attract denture-wearers who were and were not seeking implant treatment and speak with them about the study, as well as their concerns and preferences regarding new prostheses and implant retention. One cannot underestimate the difficulty in recruiting study participants for any clinical trial. Depending on the intervention, as well as any benefit an individual might gain from participating, recruitment can be anything from moderately difficult to impossible. Even when recruiting for an implant study in which participants would need to pay very low or no costs, people in the targeted study population may be reluctant to volunteer. As we have described in [151], we sought an older population in which many had concerns about surgical implant placement [152]. To retain the participants in the study, they kept in regular contact with each person, establishing a rapport and attaining their trust. We phoned them following each of their appointments to ask how they were doing, and we also reminded them of the next appointment; each participant was subsequently again phoned 1–2 days before that next appointment. We have found that personal communication has helped considerably for us to achieve trust and confidence in our study participants.

The experience and skills of the clinicians conducting the interventions in both restorative dentistry and prosthodontics also need to be considered. An efficacy study is usually conducted in the setting of a university or clinic, as well as using specific operators, e.g. specialists and GPs. However, an effectiveness study would demand a more pragmatic approach to determine the treatment performance of healthcare providers in their traditional settings. In other words, the latter kind of trial involves a broad range of operators, preferably with various levels of experience [153, 154]. The same could be expected from dental laboratories providing prosthetic care in a pragmatic trial, which would likely involve varying levels of competence [69, 130, 155].

10.4.4 Parallel or Crossover

One of the most difficult choices to make when planning an RCT is whether to perform it in a parallel or as a crossover design. Both have advantages and disadvantages, and it is sometimes difficult to decide which is most appropriate for a particular study. The advantage of a crossover design is that both interventions can be performed with the same participants. In prosthodontic research, for example, each participant would wear and rate both removable prostheses, one after the other, in a randomized order. Because both prostheses are rated by the same participant, variance is reduced; with this lower variance, the sample size needed for statistical strength can be substantially reduced. Conversely, the disadvantages of crossover designs are the potential for increased participant dropouts since they would take a longer time to complete. Furthermore, crossover studies cannot be carried out if the disease or condition is not stable over time (i.e., no symptom fluctuations), and a washout (for pharmaceuticals) or adaptation (for devices) period is often required between the interventions. Finally, the effect of the first intervention can stack (or "carry over") to the second intervention, an issue that cannot be tackled by randomization. An obvious example would be any treatment for denture stomatitis, since participants will likely have little or no inflammation when applying a second treatment. Therefore, this type of design works only for those conditions that are stable and chronic, such as tooth loss, in which the treatments aim to improve function and quality of life.

Parallel studies do not have a washout period like crossovers, so the study period can be shortened, but the number of subjects may increase. In addition, although randomized, the assurance of homogeneity between groups may be weaker than in a crossover design. On the other hand, it is useful in studies of restorative dentistry and fixed prosthodontics. Parallel-group RCTs also provide a more pragmatic approach and thus be more generalizable, since interventions can be applied in a more similar way to what real patients receive. As mentioned earlier, there are advantages and disadvantages; thus, it is necessary to decide which design to use, considering clinical questions, interventions and costs.

10.4.5 Multi-center Study

Clinical trials conducted at multiple facilities are called multi-center trials. This kind of trial engages multiple institutions around the same protocol, and these institutions recruit participants in parallel—for example, 3 institutions recruit around 100 participants simultaneously to reach a sample of 300. Multi-center trials are helpful to make participant recruitment feasible in a reasonable timeline, which would be impossible at a single institution. Extremely long recruitment periods can lead to high costs and results that may be already outdated by the time that reports are published. Although the intuitive application of a multi-center design is to achieve a large sample, these may be fundamental when eligible cases are difficult to recruit. For example, if a clinical study requires about 40–50 cases but only two to three participants/year can be recruited at a single institution (e.g., rare condition/disease), multi-center studies have the advantage of producing results in a more reasonable time period.

Another benefit of multi-center trials is their generalizability/external validity. Recruiting participants from different centers often leads to conclusions that are easier to extrapolate, since the sample is representative of a broader population. This is particularly true when the associations observed in the trial (e.g., between-group differences) seem to be the same for all subgroups of participants recruited in each research center.

Although the advantages of multi-center trials—larger sample and better external validity—are appealing, there are some caveats. Even if trial protocols are developed to ensure methodological consistency, multi-center studies may encounter problems in standardizing protocol-defined interventions. Delays in adverse event reporting may also occur. This can be critical when institutions unfamiliar with clinical research collaborate. Therefore, to conduct multi-center trials, various measures should be taken, such as appointing a principal investigator and a research /assistant/associate at each institution, organizing a committee to confirm the effectiveness and safety in handling and defining adverse events, and how to report such events. Then, networking among facilities and better communication opportunities regarding essential research procedures, such as subject selection and random assignment methods, is necessary. When conducting clinical trials in restorative dentistry and prosthodontics, issues such as the clinicians' individual skills with the intervention should also be considered, and calibration among practitioners is essential prior to the start of the trial.

10.4.6 Follow-up Period

Although longer follow-ups are better, the follow-up period depends on the risk tradeoff between follow-up adherence and dropouts; this usually relates to the subjects' age at baseline. In a removable prosthodontic study, short-term (2–3 months) and mid-term (66 months to 12 months) follow-ups are common and can reveal important differences in patient-reported outcomes. Long-term follow-up can reach 5–10 years [156–159] in implant overdenture studies, as needed to observe long-term success and survival rates of implants and prostheses [76]. Compared to conventional dentures [76], implant-retained/supported dentures may produce a greater patient commitment to their treatment (e.g., surgical procedures, treatment costs, etc.). Because of this presumed high adherence of patients to recall, the follow-up in RCTs may be more successful with the implant group than with those who receive conventional dentures [159–164]. Restorative dentistry research tends to have longer follow-ups than removable prosthodontic research. For example, research on composite restorations [24] appears to continue with annual follow-ups for 15 years following treatment [21, 24, 27, 99, 165–168].

Simple interventions are also linked to better participant adherence. Another strategy for better adherence includes a run-in period to minimize dropouts after randomization, which may be interesting in efficacy studies. This approach involves an interval between recruitment and randomization during which all participants receive the same active intervention or placebo/sham procedure. Intensive communication and reminders also improve participant attendance to follow-ups; trialists must also be attentive to patient concerns and adversities and do their best to tackle them (e.g., examining and polishing restorations and prostheses, a new clinical/radiographic exam to reassure patients who received implants). In summary, although a run-in period, short follow-up periods, and simple interventions may not always be possible, a good rapport between the participants and the research team will contribute to successful research results [169].

10.4.7 Analysis and Statistics

The analysis of prosthodontic interventional research data focuses on two areas. One is a comparison of between-group outcomes, and the other is a within-group comparison of preoperative status and postoperative outcomes. The former is important in terms of purely looking at the effect of the intervention with the assumption that the assigned groups are equivalent in most relevant characteristics. On the other hand, we often experience that the outcomes are affected by individual baseline conditions, even if they are equally assigned to individual groups. Prominent improvements may be seen with prosthetic interventions, especially in cases of low preoperative ratings. On the other hand, a high preoperative patient-reported rating may result in little improvement. Thus, exploring the effect modifier from the baseline data and the relationship between the outcomes may lead to a better informed decision-making process.

10.5 Reporting

10.5.1 CONSORT

Reporting in accordance with the CONSORT statement (http://www.consort-statement.org/) will not only standardize the article but also give the authors a sense of security as they will be able to confirm the items to be reported. The CONSORT is based on a checklist for reporting parallel-group RCTs [170]. The extensions are also available for different study designs and analysis characteristics: for cluster randomized trials [171], N-of-1 trials [172], and within-person randomized trials [173]. Most journals presently require the CONSORT checklist to be submitted by the authors, but this has not been the case in the recent past.

Specific to operative dentistry, the split-mouth design is applied [43, 166, 174–178]. In this design, the checklist must follow within-person randomized trials [173]. Identification as a within-person randomized trial in the title is to be noted; however, many do not include this in the title. RCTs (1992–2012) in eight oral health specialty journals with the highest impact factors found that only seven of 43 (16%) trials with a split-mouth design identified the trial as split mouth in the title [179]. Adherence to CONSORT facilitates searches using search engines in clinical and research settings and facilitates systematic reviews, meta-analyses, and eventual clinical application.

10.5.2 Patient Adherence and Attrition

Describing any loss to follow-up at reporting is essential. The CONSORT follow-up chart is useful to assist in conveying complete information on the trial flow. If follow-up is incomplete or interrupted, missing data at the end of the study could impact its internal validity, thus introducing systematic errors and resulting in misleading research conclusions.

Missing data is often categorized into the following three types: missing completely at random (MCAR), missing at random (MAR), and missing not at random (MNAR) [180]. Although the best medicine against lost data is to prevent it from happening, knowing possible patterns and their respective management strategies is critical to the conduct and evaluation of RCTs. MCAR relates to losses that have no relationship with participant characteristics or treatment response—they are equally likely to occur with any participant in an RCT. An example is a participant who moves to another town before a trial follow-up and cannot be examined or a participant whose tube with collected saliva falls and breaks in the laboratory. As a completely random process, this kind of missing data does not pose a threat to trial validity; the major issue comes from the widening of standard error measures when comparing trial arms.

MAR refers to losses associated with known sample characteristics. For example, participants of a specific gender or those with worse systemic conditions may be more prone to withdraw from an RCT. Another example of MAR is the removal of participants due to non-adherence or based on their performance (e.g., those who do not follow instructions in a trial about denture maintenance methods). Withdrawals driven by adverse effects would be classified as MAR if the trialists know which adversities led to each withdrawal, such as a p articipant with a lost implant in a trial in which overdenture attachments are compared. Approaches to tackle MAR data include multiple imputations and other methods, whose aim is to raise awareness on whether missing data may have led to biased outcomes. For example, results may be better for one of the trial groups if the non-compliant or unfavorable cases are lost to follow-up.

Finally, MNAR relates to missing data due to unobserved aspects. For example, consider a participant in a restorative materials trial who never returns for follow-up. If it is not possible to verify the reason for the loss, but the participant abandoned the RCT due to dissatisfaction with treatment, this can pose a major threat to the validity of the results (bias). In general, researchers should consider missing data as MNAR if potential reasons for a dropout are unknown but could be responses to treatment (for example, a dissatisfied participant) or due to any event related to the trial protocol, including adverse effects to interventions (e.g., irreversible pulpitis in the same tooth that received experimental restorative materials). When the situation is MNAR, the situation is more critical than with the MCAR and MAR; thus, the results should be carefully interpreted before they are reported.

10.5.3 Data Sharing for Meta-analysis

A systematic review is more comfortable and more accurate when data from different institutions are made available according to specific criteria. For this purpose, it is desirable to share the dataset. Even if the results of the analysis are expressed as median depending on the status of the individual studies (e.g., sample size or normality of the results obtained), we believe it is essential for researchers to submit means and standard deviations to online repositories or other sources. Also, it is even more important to describe details of the characteristics of prosthodontic and restorative dentistry, such as differences in experience between surgeons, as well as differences in surgical techniques and materials used. Researchers should be aware of the availability of raw data, which would allow them to conduct research, answer different research questions and reuse them, thus reducing research duplication and waste. At present, however, data sharing is not a widespread practice, though the problem is not limited to restorative dentistry and prosthodontics. A rigorous protocol for data sharing systems may be necessary to facilitate this point, including individual participant data. At any rate, some funding agencies and journals have increasingly recommended and/or even required data sharing. Since data sharing has been growing over the years, we recommend that researchers prepare data files and code books, considering the possibility of publishing them in the future. Researchers should consult industrial partners or intellectual property agencies in certain circumstances; however, for example, a new dental biomaterial composition tested in a trial may result in a patent deposit, thus limiting or delaying the complete disclosure of obtained data.

10.5.4 Cost Analysis

Costs are commonly assessed in health research because, even if a treatment option is shown to be significantly better than a standard treatment, its uptake is likely to be limited if the costs are high. Thus, involving an economist in an RCT team is essential. In addition to determining the costs of a specific treatment, it could also be important to understand how patients and/or the public value that treatment. Therefore, before starting the analysis, it is necessary to clarify an a priori perspective (patient, society, or funder) from which the cost analysis is being conducted. Economic assessment has been common in medical research for at least 30 years, starting before the development of two journals for the field, the Journal of Health Economics and Health Economics [181]. In fact, the International Society for Pharmacoeconomics and Outcomes Research (ISPOR) sponsored a task force and published the *Good Research Practices for Cost-Effectiveness Analysis Alongside Clinical Trials* in 2005, followed by an update in 2014 [182]. Petrou and Gray [183] describe the various types of economic assessments, including cost-effectiveness studies, that are used in randomized clinical trials.

Studies that include cost analysis can provide more clinically relevant results. Lewis [184] notes that, along with proof of the clinical effectiveness of prosthodontic interventions, comparative economic analyses should be undertaken to establish the relative value of each intervention in terms of its costs and consequences. Microcosting, a cost estimation method for all other cost items, which involves the direct enumeration and costing out of every input consumed in the treatment of a particular patient, is ideal for obtaining detailed cost analysis [184, 185].

As far as the literature review, there are not many papers that have conducted RCTs and cost analyses. Most of them are from prosthodontic studies that compared the cost of complete dentures [70, 72, 79, 186], partial dentures [128, 187], and implant overdentures [188–192]. Some papers have been published on RCTs of restorative dentistry that included a cost analysis [22, 37, 38, 193, 194]. However, few cost analyses have been implemented in RCTs in this field. Thus, we strongly suggest that cost data be collected and analyzed along with RCTs in all future prosthetic and restorative oral health research.

10.5.5 Mixed Methods Designs

Qualitative research has captured the interest of quantitative dental researchers worldwide. This type of scientific measurement approach is common in the fields of social science research, including anthropology, sociology, psychology, etc. [195]. Hearing directly from people about their perceptions of their condition(s) or treatment(s) provides a perspective and depth of understanding that cannot be attained from care providers or measurement instruments (questionnaires).

Mixed methods research combines quantitative data, for example, from an RCT, with qualitative approaches in a rigorous and prescribed manner [196]. Mixed methods results provide data not only relative to a specific hypothesis but also related participants' perspectives on the topic addressed in the quantitative part. The order in which data are gathered and the interpretation of the combined quantitative and qualitative results vary depending on the purpose of the study [197]. Unsurprisingly, mixed methods approaches have begun to appear in the dental literature [198–203], yet more studies using this method are needed.

10.6 Conclusion

Randomization in controlled clinical trials is an essential requirement in order to establish therapeutic directions in restorative dentistry [204]. RCTs are vital in producing evidence-based information to aid in decision-making on appropriate prosthetic choices that aim to maintain and increase an individual's function and quality of life. In future planning of RCTs, investigators should take into account standardized methods and outcomes, along with coherence to CONSORT for proper reporting of the study results.

10.7 Summary

Key improvements should be considered for research questions, protocol design, study implementation, and reporting on clinical research in restorative dentistry and prosthodontics.

- Search for and conduct research that is relevant and important.
- Select baseline data to identify a priori causal factors.
- Develop a clear policy on whether the research should test effectiveness or efficacy.
- Decide on the inclusion/exclusion criteria of potential study participants according to the purpose of the study.
- Select appropriate and valid outcomes in relation to the study aims and objectives.
- Consider the appropriate study endpoints.
- Plan long-term follow-up whenever possible, considering the resources and methods to be used.
- Plan an economic analysis that strengthens the potential clinical implementation of the results.
- Report results using CONSORT criteria and appropriate extensions.
- Analyze and categorize study dropouts and report according to the dropout category.
- Prepare for the possibility of providing the trial dataset for use in a meta-analysis.

10.8 Case Scenario Exercise

10.8.1 Case Scenario

Comparative evaluation of ceramic crowns made by dental technicians using ceramic-baked cast crowns and CAD/CAM. A randomized controlled trial

- Purpose: Porcelain fused metal crown, traditionally made, and fixed in the aesthetic area of the anterior teeth, have been fabricated by dental technicians for many years as an established method. On the other hand, CAD/CAM crowns, which have been used in recent years, are rapidly gaining popularity, but their effect and cost-effectiveness are unknown and will be compared.
- Study the settings: a single center.
- Method: Thirty patients who are willing to restore fixed prostheses on both sides of the maxilla were randomly assigned to either PFM or CAD for comparison. The study design will be either cross-over, parallel, or split mouth. Randomization will be based on computer-generated random numbers, and concealment of the assignment will include the use of opaque, sealed envelopes. Outcomes will be assessed at 2 weeks, 3 months, and 6 months of wearing.
- Outcomes: subjective assessment, marginal fit, as well as other validated measures. Outcomes will be analyzed in subjects who have completed follow-up and will not be subjected to ITT.

In conducting an RCT comparing the two methods using PFM and CAD, based on the points discussed in this chapter.

Questions

1. How should the protocol address the following points.
   (a) What baseline data is important to collect?
   (b) What is your strategy for recruiting participants?
   (c) What is your plan to reduce dropouts as much as possible?
   (d) What cost data is important to collect?
   (e) How will you report the results accurately and widely disseminate them?

Answers

(a) Factors that are expected to influence the outcome of the intervention will be considered as items to be collected at baseline. The selection criteria will be based on previous reports and clinical experience. In this case, it is a factor affecting fixed prostheses. Pre-treatment status, e.g., does it have a pulp or not? If the patient does not have pulp, the condition of the remaining tooth substance, root length, and status of the root canal should be covered. In addition, the occlusal state is a factor that should not be forgotten. It is also important to evaluate the periodontal condition. These factors will be collected at baseline and examined for their association with prognosis, and if significant associations are found, they will be assessed to determine whether they correspond to confounding factors for the outcome.

(b) The strategy to recruit participants for the RCT comparing PFM and CAD for fixed prostheses restoration in the maxilla involves identifying individuals who need and are willing to accept such restorations. Recruitment should target individuals open to both methods, ensuring a diverse representation. The focus should be on obtaining a balanced distribution across the chosen study design (crossover, parallel, or split mouth). Participants' commitment to completing follow-up assessments at 2 weeks, 3 months, and 6 months is crucial for meaningful outcomes analysis.

(c) To minimize dropouts in the RCT: Emphasize clear communication about the study's importance and benefits. Provide thorough information about the procedures and expectations, ensuring participants understand the commitment. Implement convenient scheduling for assessments to accommodate participants' availability. Regularly engage with participants through reminders and supportive communication. Establish a responsive and empathetic research team to address concerns promptly. Consider offering incentives to enhance motivation. Foster a positive participant experience to promote retention and commitment throughout the study duration. Assist and reach out to participants whenever they have issues or questions regarding their participation.

(d) Collecting relevant cost data is crucial for a comprehensive analysis. In the context of the RCT comparing PFM and CAD for fixed prostheses restoration, important cost data includes:
   1. Direct Costs: Expenses related to materials and procedures for both PFM and CAD methods.
   2. Labor Costs: Time and costs associated with clinicians, dental technicians, and other staff involved in the process.
   3. Indirect Costs: Overheads and facility costs associated with procedures, including utilities and maintenance.
   4. Participant Costs: Expenses incurred by participants, any out-of-pocket costs related to the prosthetic restoration.
   5. Equipment Costs: Costs of acquiring, maintaining, and operating the necessary equipment, e.g., milling machine and casting device, of both PFM and CAD methods.
   6. Follow-up Costs: Expenses associated with follow-up assessments at 2 weeks, 3, and 6 months, including staff time and materials. By systematically gathering these cost data, one can conduct a thorough economic evaluation of the PFM and CAD methods, helping to inform decision-makers on the cost-effectiveness of each approach.

(e) To ensure accurate reporting and widespread dissemination of results:
   1. Scientific Publications: Submit findings to reputable peer-reviewed journals, following rigorous scientific reporting standards.

2. Conference Presentations: Share results at relevant conferences to reach a broad audience of researchers, clinicians, and industry professionals.
3. Clinical Guidelines and Protocols: Contribute to the development or updating of clinical guidelines and protocols based on the study outcomes.
4. Online Repositories: Share data and results on publicly accessible repositories or databases to enhance transparency and accessibility.
5. Collaboration with Professional Organizations: Collaborate with dental and prosthodontic professional organizations to incorporate findings into educational materials and guidelines.
6. Collaboration with Stakeholders: Engage with key stakeholders, including healthcare providers, policymakers, and patient advocacy groups, to ensure the findings reach those who can implement or benefit from them.
7. Professional Networks: Utilize professional networks and collaborations to share findings with relevant experts and institutions.
8. Social Media and Online Platforms: Leverage social media and online platforms to share condensed versions of the results, engaging with a wider audience. By employing a multi-faceted approach, the study results can be disseminated accurately and effectively to diverse audiences, contributing to the broader understanding and application of the research findings.

References

1. Stolberg HO, Norman G, Trop I. Randomized controlled trials. AJR Am J Roentgenol. 2004;183:1539–44. https://doi.org/10.2214/ajr.183.6.01831539.
2. Anon. (n.d.-a) COVID-19 studies from the World Health Organization database. https://clinicaltrials.gov/ct2/who_table (accessed 10.23 2020).
3. Anon. (n.d.-b) Why should I register and submit results? https://clinicaltrials.gov/ct2/manage-recs/background (accessed May 11 2021).
4. Crawford JM, Briggs CL, Engeland CG. Publication bias and its implications for evidence-based clinical decision making. J Dent Educ. 2010;74:593–600. https://doi.org/10.1002/j.0022-0337.2010.74.6.tb04904.x.
5. Jokstad A, Esposito M, Coulthard P, Worthington HV. The reporting of randomized controlled trials in prosthodontics. Int J Prosthodont. 2002;15:230–42.
6. Kawai Y, Ikeguchi N, Suzuki A, Kuwashima A, Sakamoto R, Matsumaru Y, et al. A double blind randomized clinical trial comparing lingualized and fully bilateral balanced posterior occlusion for conventional complete dentures. J Prosthodont Res. 2017;61:113–22. https://doi.org/10.1016/j.jpor.2016.07.003.
7. Torres CRG, Mailart MC, Crastechini É, Feitosa FA, Esteves SRM, Di Nicoló R, et al. A randomized clinical trial of class II composite restorations using direct and semidirect techniques. Clin Oral Investig. 2020;24:1053–63. https://doi.org/10.1007/s00784-019-02999-6.
8. Kemaloğlu H, Atalayin Ozkaya C, Ergucu Z, Onal B. Follow-up of flowable resin composites performed with a universal adhesive system in noncarious cervical lesions: a randomized, controlled 24-month clinical trial. Am J Dent. 2020;33:39–42.
9. Fatma Dilsad OZ, Ergin E, Attar N, Gurgan S. Comparison of laser- and bur-prepared class I cavities restored with two different low-shrinkage composite resins: a randomized, controlled 60-month clinical trial. Clin Oral Investig. 2020;24:357–68. https://doi.org/10.1007/s00784-019-02931-y.
10. Correia A, Jurema A, Andrade MR, Borges A, Bresciani E, Caneppele T. Clinical evaluation of noncarious cervical lesions of different extensions restored with bulk-fill or conventional resin composite: preliminary results of a randomized clinical trial. Oper Dent. 2020;45:E11–e20. https://doi.org/10.2341/18-256-c.
11. Tunac AT, Celik EU, Yasa B. Two-year performance of CAD/CAM fabricated resin composite inlay restorations: a randomized controlled clinical trial. J Esthet Restor Dent. 2019;31:627–38. https://doi.org/10.1111/jerd.12534.
12. Oz FD, Ergin E, Canatan S. Twenty-four-month clinical performance of different universal adhesives in etch-and-rinse, selective etching and self-etch application modes in NCCL - a randomized controlled clinical trial. J Appl Oral Sci. 2019;27:e20180358. https://doi.org/10.1590/1678-7757-2018-0358.
13. Menezes-Silva R, Velasco SRM, Bastos RS, Molina G, Honório HM, Frencken JE, et al. Randomized clinical trial of class II restoration in permanent teeth comparing ART with composite resin after 12 months. Clin Oral Investig. 2019;23:3623–35. https://doi.org/10.1007/s00784-018-2787-1.
14. Loguercio AD, Rezende M, Gutierrez MF, Costa TF, Armas-Vega A, Reis A. Randomized 36-month follow-up of posterior bulk-filled resin composite restorations. J Dent. 2019;85:93–102. https://doi.org/10.1016/j.jdent.2019.05.018.
15. Kupietzky A, Atia Joachim D, Tal E, Moskovitz M. Long-term clinical performance of heat-cured

high-viscosity glass ionomer class II restorations versus resin-based composites in primary molars: a randomized comparison trial. Eur Arch Paediatr Dent. 2019;20:451–6. https://doi.org/10.1007/s40368-019-00423-x.
16. Balkaya H, Arslan S, Pala K. A randomized, prospective clinical study evaluating effectiveness of a bulk-fill composite resin, a conventional composite resin and a reinforced glass ionomer in Class II cavities: one-year results. J Appl Oral Sci. 2019;27:e20180678. https://doi.org/10.1590/1678-7757-2018-0678.
17. Marques IP, de Oliveira FBS, Souza JGS, Ferreira RC, Magalhães CS, França FMG, et al. Influence of surface treatment on the performance of silorane-based composite resin in class I restorations: a randomized clinical trial. Clin Oral Investig. 2018;22:2989–96. https://doi.org/10.1007/s00784-018-2390-5.
18. Dias KR, de Andrade CB, Wait TT, Chamon R, Ammari MM, Soviero VM, et al. Efficacy of sealing occlusal caries with a flowable composite in primary molars: a 2-year randomized controlled clinical trial. J Dent. 2018;74:49–55. https://doi.org/10.1016/j.jdent.2018.05.014.
19. van Dijken JW, Pallesen U. Three-year randomized clinical study of a one-step universal adhesive and a two-step self-etch adhesive in class II composite restorations. J Adhes Dent. 2017;19:287–94. https://doi.org/10.3290/j.jad.a38867.
20. Colak H, Tokay U, Uzgur R, Hamidi MM, Ercan E. A prospective, randomized, double-blind clinical trial of one nano-hybrid and one high-viscosity bulk-fill composite restorative systems in class II cavities: 12 months results. Niger J Clin Pract. 2017;20:822–31. https://doi.org/10.4103/1119-3077.212449.
21. van Dijken JW, Pallesen U. Posterior bulk-filled resin composite restorations: a 5-year randomized controlled clinical study. J Dent. 2016;51:29–35. https://doi.org/10.1016/j.jdent.2016.05.008.
22. Olegário IC, Hesse D, Bönecker M, Imparato JC, Braga MM, Mendes FM, et al. Effectiveness of conventional treatment using bulk-fill composite resin versus atraumatic restorative treatments in primary and permanent dentition: a pragmatic randomized clinical trial. BMC Oral Health. 2016;17:34. https://doi.org/10.1186/s12903-016-0260-6.
23. van Dijken JW, Pallesen U. Randomized 3-year clinical evaluation of class I and II posterior resin restorations placed with a bulk-fill resin composite and a one-step self-etching adhesive. J Adhes Dent. 2015;17:81–8. https://doi.org/10.3290/j.jad.a33502.
24. van Dijken JW, Lindberg A. A 15-year randomized controlled study of a reduced shrinkage stress resin composite. Dent Mater. 2015;31:1150–8. https://doi.org/10.1016/j.dental.2015.06.012.
25. Lawson NC, Radhakrishnan R, Givan DA, Ramp LC, Burgess JO. Two-year randomized, controlled clinical trial of a flowable and conventional composite in class I restorations. Oper Dent. 2015;40:594–602. https://doi.org/10.2341/15-038-c.
26. Franzon R, Opdam NJ, Guimarães LF, Demarco FF, Casagrande L, Haas AN, et al. Randomized controlled clinical trial of the 24-months survival of composite resin restorations after one-step incomplete and complete excavation on primary teeth. J Dent. 2015;43:1235–41. https://doi.org/10.1016/j.jdent.2015.07.011.
27. van Dijken JW, Pallesen U. A randomized 10-year prospective follow-up of class II nanohybrid and conventional hybrid resin composite restorations. J Adhes Dent. 2014;16:585–92. https://doi.org/10.3290/j.jad.a33202.
28. Rocha Gomes Torres C, Rêgo HM, Perote LC, Santos LF, Kamozaki MB, Gutierrez NC, et al. A split-mouth randomized clinical trial of conventional and heavy flowable composites in class II restorations. J Dent. 2014;42:793–9. https://doi.org/10.1016/j.jdent.2014.04.009.
29. van Dijken JW, Pallesen U. A six-year prospective randomized study of a nano-hybrid and a conventional hybrid resin composite in class II restorations. Dent Mater. 2013;29:191–8. https://doi.org/10.1016/j.dental.2012.08.013.
30. Fron Chabouis H, Prot C, Fonteneau C, Nasr K, Chabreron O, Cazier S, et al. Efficacy of composite versus ceramic inlays and onlays: study protocol for the CECOIA randomized controlled trial. Trials. 2013;14:278. https://doi.org/10.1186/1745-6215-14-278.
31. Efes BG, Yaman BC, Gurbuz O, Gumuştaş B. Randomized controlled trial of the 2-year clinical performance of a silorane-based resin composite in class 1 posterior restorations. Am J Dent. 2013;26:33–8.
32. Banomyong D, Harnirattisai C, Burrow MF. Posterior resin composite restorations with or without resin-modified, glass-ionomer cement lining: a 1-year randomized, clinical trial. J Investig Clin Dent. 2011;2:63–9. https://doi.org/10.1111/j.2041-1626.2010.00036.x.
33. Coelho-de-Souza FH, Klein-Júnior CA, Camargo JC, Beskow T, Balestrin MD, Demarco FF. Double-blind randomized clinical trial of posterior composite restorations with or without bevel: 6-month follow-up. J Contemp Dent Pract. 2010;11:001–8.
34. dos Santos MP, Passos M, Luiz RR, Maia LC. A randomized trial of resin-based restorations in class I and class II beveled preparations in primary molars: 24-month results. J Am Dent Assoc. 2009;140:156–66.; quiz 247-8. https://doi.org/10.14219/jada.archive.2009.0129.
35. Kuijs RH, Fennis WM, Kreulen CM, Roeters FJ, Creugers NH, Burgersdijk RC. A randomized clinical trial of cusp-replacing resin composite restorations: efficiency and short-term effectiveness. Int J Prosthodont. 2006;19:349–54.
36. Kang YG, Kim JY, Kim J, Won PJ, Nam JH. Release of bisphenol A from resin composite used to bond orthodontic lingual retainers. Am J Orthod Dentofac Orthop. 2011;140:779–89. https://doi.org/10.1016/j.ajodo.2011.04.022.

37. Muñoz-Sandoval C, Gambetta-Tessini K, Giacaman RA. Microcavitated (ICDAS 3) carious lesion arrest with resin or glass ionomer sealants in first permanent molars: a randomized controlled trial. J Dent. 2019;88:103163. https://doi.org/10.1016/j.jdent.2019.07.001.
38. Liu BY, Xiao Y, Chu CH, Lo EC. Glass ionomer ART sealant and fluoride-releasing resin sealant in fissure caries prevention--results from a randomized clinical trial. BMC Oral Health. 2014;14:54. https://doi.org/10.1186/1472-6831-14-54.
39. Chen X, Du MQ, Fan MW, Mulder J, Huysmans MC, Frencken JE. Caries-preventive effect of sealants produced with altered glass-ionomer materials, after 2 years. Dent Mater. 2012;28:554–60. https://doi.org/10.1016/j.dental.2012.01.001.
40. Chen X, Cuijpers V, Fan M, Frencken JE. Marginal leakage of two newer glass-ionomer-based sealant materials assessed using micro-CT. J Dent. 2010;38:731–5. https://doi.org/10.1016/j.jdent.2010.05.018.
41. Baseggio W, Naufel FS, Davidoff DC, Nahsan FP, Flury S, Rodrigues JA. Caries-preventive efficacy and retention of a resin-modified glass ionomer cement and a resin-based fissure sealant: a 3-year split-mouth randomised clinical trial. Oral Health Prev Dent. 2010;8:261–8.
42. Kervanto-Seppälä S, Lavonius E, Pietilä I, Pitkäniemi J, Meurman JH, Kerosuo E. Comparing the caries-preventive effect of two fissure sealing modalities in public health care: a single application of glass ionomer and a routine resin-based sealant programme. A randomized split-mouth clinical trial. Int J Paediatr Dent. 2008;18:56–61. https://doi.org/10.1111/j.1365-263X.2007.00855.x.
43. Poulsen S, Beiruti N, Sadat N. A comparison of retention and the effect on caries of fissure sealing with a glass-ionomer and a resin-based sealant. Community Dent Oral Epidemiol. 2001;29:298–301. https://doi.org/10.1034/j.1600-0528.2001.290409.x.
44. Ferreira JM, Pinheiro SL, Sampaio FC, Menezes VA. Use of glass ionomer cement containing antibiotics to seal off infected dentin: a randomized clinical trial. Braz Dent J. 2013;24:68–73. https://doi.org/10.1590/0103-6440201301925.
45. Amaral MT, Guedes-Pinto AC, and Chevitarese O. Effects of a glass-ionomer cement on the remineralization of occlusal caries--an in situ study. Braz Oral Res 2006; 20: 91–96. doi: https://doi.org/10.1590/s1806-83242006000200001
46. Donly KJ, Segura A. Fluoride release and caries inhibition associated with a resin-modified glass-ionomer cement at varying fluoride loading doses. Am J Dent. 2002;15:8–10.
47. ten Cate JM, van Duinen RN. Hypermineralization of dentinal lesions adjacent to glass-ionomer cement restorations. J Dent Res. 1995;74:1266–71. https://doi.org/10.1177/00220345950740060501.
48. Valério RA, Borsatto MC, Serra MC, Polizeli SA, Nemezio MA, Galo R, et al. Caries removal in deciduous teeth using an Er:YAG laser: a randomized split-mouth clinical trial. Clin Oral Investig. 2016;20:65–73. https://doi.org/10.1007/s00784-015-1470-z.
49. Hadley J, Young DA, Eversole LR, Gornbein JA. A laser-powered hydrokinetic system for caries removal and cavity preparation. J Am Dent Assoc. 2000;131:777–85. https://doi.org/10.14219/jada.archive.2000.0277.
50. Franzon R, Guimarães LF, Magalhães CE, Haas AN, Araujo FB. Outcomes of one-step incomplete and complete excavation in primary teeth: a 24-month randomized controlled trial. Caries Res. 2014;48:376–83. https://doi.org/10.1159/000357628.
51. Bressani AE, Mariath AA, Haas AN, Garcia-Godoy F, de Araujo FB. Incomplete caries removal and indirect pulp capping in primary molars: a randomized controlled trial. Am J Dent. 2013;26:196–200.
52. Hevinga MA, Opdam NJ, Frencken JE, Truin GJ, Huysmans MC. Does incomplete caries removal reduce strength of restored teeth? J Dent Res. 2010;89:1270–5. https://doi.org/10.1177/0022034510377790.
53. Yildiz E, Sirinkaraarslan E, Yegin Z, Cebe MA, Tosun G. Effect of caries removal techniques on the bond strength of adhesives to caries-affected primary dentin in vitro. Eur J Paediatr Dent. 2013;14:209–14.
54. Hesse D, Bonifácio CC, Mendes FM, Braga MM, Imparato JC, Raggio DP. Sealing versus partial caries removal in primary molars: a randomized clinical trial. BMC Oral Health. 2014;14:58. https://doi.org/10.1186/1472-6831-14-58.
55. Viral PM, Nagarathna C, Shakuntala BS. Chemomechanical caries removal in primary molars : evaluation of marginal leakage and shear bond strength in bonded restorations--an in vitro study. J Clin Pediatr Dent. 2013;37:269–74. https://doi.org/10.17796/jcpd.37.3.a56x8502133706nq.
56. Maltz M, Jardim JJ, Mestrinho HD, Yamaguti PM, Podestá K, Moura MS, et al. Partial removal of carious dentine: a multicenter randomized controlled trial and 18-month follow-up results. Caries Res. 2013;47:103–9. https://doi.org/10.1159/000344013.
57. Sirin Karaarslan E, Yildiz E, Cebe MA, Yegin Z, Ozturk B. Evaluation of micro-tensile bond strength of caries-affected human dentine after three different caries removal techniques. J Dent. 2012;40:793–801. https://doi.org/10.1016/j.jdent.2012.05.013.
58. Dalpian DM, Casagrande L, Franzon R, Dutra GM, de Araujo FB. Dentin microhardness of primary teeth undergoing partial carious removal. J Clin Pediatr Dent. 2012;36:363–7.
59. Shabzendedar M, Moosavi H, Talbi M, Sharifi M. Permeability evaluation after decay removal in primary teeth with current caries-excavation techniques. J Contemp Dent Pract. 2011;12:441–6. https://doi.org/10.5005/jp-journals-10024-1073.
60. Orhan AI, Oz FT, Orhan K. Pulp exposure occurrence and outcomes after 1- or 2-visit indirect pulp therapy vs complete caries removal in primary and permanent molars. Pediatr Dent. 2010;32:347–55.

61. Bjørndal L, Reit C, Bruun G, Markvart M, Kjaeldgaard M, Näsman P, et al. Treatment of deep caries lesions in adults: randomized clinical trials comparing stepwise vs. direct complete excavation, and direct pulp capping vs. partial pulpotomy. Eur J Oral Sci. 2010;118:290–7. https://doi.org/10.1111/j.1600-0722.2010.00731.x.
62. Peric T, Markovic D, Petrovic B. Clinical evaluation of a chemomechanical method for caries removal in children and adolescents. Acta Odontol Scand. 2009;67:277–83. https://doi.org/10.1080/00016350902976779.
63. Lula EC, Monteiro-Neto V, Alves CM, Ribeiro CC. Microbiological analysis after complete or partial removal of carious dentin in primary teeth: a randomized clinical trial. Caries Res. 2009;43:354–8. https://doi.org/10.1159/000231572.
64. Kirzioglu Z, Gurbuz T, Yilmaz Y. Clinical evaluation of chemomechanical and mechanical caries removal: status of the restorations at 3, 6, 9 and 12 months. Clin Oral Investig. 2007;11:69–76. https://doi.org/10.1007/s00784-006-0072-1.
65. Peters MC, Flamenbaum MH, Eboda NN, Feigal RJ, Inglehart MR. Chemomechanical caries removal in children: efficacy and efficiency. J Am Dent Assoc. 2006;137:1658–66. quiz 729-30. https://doi.org/10.14219/jada.archive.2006.0111.
66. Alabdullah MM, Nabawia A, Ajaj MA, Saltaji H. Effect of fluoride-releasing resin composite in white spot lesions prevention: a single-centre, split-mouth, randomized controlled trial. Eur J Orthod. 2017;39:634–40. https://doi.org/10.1093/ejo/cjx010.
67. Erdemir U, Sancakli HS, Yaman BC, Ozel S, Yucel T, Yıldız E. Clinical comparison of a flowable composite and fissure sealant: a 24-month split-mouth, randomized, and controlled study. J Dent. 2014;42:149–57. https://doi.org/10.1016/j.jdent.2013.11.015.
68. Lira-Oetiker M, Seguel-Galdames F, Quero-Vallejos I, Uribe SE. Randomised clinical trial of patient satisfaction with traditional and simplified complete dentures. J Oral Rehabil. 2018;45:386–92. https://doi.org/10.1111/joor.12617.
69. Ceruti P, Mobilio N, Bellia E, Borracchini A, Catapano S, Gassino G. Simplified edentulous treatment: a multicenter randomized controlled trial to evaluate the timing and clinical outcomes of the technique. J Prosthet Dent. 2017;118:462–7. https://doi.org/10.1016/j.prosdent.2017.01.024.
70. Vecchia MP, Regis RR, Cunha TR, de Andrade IM, da Matta JC, de Souza RF. A randomized trial on simplified and conventional methods for complete denture fabrication: cost analysis. J Prosthodont. 2014;23:182–91. https://doi.org/10.1111/jopr.12090.
71. Cunha TR, Della Vecchia MP, Regis RR, Ribeiro AB, Muglia VA, Mestriner W Jr, et al. A randomised trial on simplified and conventional methods for complete denture fabrication: masticatory performance and ability. J Dent. 2013;41:133–42. https://doi.org/10.1016/j.jdent.2012.09.008.
72. Kawai Y, Murakami H, Takanashi Y, Lund JP, Feine JS. Efficient resource use in simplified complete denture fabrication. J Prosthodont. 2010;19:512–6. https://doi.org/10.1111/j.1532-849X.2010.00628.x.
73. Heydecke G, Vogeler M, Wolkewitz M, Türp JC, Strub JR. Simplified versus comprehensive fabrication of complete dentures: patient ratings of denture satisfaction from a randomized crossover trial. Quintessence Int. 2008;39:107–16.
74. Kawai Y, Murakami H, Shariati B, Klemetti E, Blomfield JV, Billette L, et al. Do traditional techniques produce better conventional complete dentures than simplified techniques? J Dent. 2005;33:659–68. https://doi.org/10.1016/j.jdent.2005.01.005.
75. Mengatto CM, Gameiro GH, Brondani M, Owen CP, MacEntee MI. A randomized controlled trial of mastication with complete dentures made by a conventional or an abbreviated technique. Int J Prosthodont. 2017;30:439–44. https://doi.org/10.11607/ijp.4741.
76. Kawai Y, Muarakami H, Feine JS. Do traditional techniques produce better conventional complete dentures than simplified techniques? A 10-year follow-up of a randomized clinical trial. J Dent. 2018;74:30–6. https://doi.org/10.1016/j.jdent.2018.04.027.
77. de Villa CG, Armenine TE, Paleari AG, Nascimento GMO, Munhoz MFV. Teaching complete denture procedures to dental students by conventional or simplified methods: a randomized clinical trial. J Dent Educ. 2019;83:303–13. https://doi.org/10.21815/jde.019.023.
78. Komagamine Y, Kanazawa M, Sato Y, Iwaki M, Jo A, Minakuchi S. Masticatory performance of different impression methods for complete denture fabrication: a randomized controlled trial. J Dent. 2019;83:7–11. https://doi.org/10.1016/j.jdent.2019.01.009.
79. Miyayasu A, Kanazawa M, Jo A, Sato Y, Minakuchi S. Cost-effectiveness analysis of two impression methods for the fabrication of mandibular complete dentures. J Dent. 2018;68:98–103. https://doi.org/10.1016/j.jdent.2017.10.006.
80. Jo A, Kanazawa M, Sato Y, Iwaki M, Akiba N, Minakuchi S. A randomized controlled trial of the different impression methods for the complete denture fabrication: Patient reported outcomes. J Dent. 2015;43:989–96. https://doi.org/10.1016/j.jdent.2015.05.007.
81. Hyde TP, Craddock HL, Gray JC, Pavitt SH, Hulme C, Godfrey M, et al. A randomised controlled trial of complete denture impression materials. J Dent. 2014;42:895–901. https://doi.org/10.1016/j.jdent.2014.02.005.
82. Hyde TP, Craddock HL, Blance A, Brunton PA. A cross-over randomised controlled trial of selective pressure impressions for lower complete dentures. J Dent. 2010;38:853–8. https://doi.org/10.1016/j.jdent.2010.07.003.
83. Brandt S, Danielczak R, Kunzmann A, Lauer HC, Molzberger M. Prospective clinical study of bilateral balanced occlusion (BBO) versus canine-guided occlusion (CGO) in complete denture wearers. Clin Oral Investig. 2019;23:4181–8. https://doi.org/10.1007/s00784-019-02857-5.

84. Farias Neto A, Mestriner Junior W, Carreiro AF. Masticatory efficiency in denture wearers with bilateral balanced occlusion and canine guidance. Braz Dent J. 2010;21:165–9. https://doi.org/10.1590/s0103-64402010000200013.
85. Heydecke G, Akkad AS, Wolkewitz M, Vogeler M, Türp JC, Strub JR. Patient ratings of chewing ability from a randomised crossover trial: lingualised vs. first premolar/canine-guided occlusion for complete dentures. Gerodontology. 2007;24:77–86. https://doi.org/10.1111/j.1741-2358.2007.00153.x.
86. Komagamine Y, Kanazawa M, Iwaki M, Jo A, Suzuki H, Amagai N, et al. Combined effect of new complete dentures and simple dietary advice on nutritional status in edentulous patients: study protocol for a randomized controlled trial. Trials. 2016;17:539. https://doi.org/10.1186/s13063-016-1664-y.
87. Valentini-Mioso F, Maske TT, Cenci MS, Boscato N, Pereira-Cenci T. Chemical hygiene protocols for complete dentures: a crossover randomized clinical trial. J Prosthet Dent. 2019;121:83–9. https://doi.org/10.1016/j.prosdent.2017.12.022.
88. Ribeiro AB, de Araújo CB, Silva LEV, Fazan-Junior R, Salgado HC, Ribeiro AB, et al. Hygiene protocols for the treatment of denture-related stomatitis: local and systemic parameters analysis—a randomized, double-blind trial protocol. Trials. 2019;20:661. https://doi.org/10.1186/s13063-019-3854-x.
89. Ramage G, O'Donnell L, Sherry L, Culshaw S, Bagg J, Czesnikiewicz-Guzik M, et al. Impact of frequency of denture cleaning on microbial and clinical parameters—a bench to chairside approach. J Oral Microbiol. 2019;11:1538437. https://doi.org/10.1080/20002297.2018.1538437.
90. Arruda CNF, Salles MM, Badaro MM, de Cassia OV, Macedo AP, Silva-Lovato CH, et al. Effect of sodium hypochlorite and Ricinus communis solutions on control of denture biofilm: a randomized crossover clinical trial. J Prosthet Dent. 2017;117:729–34. https://doi.org/10.1016/j.prosdent.2016.08.035.
91. Peracini A, Regis RR, Souza RF, Pagnano VO, Silva CH, Paranhos HF. Alkaline peroxides versus sodium hypochlorite for removing denture biofilm: a crossover randomized trial. Braz Dent J. 2016;27:700–4. https://doi.org/10.1590/0103-6440201600913.
92. Moffa EB, Izumida FE, Jorge JH, Mussi MC, Siqueira WL, Giampaolo ET. Effectiveness of chemical disinfection on biofilms of relined dentures: a randomized clinical trial. Am J Dent. 2016;29:15–9.
93. Salles MM, Badaró MM, Arruda CN, Leite VM, Silva CH, Watanabe E, et al. Antimicrobial activity of complete denture cleanser solutions based on sodium hypochlorite and Ricinus communis—a randomized clinical study. J Appl Oral Sci. 2015;23:637–42. https://doi.org/10.1590/1678-775720150204.
94. Aoun G, Cassia A, Berberi A. Effectiveness of a chlorhexidine Digluconate 0.12% and Cetylpyridinium chloride 0.05% solution in eliminating Candida albicans colonizing dentures: a randomized clinical in vivo study. J Contemp Dent Pract. 2015;16:433–6. https://doi.org/10.5005/jp-journals-10024-1702.
95. Nishi Y, Seto K, Kamashita Y, Kaji A, Kurono A, Nagaoka E. Survival of microorganisms on complete dentures following ultrasonic cleaning combined with immersion in peroxide-based cleanser solution. Gerodontology. 2014;31:202–9. https://doi.org/10.1111/ger.12027.
96. Duyck J, Vandamme K, Muller P, Teughels W. Overnight storage of removable dentures in alkaline peroxide-based tablets affects biofilm mass and composition. J Dent. 2013;41:1281–9. https://doi.org/10.1016/j.jdent.2013.08.002.
97. de Andrade IM, Cruz PC, da Silva CH, de Souza RF, Paranhos Hde F, Candido RC, et al. Effervescent tablets and ultrasonic devices against Candida and mutans streptococci in denture biofilm. Gerodontology. 2011;28:264–70. https://doi.org/10.1111/j.1741-2358.2010.00378.x.
98. Paranhos HF, Silva-Lovato CH, Souza RF, Cruz PC, Freitas KM, Peracini A. Effects of mechanical and chemical methods on denture biofilm accumulation. J Oral Rehabil. 2007;34:606–12. https://doi.org/10.1111/j.1365-2842.2007.01753.x.
99. Koc Vural U, Gokalp S, Kiremitci A. Effect of cavity lining on the restoration of root surface carious lesions: a split-mouth, 5-year randomized controlled clinical trial. Clin Oral Investig. 2020;24:979–89. https://doi.org/10.1007/s00784-019-03001-z.
100. Stafuzza TC, Vitor LLR, Rios D, Cruvinel T, Loureço Neto N, Sakai VT, et al. A randomized clinical trial of cavity liners after selective caries removal: one-year follow-up. J Appl Oral Sci. 2019;27:e20180700. https://doi.org/10.1590/1678-7757-2018-0700.
101. Schenkel AB, Veitz-Keenan A. Dental cavity liners for Class I and Class II resin-based composite restorations. Cochrane Database Syst Rev. 2019;3:CD010526. https://doi.org/10.1002/14651858.CD010526.pub3.
102. Pereira MA, Santos-Júnior RBD, Tavares JA, Oliveira AH, Leal PC, Takeshita WM, et al. No additional benefit of using a calcium hydroxide liner during stepwise caries removal: a randomized clinical trial. J Am Dent Assoc. 2017;148:369–76. https://doi.org/10.1016/j.adaj.2017.02.019.
103. Schenkel AB, Peltz I, Veitz-Keenan A. Dental cavity liners for class I and class II resin-based composite restorations. Cochrane Database Syst Rev. 2016;10:Cd010526. https://doi.org/10.1002/14651858.CD010526.pub2.
104. Schwendicke F, Göstemeyer G, Gluud C. Cavity lining after excavating caries lesions: meta-analysis and trial sequential analysis of randomized clinical trials. J Dent. 2015;43:1291–7. https://doi.org/10.1016/j.jdent.2015.07.017.
105. Duque C, Negrini Tde C, Sacono NT, Spolidorio DM, de Souza Costa CA, Hebling J. Clinical and microbiological performance of resin-modified glass-ionomer liners after incomplete dentine caries removal. Clin Oral Investig. 2009;13:465–71. https://doi.org/10.1007/s00784-009-0304-2.
106. von Fraunhofer JA, Marshall KR, Holman BG. The effect of base/liner use on restoration leakage. Gen Dent. 2006;54:106–9.

107. Kucuk EB, Malkoc S, Demir A. Microcomputed tomography evaluation of white spot lesion remineralization with various procedures. Am J Orthod Dentofac Orthop. 2016;150:483–90. https://doi.org/10.1016/j.ajodo.2016.02.026.
108. Liu Y, Li N, Qi Y, Niu LN, Elshafiy S, Mao J, et al. The use of sodium trimetaphosphate as a biomimetic analog of matrix phosphoproteins for remineralization of artificial caries-like dentin. Dent Mater. 2011;27:465–77. https://doi.org/10.1016/j.dental.2011.01.008.
109. Geraldo-Martins V, Thome T, Mayer M, Marques M. The use of bur and laser for root caries treatment: a comparative study. Oper Dent. 2013;38:290–8. https://doi.org/10.2341/11-345-l.
110. Rolland SL, McCabe JF, Imazato S, Walls AW. A randomised trial comparing the antibacterial effects of dentine primers against bacteria in natural root caries. Caries Res. 2011;45:574–80. https://doi.org/10.1159/000334623.
111. Lucchesi JA, Santos VR, Amaral CM, Peruzzo DC, Duarte PM. Coronally positioned flap for treatment of restored root surfaces: a 6-month clinical evaluation. J Periodontol. 2007;78:615–23. https://doi.org/10.1902/jop.2007.060380.
112. Minakuchi S, Munoz CA, Jessop N. Effect of flexural load cycling on microleakage of extended root caries restorations. Oper Dent. 2005;30:234–8.
113. Hara AT, Magalhães CS, Serra MC, Rodrigues AL Jr. Cariostatic effect of fluoride-containing restorative systems associated with dentifrices on root dentin. J Dent. 2002;30:205–12. https://doi.org/10.1016/s0300-5712(02)00017-9.
114. Skupien JA, Cenci MS, Opdam NJ, Kreulen CM, Huysmans MC, Pereira-Cenci T. Crown vs. composite for post-retained restorations: a randomized clinical trial. J Dent. 2016;48:34–9. https://doi.org/10.1016/j.jdent.2016.03.007.
115. Mannocci F, Bertelli E, Sherriff M, Watson TF, Ford TR. Three-year clinical comparison of survival of endodontically treated teeth restored with either full cast coverage or with direct composite restoration. J Prosthet Dent. 2002;88:297–301. https://doi.org/10.1067/mpr.2002.128492.
116. Meijering AC, Roeters FJ, Mulder J, Creugers NH. Patients' satisfaction with different types of veneer restorations. J Dent. 1997a;25:493–7. https://doi.org/10.1016/s0300-5712(96)00067-x.
117. Meijering AC, Roeters FJ, Mulder J, Creugers NH. Recognition of veneer restorations by dentists and beautician students. J Oral Rehabil. 1997b;24:506–11. https://doi.org/10.1046/j.1365-2842.1997.00525.x.
118. Meijering AC, Creugers NH, Roeters FJ, Mulder J. Survival of three types of veneer restorations in a clinical trial: a 2.5-year interim evaluation. J Dent. 1998;26:563–8. https://doi.org/10.1016/s0300-5712(97)00032-8.
119. Meijering AC, Creugers NH, Mulder J, Roeters FJ. Treatment times for three different types of veneer restorations. J Dent. 1995;23:21–6. https://doi.org/10.1016/0300-5712(95)90656-3.
120. Naumann M, Sterzenbach G, Dietrich T, Bitter K, Frankenberger R, von Stein-Lausnitz M. Dentin-like versus rigid endodontic post: 11-year randomized controlled pilot trial on no-wall to 2-wall defects. J Endod. 2017;43:1770–5. https://doi.org/10.1016/j.joen.2017.06.030.
121. Monaco C, Llukacej A, Baldissara P, Arena A, Scotti R. Zirconia-based versus metal-based single crowns veneered with overpressing ceramic for restoration of posterior endodontically treated teeth: 5-year results of a randomized controlled clinical study. J Dent. 2017;65:56–63. https://doi.org/10.1016/j.jdent.2017.07.004.
122. Tunjan R, Rosentritt M, Sterzenbach G, Happe A, Frankenberger R, Seemann R, et al. Are endodontically treated incisors reliable abutments for zirconia-based fixed partial dentures in the esthetic zone? J Endod. 2012;38:519–22. https://doi.org/10.1016/j.joen.2011.12.027.
123. Schneider BJ, Freitag-Wolf S, Kern M. Tactile sensitivity of vital, and endodontically treated teeth. J Dent. 2014;42:1422–7. https://doi.org/10.1016/j.jdent.2014.08.016.
124. Kiatsirirote K, Sitthisettapong T, Phantumvanit P, Chan DCN. Fluoride-releasing effect of a modified resin denture containing S-PRG fillers on salivary fluoride retention: a randomized clinical study. Caries Res. 2019;53:137–44. https://doi.org/10.1159/000490627.
125. Walter MH, Dreyhaupt J, Hannak W, Wolfart S, Luthardt RG, Stark H, et al. The randomized shortened dental arch study: tooth loss over 10 years. Int J Prosthodont. 2018;31:77–84. https://doi.org/10.11607/ijp.5368.
126. Khan S, Chikte UM, Omar R. Outcomes with a posterior reduced dental arch: a randomised controlled trial. J Oral Rehabil. 2017;44:870–8. https://doi.org/10.1111/joor.12549.
127. McKenna G, Allen PF, O'Mahony D, Cronin M, DaMata C, Woods N. The impact of rehabilitation using removable partial dentures and functionally orientated treatment on oral health-related quality of life: a randomised controlled clinical trial. J Dent. 2015;43:66–71. https://doi.org/10.1016/j.jdent.2014.06.006.
128. McKenna G, Allen F, Woods N, O'Mahony D, Cronin M, DaMata C, et al. Cost-effectiveness of tooth replacement strategies for partially dentate elderly: a randomized controlled clinical trial. Community Dent Oral Epidemiol. 2014a;42:366–74. https://doi.org/10.1111/cdoe.12085.
129. Almufleh B, Emami E, Alageel O, de Melo F, Seng F, Caron E, et al. Patient satisfaction with laser-sintered removable partial dentures: a crossover pilot clinical trial. J Prosthet Dent. 2018;119:560–67.e1. https://doi.org/10.1016/j.prosdent.2017.04.021.
130. Sampaio-Fernandes MA, Sampaio-Fernandes MM, Fonseca PA, Almeida PR, Reis-Campos JC, Figueiral MH. Evaluation of occlusal rest seats with 3D technology in dental education. J Dent Educ. 2015;79:166–76.
131. Stober T, Bermejo JL, Beck-Mussoter J, Seche AC, Lehmann F, Koob J, et al. Clinical performance of conical and electroplated telescopic double crown-

retained partial dentures: a randomized clinical study. Int J Prosthodont. 2012;25:209–16.
132. Wallace S, Samietz S, Abbas M, McKenna G, Woodside JV, Schimmel M. Impact of prosthodontic rehabilitation on the masticatory performance of partially dentate older patients: can it predict nutritional state? Results from a RCT. J Dent. 2018;68:66–71. https://doi.org/10.1016/j.jdent.2017.11.003.
133. Amagai N, Komagamine Y, Kanazawa M, Iwaki M, Jo A, Suzuki H, et al. The effect of prosthetic rehabilitation and simple dietary counseling on food intake and oral health related quality of life among the edentulous' individuals: a randomized controlled trial. J Dent. 2017;65:89–94. https://doi.org/10.1016/j.jdent.2017.07.011.
134. Tanasić I, Radaković T, Šojić LT, Lemić AM, Soldatović I. Association between dentition status and malnutrition risk in Serbian elders. Int J Prosthodont. 2016;29:484–6. https://doi.org/10.11607/ijp.4752.
135. McKenna G, Allen PF, O'Mahony D, Flynn A, Cronin M, DaMata C, et al. Comparison of functionally orientated tooth replacement and removable partial dentures on the nutritional status of partially dentate older patients: a randomised controlled clinical trial. J Dent. 2014b;42:653–9. https://doi.org/10.1016/j.jdent.2014.03.005.
136. McKenna G, Allen PF, Flynn A, O'Mahony D, DaMata C, Cronin M, et al. Impact of tooth replacement strategies on the nutritional status of partially-dentate elders. Gerodontology. 2012;29:e883–90. https://doi.org/10.1111/j.1741-2358.2011.00579.x.
137. Gray JC, Navarro-Coy N, Pavitt SH, Hulme C, Godfrey M, Craddock HL, et al. IMPROVDENT: improving dentures for patient benefit. A crossover randomised clinical trial comparing impression materials for complete dentures. BMC Oral Health. 2012;12:37. https://doi.org/10.1186/1472-6831-12-37.
138. Arija V, Martin N, Canela T, Anguera C, Castelao AI, Garcia-Barco M, et al. Nutrition education intervention for dependent patients: protocol of a randomized controlled trial. BMC Public Health. 2012;12:373. https://doi.org/10.1186/1471-2458-12-373.
139. McGarry TJ, Nimmo A, Skiba JF, Ahlstrom RH, Smith CR, Koumjian JH. Classification system for complete edentulism. The American College of Prosthodontics. J Prosthodont. 1999;8:27–39. https://doi.org/10.1111/j.1532-849x.1999.tb00005.x.
140. McGarry TJ, Nimmo A, Skiba JF, Ahlstrom RH, Smith CR, Koumjian JH, et al. Classification system for partial edentulism. J Prosthodont. 2002;11:181–93. https://doi.org/10.1053/jopr.2002.126094.
141. McGarry TJ, Nimmo A, Skiba JF, Ahlstrom RH, Smith CR, Koumjian JH, et al. Classification system for the completely dentate patient. J Prosthodont. 2004;13:73–82. https://doi.org/10.1111/j.1532-849X.2004.04019.x.
142. Ikebe K, Matsuda K, Murai S, Maeda Y, Nokubi T. Validation of the Eichner index in relation to occlusal force and masticatory performance. Int J Prosthodont. 2010;23:521–4.
143. Schuster AJ, Marcello-Machado RM, Bielemann AM, Pinto LR, Faot F. Is predicting masticatory function based on mandibular bone atrophy as defined by clinical and radiographic parameters possible? A clinical study. J Prosthet Dent. 2019;121:432–9. https://doi.org/10.1016/j.prosdent.2018.05.018.
144. Eufinger H, Gellrich NC, Sandmann D, Dieckmann J. Descriptive and metric classification of jaw atrophy. Int J Oral Maxillofac Surg. 1997;26:23–8. https://doi.org/10.1016/s0901-5027(97)80841-7.
145. Locker D, Slade G. Oral health and the quality of life among older adults: the oral health impact profile. J Can Dent Assoc. 1993;59(830–33):37–8.
146. Atchison KA, Dolan TA. Development of the geriatric oral health assessment index. J Dent Educ. 1990;54:680–7. https://doi.org/10.1002/j.0022-0337.1990.54.11.tb02481.x.
147. de Souza RF, Ribeiro AB, Oates TW, Feine JS. The McGill Denture satisfaction questionnaire revisited: exploratory factor analysis of a binational sample. Gerodontology. 2020;37:233–43. https://doi.org/10.1111/ger.12477.
148. Awad MA, Feine JS. Measuring patient satisfaction with mandibular prostheses. Community Dent Oral Epidemiol. 1998;26:400–5. https://doi.org/10.1111/j.1600-0528.1998.tb01978.x.
149. Komagamine Y, Kanazawa M, Kaiba Y, Sato Y, Minakuchi S. Reliability and validity of a questionnaire for self-assessment of complete dentures. BMC Oral Health. 2014;14:45. https://doi.org/10.1186/1472-6831-14-45.
150. Rooshenas L, Elliott D, Wade J, Jepson M, Paramasivan S, Strong S, et al. Conveying equipoise during recruitment for clinical trials: qualitative synthesis of clinicians' practices across six randomised controlled trials. PLoS Med. 2016;13:e1002147. https://doi.org/10.1371/journal.pmed.1002147.
151. Perri R, Wollin S, Drolet N, Mai S, Awad M, Feine J. Monitoring recruitment success and cost in a randomized clinical trial. Eur J Prosthodont Restor Dent. 2006;14:126–30.
152. Ellis JS, Levine A, Bedos C, Mojon P, Rosberger Z, Feine J, et al. Refusal of implant supported mandibular overdentures by elderly patients. Gerodontology. 2011;28:62–8. https://doi.org/10.1111/j.1741-2358.2009.00348.x.
153. Scotti N, Comba A, Gambino A, Manzon E, Breschi L, Paolino D, et al. Influence of operator experience on non-carious cervical lesion restorations: clinical evaluation with different adhesive systems. Am J Dent. 2016;29:33–8.
154. Nissan J, Oz-Ari B, Gross O, Ghelfan O, Chaushu G. Long-term prosthetic aftercare of direct vs. indirect attachment incorporation techniques to mandibular implant-supported overdenture. Clin Oral Implants Res. 2011;22:627–30. https://doi.org/10.1111/j.1600-0501.2010.02026.x.
155. Omar R, Al-Tarakemah Y, Akbar J, Al-Awadhi S, Behbehani Y, Lamontagne P. Influence of procedural variations during the laboratory phase of complete denture fabrication on patient satisfaction and den-

ture quality. J Dent. 2013;41:852–60. https://doi.org/10.1016/j.jdent.2013.07.013.
156. Slot W, Raghoebar GM, Cune MS, Vissink A, Meijer HJA. Four or six implants in the maxillary posterior region to support an overdenture: 5-year results from a randomized controlled trial. Clin Oral Implants Res. 2019;30:169–77. https://doi.org/10.1111/clr.13403.
157. Ma S, Tawse-Smith A, De Silva RK, Atieh MA, Alsabeeha NH, Payne AG. Maxillary three-implant overdentures opposing mandibular two-implant overdentures: 10-year surgical outcomes of a randomized controlled trial. Clin Implant Dent Relat Res. 2016;18:527–44. https://doi.org/10.1111/cid.12325.
158. Müller F, Al-Nawas B, Storelli S, Quirynen M, Hicklin S, Castro-Laza J, et al. Small-diameter titanium grade IV and titanium-zirconium implants in edentulous mandibles: five-year results from a double-blind, randomized controlled trial. BMC Oral Health. 2015;15:123. https://doi.org/10.1186/s12903-015-0107-6.
159. Naert I, Alsaadi G, van Steenberghe D, Quirynen M. A 10-year randomized clinical trial on the influence of splinted and unsplinted oral implants retaining mandibular overdentures: peri-implant outcome. Int J Oral Maxillofac Implants. 2004;19:695–702.
160. Vroom MG, Sipos P, de Lange GL, Gründemann LJ, Timmerman MF, Loos BG, et al. Effect of surface topography of screw-shaped titanium implants in humans on clinical and radiographic parameters: a 12-year prospective study. Clin Oral Implants Res. 2009;20:1231–9. https://doi.org/10.1111/j.1600-0501.2009.01768.x.
161. Meijer HJ, Raghoebar GM, Batenburg RH, Vissink A. Mandibular overdentures supported by two Brånemark, IMZ or ITI implants: a ten-year prospective randomized study. J Clin Periodontol. 2009;36:799–806. https://doi.org/10.1111/j.1600-051X.2009.01442.x.
162. Visser A, Meijer HJ, Raghoebar GM, Vissink A. Implant-retained mandibular overdentures versus conventional dentures: 10 years of care and aftercare. Int J Prosthodont. 2006;19:271–8.
163. Meijer HJ, Raghoebar GM, Van't Hof MA, Visser A. A controlled clinical trial of implant-retained mandibular overdentures: 10 years' results of clinical aspects and aftercare of IMZ implants and Brånemark implants. Clin Oral Implants Res. 2004;15:421–7. https://doi.org/10.1111/j.1600-0501.2004.01024.x.
164. Meijer HJ, Raghoebar GM, Van't Hof MA. Comparison of implant-retained mandibular overdentures and conventional complete dentures: a 10-year prospective study of clinical aspects and patient satisfaction. Int J Oral Maxillofac Implants. 2003;18:879–85.
165. Pummer A, Cieplik F, Nikolić M, Buchalla W, Hiller KA, Schmalz G. Longevity of posterior composite and compomer restorations in children placed under different types of anesthesia: a retrospective 5-year study. Clin Oral Investig. 2020;24:141–50. https://doi.org/10.1007/s00784-019-02911-2.
166. Barabanti N, Gagliani M, Roulet JF, Testori T, Ozcan M, Cerutti A. Marginal quality of posterior microhybrid resin composite restorations applied using two polymerisation protocols: 5-year randomised split mouth trial. J Dent. 2013;41:436–42. https://doi.org/10.1016/j.jdent.2013.02.009.
167. Casagrande L, Falster CA, Di Hipolito V, De Góes MF, Straffon LH, Nör JE, et al. Effect of adhesive restorations over incomplete dentin caries removal: 5-year follow-up study in primary teeth. J Dent Child (Chic). 2009;76:117–22.
168. Heck K, Manhart J, Hickel R, Diegritz C. Clinical evaluation of the bulk fill composite QuiXfil in molar class I and II cavities: 10-year results of a RCT. Dent Mater. 2018;34:e138–e47. https://doi.org/10.1016/j.dental.2018.03.023.
169. Friedman LM, Furberg CD, DeMets DL, Reboussin DM, Granger CB. Fundamentals of clinical trials. 5th ed. Springer International Publishing; 2015.
170. Schulz KF, Altman DG, Moher D, Group C. CONSORT 2010 statement: updated guidelines for reporting parallel group randomised trials. BMJ. 2010;340:c332. https://doi.org/10.1136/bmj.c332.
171. Campbell MK, Piaggio G, Elbourne DR, Altman DG, Group C. Consort 2010 statement: extension to cluster randomised trials. BMJ. 2012;345:e5661. https://doi.org/10.1136/bmj.e5661.
172. Shamseer L, Sampson M, Bukutu C, Schmid CH, Nikles J, Tate R, et al. CONSORT extension for reporting N-of-1 trials (CENT) 2015: explanation and elaboration. BMJ. 2015;350:h1793. https://doi.org/10.1136/bmj.h1793.
173. Pandis N, Chung B, Scherer RW, Elbourne D, Altman DG. CONSORT 2010 statement: extension checklist for reporting within person randomised trials. BMJ. 2017;357:j2835. https://doi.org/10.1136/bmj.j2835.
174. Oliveira CA, Dias PF, Dos Santos MP, Maia LC. Split mouth randomized controlled clinical trial of beveled cavity preparations in primary molars: an 18-Month follow up. J Dent. 2008;36:754–8. https://doi.org/10.1016/j.jdent.2008.05.006.
175. Gorseta K, Glavina D, Borzabadi-Farahani A, Van Duinen RN, Skrinjaric I, Hill RG, et al. One-year clinical evaluation of a Glass Carbomer fissure sealant, a preliminary study. Eur J Prosthodont Restor Dent. 2014;22:67–71.
176. Sartori N, Stolf SC, Silva SB, Lopes GC, Carrilho M. Influence of chlorhexidine digluconate on the clinical performance of adhesive restorations: a 3-year follow-up. J Dent. 2013;41:1188–95. https://doi.org/10.1016/j.jdent.2013.09.004.
177. Ernst CP, Brandenbusch M, Meyer G, Canbek K, Gottschalk F, Willershausen B. Two-year clinical performance of a nanofiller vs a fine-particle hybrid resin composite. Clin Oral Investig. 2006;10:119–25. https://doi.org/10.1007/s00784-006-0041-8.
178. Kotsanos N, Dionysopoulos P. Lack of effect of fluoride releasing resin modified glass ionomer restorations on the contacting surface of adjacent primary molars. a clinical prospective study. Eur J Paediatr Dent. 2004;5:136–42.
179. Koletsi D, Fleming PS, Seehra J, Bagos PG, Pandis N. Are sample sizes clear and justified in RCTs published in dental journals? PLoS One. 2014;9:e85949. https://doi.org/10.1371/journal.pone.0085949.

180. Pedersen AB, Mikkelsen EM, Cronin-Fenton D, Kristensen NR, Pham TM, Pedersen L, et al. Missing data and multiple imputation in clinical epidemiological research. Clin Epidemiol. 2017;9:157–66. https://doi.org/10.2147/CLEP.S129785.
181. Coast J. A history that goes hand in hand: Reflections on the development of health economics and the role played by Social Science & Medicine, 1967–2017. Soc Sci Med. 2018;196:227–32. https://doi.org/10.1016/j.socscimed.2017.10.032.
182. Ramsey SD, Willke RJ, Glick H, Reed SD, Augustovski F, Jonsson B, et al. Cost-effectiveness analysis alongside clinical trials II-An ISPOR Good Research Practices Task Force report. Value Health. 2015;18:161–72. https://doi.org/10.1016/j.jval.2015.02.001.
183. Petrou S, Gray A. Economic evaluation alongside randomised controlled trials: design, conduct, analysis, and reporting. Br Med J 2011; 342: d1548. doi: https://doi.org/10.1136/bmj.d1548.
184. Diana B. Methods for quantitative synthesis in medicine, meta-analysis, decision analysis and cost-effectiveness analysis. 2nd ed. USA: Oxford University Press; 2000.
185. Frick KD. Microcosting quantity data collection methods. Med Care. 2009;47:S76–81. https://doi.org/10.1097/MLR.0b013e31819bc064.
186. Hulme C, Yu G, Browne C, O'Dwyer J, Craddock H, Brown S, et al. Cost-effectiveness of silicone and alginate impressions for complete dentures. J Dent. 2014;42:902–7. https://doi.org/10.1016/j.jdent.2014.03.001.
187. Hofmann E, Behr M, Handel G. Frequency and costs of technical failures of clasp- and double crown-retained removable partial dentures. Clin Oral Investig. 2002;6:104–8. https://doi.org/10.1007/s00784-002-0160-9.
188. Della Vecchia MP, Leles CR, Cunha TR, Ribeiro AB, Sorgini DB, Muglia VA, et al. Mini-implants for mandibular overdentures: cost-effectiveness analysis alongside a randomized trial. JDR Clin Trans Res. 2018;3:47–56. https://doi.org/10.1177/2380084417741446.
189. Heydecke G, Penrod JR, Takanashi Y, Lund JP, Feine JS, Thomason JM. Cost-effectiveness of mandibular two-implant overdentures and conventional dentures in the edentulous elderly. J Dent Res. 2005;84:794–9. https://doi.org/10.1177/154405910508400903.
190. Takanashi Y, Penrod JR, Lund JP, Feine JS. A cost comparison of mandibular two-implant overdenture and conventional denture treatment. Int J Prosthodont. 2004;17:181–6.
191. Takanashi Y, Penrod JR, Chehade A, Klemetti E, Savard A, Lund JP, et al. Does a prosthodontist spend more time providing mandibular two-implant overdentures than conventional dentures? Int J Prosthodont. 2002;15:397–403.
192. van der Wijk P, Bouma J, van Waas MA, van Oort RP, Rutten FF. The cost of dental implants as compared to that of conventional strategies. Int J Oral Maxillofac Implants. 1998;13:546–53.
193. Ladewig NM, Sahiara CS, Yoshioka L, Olegário IC, Floriano I, Tedesco TK, et al. Efficacy of conventional treatment with composite resin and atraumatic restorative treatment in posterior primary teeth: study protocol for a randomised controlled trial. BMJ Open. 2017;7:e015542. https://doi.org/10.1136/bmjopen-2016-015542.
194. Goldman AS, Chen X, Fan M, Frencken JE. Methods and preliminary findings of a cost-effectiveness study of glass-ionomer-based and composite resin sealant materials after 2 yr. Eur J Oral Sci. 2014;122:230–7. https://doi.org/10.1111/eos.12129.
195. Sawatsky AP, Ratelle JT, Beckman TJ. Qualitative research methods in medical education. Anesthesiology. 2019;131:14–22. https://doi.org/10.1097/ALN.0000000000002728.
196. Gaglio B, Henton M, Barbeau A, Evans E, Hickam D, Newhouse R, et al. Methodological standards for qualitative and mixed methods patient centered outcomes research. BMJ. 2020;371:m4435. https://doi.org/10.1136/bmj.m4435.
197. Shneerson CL, Gale NK. Using mixed methods to identify and answer clinically relevant research questions. Qual Health Res. 2015;25:845–56. https://doi.org/10.1177/1049732315580107.
198. Macdonald ME, Keboa MT, Nurelhuda NM, Lawrence HP, Carnevale F, McNally M, et al. The oral health of refugees and asylum seekers in Canada: a mixed methods study protocol. Int J Environ Res Public Health. 2019;16 https://doi.org/10.3390/ijerph16040542.
199. Templeton AR, Young L, Bish A, Gnich W, Cassie H, Treweek S, et al. Patient-, organization-, and system-level barriers and facilitators to preventive oral health care: a convergent mixed-methods study in primary dental care. Implement Sci. 2016;11:5. https://doi.org/10.1186/s13012-015-0366-2.
200. Ahmad B, Landes D, Moffatt S. Dental public health in action: barriers to oral healthcare provision for older people in residential and nursing care homes: a mixed method evaluation and strategy development in County Durham. North East England Community Dent Health. 2018;35:136–9. https://doi.org/10.1922/CDH_4143Ahmad04.
201. Masood M, Newton T, Kharbanda OP, Masood Y, Feine J, Gussy M, et al. Building oral health research capacity in India: identifying barriers and enablers using mixed methods. JDR Clin Trans Res. 2017;2:106–8. https://doi.org/10.1177/2380084417691722.
202. Zelig R, Jones VM, Touger-Decker R, Hoskin ER, Singer SR, Byham-Gray L, et al. The eating experience: adaptive and maladaptive strategies of older adults with tooth loss. JDR Clin Trans Res. 2019;4:217–28. https://doi.org/10.1177/2380084419827532.
203. Porritt J, Rodd H, Morgan A, Williams C, Gupta E, Kirby J, et al. Development and testing of a cognitive behavioral therapy resource for children's dental anxiety. JDR Clin Trans Res. 2017;2:23–37. https://doi.org/10.1177/2380084416673798.
204. Mickenautsch S, Berger VW. The role of the randomised controlled trial in restorative dentistry and the correct purpose of observational data. Br Dent J. 2019; https://doi.org/10.1038/sj.bdj.2019.43.

Randomized Controlled Trials in Geriatric Dentistry

11

Jhanvi Desai, Leonardo Marchini, Christopher Childs, and Richie Kohli

11.1 Introduction

The global population is aging. There has been a striking increase in the average life expectancy during the twentieth century. At the same time, there has been a decrease in fertility rates, which has brought about a shift in worldwide demographics. Between 2015 and 2050, the proportion of the world's population over 60 years of age will nearly double from 12% to 22% [1].

As lifespan increases, chronic illnesses are replacing acute health issues as the main health concern for older adults. Some of the leading causes of death among older adults are chronic diseases like heart disease, cancer, Alzheimer's disease, etc. In turn, these chronic diseases can cause long-term disabilities, including mobility and cognitive impairments, that prevent people from caring for themselves. The Center for Disease Control and Prevention (CDC) reports that 20% of older adults have a disability [2].

Chronic diseases and disabilities are associated with an increased risk for falls, polypharmacy, and behavioral health issues, and they can reduce the chances of living independently for older adults. Another outcome of the mounting systemic health challenges is an increased risk for rapid oral health deterioration (ROHD) among older adults [3]. Many aging-related conditions, such as polypharmacy-induced xerostomia, lack of dental pain perception, high prevalence of caries and periodontal disease, sensory deterioration, and reduced manual dexterity, can contribute to a higher risk of ROHD among older adults. When older adults become frail and institutionalized, access to oral health care and maintenance becomes even more challenging [4]. Their daily oral hygiene is generally performed by caregivers, which is inadequate [3, 4].

Developing clinical research programs in geriatric dentistry requires that we understand the needs of our aging population and provide appropriate evidence-based dental care for this population. This research provides empirical evidence for best clinical practices and informs decision-making processes for developing appropriate public policies. This chapter investigates the current trends of randomized clinical trials (RCT) in geriatric dentistry, providing a synthesis of what has been done thus far, what gaps still exist, and

J. Desai (✉) · L. Marchini
Department of Preventive and Community Dentistry, College of Dentistry, University of Iowa, Iowa City, IA, USA
e-mail: jhanvi-desai@uiowa.edu; leonardo-marchini@uiowa.edu

C. Childs
Hardin Library for the Health Sciences, University of Iowa, Iowa City, IA, USA
e-mail: chris-childs@uiowa.edu

R. Kohli
Division of Dental Public Health, School of Dentistry, Oregon Health & Science University, Portland, OR, USA
e-mail: kohli@ohsu.edu

R. Kohli et al. (eds.), *Randomized Controlled Trials in Evidence-Based Dentistry*,
https://doi.org/10.1007/978-3-031-47651-8_11

opportunities for future research in the field. The chapter first provides a critical analysis of gaps in existing randomized controlled trials and then addresses ongoing methodological issues.

11.2 Critical Analysis and Gaps in Existing Randomized Controlled Trials by Outcomes

A health sciences librarian performed literature searches in four electronic databases, namely, MEDLINE via PubMed interface, Embase, Cumulative Index to Nursing and Allied Health Literature (CINAHL), and AgeLine. The searches were performed over 4 weeks from October 17, 2019, through November 11, 2019, starting with PubMed and progressing in order as listed. The search terms (Box 11.1) were developed by a dentist with 20+ years of training in geriatric dentistry research (LM) and the health sciences librarian (CC), who combined the terms to create a comprehensive search strategy. The health sciences librarian then adapted the original search strategy for the other databases listed. An English language and human studies filter were applied to all database searches, except for the Cochrane Library, where those filters are not available.

The search process and selection of articles used in this scoping review can be found in the Preferred Reporting Items for Systematic Reviews and Meta-Analyses (PRISMA) diagram (Fig. 11.1). A total of 405 citations were retrieved from four databases: 221 in PubMed, 92 in Embase, 69 in CINAHL, and 23 in AgeLine. After duplicates were removed, 336 citations remained. Initial screening based on abstract and title alone yielded 81 citations. After full-text reviews, 76 articles were selected and used to create the content for this chapter. The 76 articles included 74 RCTs and 2 proposed study protocols for conducting a randomized controlled trial. These latter two were proposed studies with directives about how to carry out the trial without actually performing the steps; thus, no outcomes were reported.

The structure and syntax of the database searches are commonly used in systematic reviews. All the terms in the search strategy were divided into three groups, as described in Box 11.1.

Box 11.1 Terms Used for the Database Search

Group 1: Population.

"Aged, 80 and over"[MeSH] OR Aged 80 and over [tw] OR Oldest Old [tw] OR Nonagenarians [tw] OR Nonagenarian [tw] OR Octogenarians [tw] OR Octogenarian [tw] OR Centenarians [tw] OR Centenarian [tw] OR **"Frail Elderly"[MeSH]** OR Frail Elderly [tw] OR Frail Elders [tw] OR Frail Elder [tw] OR Functionally-Impaired Elderly [tw] OR Functionally Impaired Elderly [tw] OR Frail Older Adults [tw] OR Frail Older Adult [tw] OR community-dwelling elders [tw] OR independently-living older adults [tw] OR institutionalized elders [tw] OR medically complex patients [tw].

AND

Group 2: Geriatric Dentistry.

"Dental Care"[MeSH] OR Dental Care [tw] OR **"Geriatric Dentistry"[MeSH]** OR Geriatric Dentistry [tw] OR **"Oral Health"[MeSH]** OR Oral Health [tw] OR **"Oral Hygiene"[MeSH]** OR Oral Hygiene [tw] OR Dental Hygiene [tw].

AND

RCT Filter #1.

Randomized Controlled Trial*[tw] OR Randomised Controlled Trial*[tw] OR RCT*[tw] OR "Randomized Controlled Trial" [Publication Type] OR "Randomized Controlled Trials as Topic"[MeSH].

Based on the findings of our database search analysis on existing RCTs in geriatric dentistry as explained above, the RCTs ($N = 76$ articles) were categorized as: (1) oral hygiene routines and/or caregivers' education (27 articles), (2) mechanical

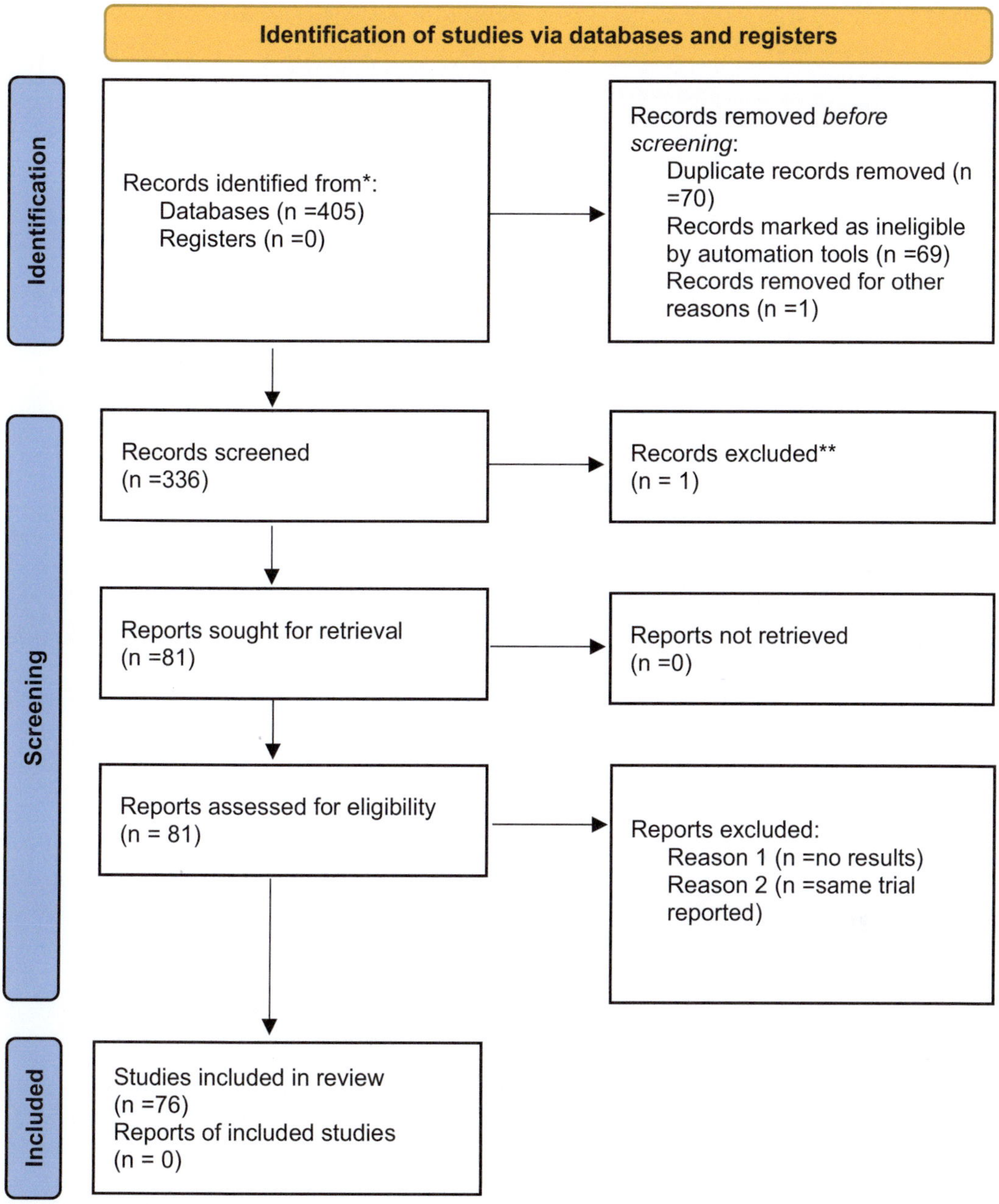

Fig. 11.1 Preferred reporting items for systematic reviews and meta-analyses (PRISMA) flow diagram- *From:* Page MJ, McKenzie JE, Bossuyt PM, Boutron I, Hoffmann TC, Mulrow CD, et al. The PRISMA 2020 statement: an updated guideline for reporting systematic reviews. BMJ 2021; 372: n71. doi: 10.1136/bmj.n71

or chemotherapeutic agents to prevent oral diseases (29 articles), (3) restorative techniques and materials (14 articles), and (4) miscellaneous (6 articles). Table 11.1 provides a summary of the outcomes of the reviewed articles and their strength of evidence. Table 11.2 provides examples of gaps in research and future recommendations for research related to RCTs in geriatric dentistry.

Table 11.1 Summary of the outcomes of the reviewed articles and their strength of evidence

Topic with references		
(1) Prevention (OH routine and caregivers' education)	Study outcomes	Strength of evidence
Professional oral care [5–10]	Tooth-brushing by dentists, hygienists, and dental nurses on a weekly/bi-weekly basis showed improvement in oral health outcomes like oral health indices, plaque index, nutritional status, oral function, and incidence of influenza among older adults.	Moderate
Motivation-education [11, 12]	In community-dwelling older adults, there was increased self-efficacy in-home care with improvements in periodontal parameters such as plaque scores and gingival indices. This study also coupled the use of chlorhexidine and fluoride varnish; however, there was a negligible anti-caries effect of the intervention.	Moderate
Caregiver education: setting up hygiene protocols [13–19]	Setting daily oral hygiene protocols and educating caregivers in nursing homes to deliver care had conflicting results across the 7 studies that were evaluated. Two studies showed a reduction in plaque levels, and one study reported a reduction in pneumonia among nursing home residents who received daily oral care by a nurse. Four studies showed no difference in oral health post-intervention.	Conflicting results
Supervised oral health care [20, 21]	Supervised oral health care in nursing home populations showed a reduction in denture plaque but not in dental plaque.	Moderate
Tongue cleaning [22, 23]	In the 2 studies where oral care was complemented with tongue cleaning, there was improved coughing ability and a reduction in candida scores in institutionalized older adults.	Low
Daily oral care for hospitalized frail patients [24, 25]	There was a reduction in dental and denture plaque in the admitted frail older patients.	Low
(2) Mechanical or chemotherapeutic agents to prevent oral diseases		
Fluoride [26–31]	Use of silver diamine fluoride (SDF) every 6 months and rinsing with 10 ml of 0.05% NaF twice daily (as compared to the use of fluoride tablets, toothpaste, and slurry) were found to be effective in caries prevention. In a nursing home-based study, lesser progression in root caries was reported with the use of 5000 ppm fluoride toothpaste. An OHRQoL study in community-dwelling adults reported that patients did not perceive any difference between the use of two fluoridated toothpaste (1450 ppm vs. 5000 ppm).	Moderate
Chlorhexidine [32–37]	Chlorhexidine in the form of 0.2% spray (varnish) had an anti-caries effect, while that in the form of chewing gum and daily mouth-rinse (concentration 0.12–0.2%) showed improvement in the plaque and gingival indices as well as caries reduction. A study found that daily 0.05% chlorhexidine rinse application in patients with dysphagia did not show significant improvement in the incidence of pneumonia.	Moderate
Fluoride+CHX [31, 38]	The use of SDF, fluoride varnish, and chlorhexidine varnish was more effective in root caries prevention in institutionalized older adults.	High
Electric toothbrush [39–42]	No difference was reported in the effectiveness of the use of an electric toothbrush when compared with a manual toothbrush.	Moderate
(3) Restorative (techniques and materials)		
ART [43–47]	ART restoration survival rates were comparable to conventional restorations; it was more cost-effective; and patient perception was good for this technique. ART, when coupled with Cariosolv gel, did not have any better outcomes than ART alone.	High

Table 11.1 (continued)

Topic with references		
(1) Prevention (OH routine and caregivers' education)	Study outcomes	Strength of evidence
(3) Restorative (techniques and materials)		
RPD vs. SDA [48–52]	Shortened dental arch (SDA) was found to be more cost-effective, and patients with SDA were perceived to have better OHRQoL. Nutritionally, SDA and removable partial dentures had similar outcomes.	Moderate
Implants [53–55]	Implant-retained mandibular overdentures had better denture satisfaction and OHRQoL than conventional mandibular dentures while chewing efficiency was found to be no different between the two groups. The chewing efficiency of implant-retained mandibular overdentures that were loaded immediately vs. conventionally was found to be similar.	Moderate
(4) Miscellaneous		
Reflexes and aspiration pneumonia [56–58]	Daily oral care improves cough reflex sensitivity. Resistance training of swallowing muscles did not improve dysphagia. Daily oral care and upright feeding posture did not significantly reduce the incidence of aspiration pneumonia.	Low

Table 11.2 Examples of knowledge gaps in RCTs in geriatric dentistry

Topic	Knowledge gaps
(1) Prevention (OH routine and caregivers' education)	Clinical outcome measures for professional oral care in patients with dementia Clinical effectiveness of professional oral health care in reducing the risk of influenza and aspiration pneumonia Standardization and effectiveness of oral hygiene protocols for geriatric patients by dental disease risk Clinical effectiveness and cost-effectiveness of caregivers vs. dental professionals who provided oral hygiene for nursing home residents Effective protocols for oral cancer prevention
(2) Mechanical or chemotherapeutic agents to prevent oral diseases	Effectiveness of SDF to prevent and arrest root caries when not used in conjunction with oral hygiene instruction/education Effectiveness of SDF on coronal caries and long-term effects in the elderly with varying levels of dependency Long-term effectiveness of high-fluoride toothpaste in preventing root caries Protocol for chlorhexidine-thymol varnish to decrease the incidence of root caries Comparative effectiveness of different fluoride modalities to decrease the incidence and progression of coronal and root caries Comparative effectiveness of a manual vs. electric toothbrush Effect of oral disease preventive modalities on OHQoL
(3) Restorative (techniques and materials)	Long-term survival rates of ART vs. conventional restorations Functional outcomes for patients with treated and untreated shortened dental arches Effectiveness of different treatment regimens for peri-implantitis
(4) Miscellaneous	Clinical effectiveness of professional oral health care in reducing the risk of aspiration pneumonia Effect of improved oral health on OHQoL Comparative effectiveness of nickel-titanium (NiTi) rotary files compared to stainless-steel (SST) hand files in geriatric patients Effect of novel painless single tooth anesthesia (STA) vs. conventional anesthesia on elderly patients' clinical outcomes Effect of improved social determinants of health on oral health and quality of life Effect of the use of teledentistry and/or allied health professions on dental access for geriatric patients

The next section of this chapter discusses the details of the articles centered around the four main categories.

11.2.1 Oral Hygiene Routines and/or Caregivers' Education: 27 Articles

This category consists of articles about preventive measures for improving oral hygiene among older adults. The interventions range from educating older adults, providing professional oral care, or introducing oral hygiene protocols for them to follow, and they were applied to both community-dwelling older adults and residents in long-term care facilities. For community-dwelling older adults, preventive measures included outcomes of weekly oral care delivered at a daycare facility by dental hygienists [5], customized oral hygiene instructions for patients visiting a community-based health center [59], and oral hygiene education and preventive protocols for evaluating caries prevention and periodontal outcomes in older adult patients [11, 12]. For those in long-term care facilities, preventive measures included educating support staff, introducing oral hygiene protocols, and evaluating outcomes for these interventions.

The majority of the randomized controlled trials included only patients in long-term care facilities. About 20 articles were identified, and the research topics for these articles were then divided into sub-categories. The first sub-category concerned the delivery of professional oral care (5 studies). Two of these five studies examined the effects of weekly tooth brushing by dental hygienists/nurses on the oral health of institutionalized older adults [6, 7]. Two Danish studies determined whether professional oral care, nutritional supplements, and exercise resulted in improved social and functional abilities among nursing home residents [8, 9]. The fifth study, conducted in Japan, identified nutritional outcomes associated with professional oral care delivered by a dentist to nursing home residents three times a week [10].

The second sub-category includes studies about implementing oral care protocols in long-term care facilities, educating caregivers in those facilities, and measuring outcomes for these interventions based on plaque scores, risk of pneumonia, etc. (7 studies) [13–19].

Supervised versus non-supervised mouth care was a third sub-category, but only two of the three studies in this sub-category included interventions [20, 21, 60].

The final sub-category includes studies with interventions such as using occupational therapy to improve oral hygiene, using functional therapy with oral care to improve nutritional status, and using strategies to provide oral hygiene to patients with dementia; this category also includes studies evaluating outcomes of tongue cleaning to improve oral hygiene among institutionalized older adults [22, 23, 61–63].

Of these studies, two focused on oral hygiene as an important parameter for recovery after surgery and pneumonia for frail, hospitalized older adults [24, 64], and another study discussed improving dental and denture hygiene among older adults under long-term hospital care by educating their caregivers [25].

There is low to moderate evidence about the effectiveness of oral hygiene routines and/or caregivers' education, as described below:

1. Tooth-brushing by dentists, hygienists, and dental nurses on a weekly/bi-weekly basis showed improvement in oral health outcomes like oral health indices, plaque index, nutritional status, oral function, and the incidence of influenza among older adults.
2. In community-dwelling older adults, there was increased self-efficacy in-home care with improvements in periodontal parameters such as plaque scores and gingival indices. This study also coupled the use of chlorhexidine and fluoride varnish; however, there was a negligible anti-caries effect of the intervention.
3. Setting daily oral hygiene protocols and educating caregivers in nursing homes to deliver care had conflicting results across the seven studies evaluated. Two studies showed a reduction in plaque levels, and another study reported a reduction in pneumonia among nursing home residents who received daily

oral care by a nurse. Four studies showed no difference in oral health post-intervention. Supervised oral health care in nursing home populations showed a reduction in denture plaque but not in dental plaque.

4. In the two studies where oral care was complemented with tongue cleaning, there was improved coughing ability and a reduction in candida scores measuring institutionalized older adults' tongue coating. There was a reduction in dental and denture plaque for frail older adults admitted to the hospital.

There were gaps in research particularly related to (1) clinical outcome measures for professional oral care in patients with dementia; (2) clinical effectiveness of professional oral health care in reducing the risk of influenza and aspiration pneumonia; (3) standardization and effectiveness of oral hygiene protocols for geriatric patients by dental disease risk; (4) clinical effectiveness and cost-effectiveness of caregiver vs. dental professional provided oral hygiene for nursing home residents; and (5) oral cancer prevention in geriatric patients.

11.2.2 Mechanical or Chemotherapeutic Agents to Prevent Oral Diseases: 29 Articles

Preventive studies in this category evaluate the use of different mechanical or chemotherapeutic agents to prevent oral diseases. The research topics were further subdivided according to the purpose of the chemotherapeutic or mechanical agents used to bring about preventive outcomes in the geriatric population.

For the studies examining chemotherapeutic agents or materials, 16 used various materials in a nursing home setting to lower plaque and microbial counts. Some preventive materials used in these 16 studies included lactoferrin and lactoperoxidase-containing foods; gel and mouth-rinse; moisturizing gel and mouthwash [65–67]; chlorhexidine (CHX)/xylitol chewing gum [32, 68], CHX spray [33], CHX swabs [34], probiotic lozenges [69], stannous fluoride-based toothpaste [26], and alcohol-free mouth rinses; and gels [35, 70–73]. A hospital ward-based study explored the use of CHX mouth rinse among older patients [36], and a community-based study investigated the effect of inorganic pyrophosphate as a treatment for older adults with periodontitis [74]. These studies used various materials to prevent root caries in community-dwelling residents, including CHX/Xylitol chewing gum [75], silver diamine fluoride (SDF) [27], and higher-concentration fluoride toothpastes [28]. Five studies conducted in nursing home settings explored oral health outcomes resulting from the use of fluoride varnish, CHX varnish, silver diamine fluoride (SDF), and higher concentration fluoride toothpaste [29–31, 37, 38]. A recent case-based series that enrolled independent community-dwelling adults also showed arrested root lesions and crown margins with repeated application of 38% SDF at 6-month intervals [76]. Another study discussed the effects of alcohol-containing mouth rinse on xerostomia in community-based older adults [77].

The remaining studies used mechanical agents or instruments to deliver preventive care, including four studies that examined outcomes associated with using electric toothbrushes, three of which were for nursing home residents [39–41], and another that determined the effectiveness of implant-supported mandibular overdentures [42]. There is moderate to high evidence for the effectiveness of different chemotherapeutic or mechanical agents in preventing oral diseases, as described below:

1. Chlorhexidine, in the form of a 0.2% spray had an anti-caries effect as chewing gum, and as a daily mouth-rinse (concentration 0.12–0.2%), plaque and gingival indices improved and caries incidence was reduced. A study with a daily 0.05% chlorhexidine rinse application in patients with dysphagia did not show significant improvement in the incidence of pneumonia.
2. Use of SDF every 6 months and rinse with 10 ml of 0.05% NaF twice daily were more effective at caries prevention than was the use of a fluoride tablet, toothpaste, and slurry.

3. In a nursing home-based study, the use of 5000 ppm fluoride toothpaste slowed root caries progression.
4. An OHRQoL study reported that community-dwelling patients did not perceive any difference between the use of two fluoridated toothpaste (1450 ppm vs. 5000 ppm).
5. The use of SDF, fluoride varnish, and chlorhexidine varnish was more effective in root caries prevention in institutionalized older adults when compared to routine oral hygiene practices.
6. The use of an electric toothbrush was no more effective than a manual toothbrush in improving oral hygiene status.

The gaps in this research topic on prevention could be identified as (1) the effectiveness of SDF to prevent and arrest root caries when used independently of oral hygiene instruction/education; (2) effectiveness of SDF on coronal caries and long-term effects among older adults with varying levels of dependency; (3) long-term effectiveness of high-fluoride toothpaste in preventing root caries; (4) protocols for the use of chlorhexidine-thymol varnish to decrease the incidence of root caries; (5) comparative effectiveness of different fluoride modalities to decrease the incidence and progression of coronal and root caries; (6) comparative effectiveness of a manual versus an electric toothbrush; and (7) effect of oral disease preventive modalities on OHQoL.

11.2.3 Restorative (Techniques and Materials): 14 Articles

This category included studies dealing with restorative and rehabilitative measures.

In the restorative sub-category, all studies involved the use of ART (atraumatic restorative treatment). Two studies examined the survival rates of restorations placed using the ART technique on community-dwelling older adults and institutionalized adults [43, 44], while one study used ART with Cariosolv to treat root caries in institutionalized older adults, measuring survival rate outcomes [45]. One study focused on patient perceptions of minimally invasive dentistry among community-dwelling older adults [46], while another investigated the cost-effectiveness of ART restorations for older adults treated at a day hospital and a dental school [47].

In the rehabilitative sub-category, the studies discussed tooth/teeth replacement strategies using removable prostheses. Two studies investigated masticatory efficiency and patient-perceived oral health-related quality of life (OHRQoL) with implant-retained mandibular overdentures [53, 54]. Passia et al. (2017) compared the loading protocol of implants and the chewing efficiency of mandibular implant overdentures [55]. In a series of five articles, McKenna et al. explored cost-effectiveness, OHRQoL, and nutritional status in partially edentulous older adults using either removable partial dentures or maintaining a shortened dental arch (SDA) [48–52]. A study to understand the effect of a domiciliary denture service on oral health-related quality of life showed improvement in the study group when they received home visits from a denture team for denture adjustments [78]. There is moderate to high evidence for the effectiveness of different restorative and rehabilitative measures, as described below:

1. ART restoration survival rates were comparable to conventional restorations, but it was more cost-effective, and patient's perceptions of the technique were favorable. ART when coupled with Cariosolv gel, did not have any better outcomes than ART alone.
2. A shortened dental arch (SDA) was found to be more cost-effective, and patients with an SDA saw their OHRQoL in more favorable terms. Nutritionally, SDA and removable partial dentures had similar outcomes.
3. An implant-retained mandibular overdenture resulted in better denture satisfaction and OHRQoL than conventional mandibular dentures while chewing efficiency was no different between the two groups. The chewing efficiency of implant-retained mandibular overdentures, which were loaded immediately rather than conventionally, had similar results.

4. Domiciliary denture service improved the oral health-related quality of life in older adults.

   The gaps in this research area could be identified as 1) long-term survival rates of ART versus conventional restorations; 2) functional outcomes for patients with treated and untreated SDA; and 3) effectiveness of different treatment regimens for peri-implantitis.

11.2.4 Miscellaneous: (6 Articles)

This category includes studies in which the subject of the research does not conform to the other categories. Two studies discuss interventions like daily oral care to improve cough reflex sensitivity and oral care with an upright feeding posture to reduce the incidence of pneumonia [56, 57]. Wakabayashi et al. (2018) discussed resistance training of the oral musculature and dysphagia [58]. Two investigations explored patient perceptions—of sleep quality in edentulous patients [79] and of having oral exams as part of their general health checkups at medical centers [80]. Weijenberg et al. (2013) put forward a study protocol aimed at evaluating masticatory efficiency and OHRQoL in older adults with dementia [81].

The findings related to these studies provide low evidence as follows: (1) Daily oral care improved cough reflex sensitivity; (2) Resistance training of swallowing muscles did not improve dysphagia; (3) Daily oral care and upright feeding posture did not significantly reduce the incidence of aspiration pneumonia.

The research gap in this area was related to (1) the clinical effectiveness of professional oral health care in reducing the risk of aspiration pneumonia and (2) the effect of oral health on quality of life.

In addition to the gaps reported above, research is lacking in many other areas of oral care for older adults, such as endodontics, oral surgery, esthetic dentistry, orthodontics, teledentistry, and dental quality measures. Some examples are (1) the comparative effectiveness of nickel-titanium (NiTi) rotary files compared to stainless-steel (SST) hand files for older patients; (2) the effect of novel painless single-tooth anesthesia (STA) versus conventional anesthesia on clinical outcomes for older patients; and (3) the effect of the use of teledentistry and/or allied health professions on dental access for older patients. Geriatric dental care and research also need to encompass medical as well as social health modifiers to improve the overall health and quality of life of the elderly.

Any randomized controlled trial needs a rigorous, valid methodology. The following section provides a comprehensive sketch of the methodology protocols that have been followed by the studies mentioned previously. Apart from the trends that have been followed so far, some troubleshooting recommendations have also been included to encourage new researchers.

11.3 Critical Analysis of Existing Randomized Controlled Trials by Methodological Issues and Risk of Bias, with Future Recommendations

11.3.1 Study Setting

For the RCTs identified, the greatest number was conducted in Japan (15), followed by the UK (7), Ireland (7), the United States (6), and Canada (5). Approximately 62% of the studies were conducted in nursing homes or long-term care (LTC) facilities, and 33% were carried out among community-dwelling older adults. The remaining 5% of the studies were conducted in hospital settings or medical wards.

Any change in sensory, cognitive, or musculoskeletal status can render independent, community-living older adults frail. This drastic turn of events can render them incapacitated to participate and/or comply with the guidelines of a research study; thus, ease of access to care is vitally important. Thus, for example, during the planning process for the trial, community-based transportation to and from the dental center must be part of the study protocol to maximize patient attendance. Nursing home-based studies have the advantage of having a large target population available at a single site, but such studies have a range of issues, including concerns about a lack of autonomy and using third parties to help conduct the study. As such, there are no ideal settings when it comes to conducting geriatric research, but a deeper understanding of the community and increased social support for older adults can improve the feasibility of studies.

11.3.2 Study Duration

Study duration ranged from 5 days in a hospital-based study to a 5-year study based in a nursing home. Sixteen RCTs were for 1 year, and another six were for more than 1 year. The remaining studies lasted less than 1 year.

The cost and attrition of research subjects from the sample population pose challenges for conducting longitudinal studies with older adults. Since the attrition rates are higher in geriatric research than in the general population, conducting long-term studies in this field is significantly more challenging. This fact is likely one of the primary reasons for the limited study duration of most of the studies.

11.3.3 Study Funding

Forty-nine studies of the 76 reviewed articles were partly or completely funded. The majority of the funding was from public research funds, i.e., universities, local governing bodies, and federal funding sources. Around 12 studies had dental products or experimental products donated by the manufacturing companies.

The study conducted by Kraft et al. (2015) not only had the experimental product but also a grant funded by a probiotic manufacturing company [69]. Two other studies (Morita et al. 2017; Nakano et al. 2017) had a potential conflict of interest as the majority of the authors were employees of the milk industry, which sponsored the experimental product as well as the study [65, 66].

Funding consortiums that involve a combination of public agencies, non-profit foundations, and corporations can help dental geriatric research, improve collaboration with other fields such as geriatric medicine, nursing, etc., and broaden the scope of available funds for furthering dental research in older adults.

11.3.4 Recruitment of the Sample Population

For 74 of the articles, sample sizes ranged from 13 individuals in 1987 to a minimum of 13 individuals across 74 articles. In the remaining two studies, the number of restorations was reported rather than the number of patients. Twelve studies reported challenges in recruiting study participants. Some of the challenges mentioned included patients not being able to include persons with cognitive impairments [7], facilities refusing to participate, facilities having too few residents for the study [12, 19], and communication or language barriers [22]. Additionally, for many microbiological studies, frequent use of antibiotics and anti-fungal materials among older adults resulted in the exclusion of multiple participants from studies [7, 34, 69]. Kraft et al. (2015) indicated that severe chronic diseases, malignancies, and/or terminal diseases reduced the pool of participants to recruit from and reduced subject retention [69]. They also showed that a significant number of older adults were reluctant to enroll in research studies. Muller et al. (2013) also indicated that patients were reluctant to participate in their free-implant study because of fears pertaining to surgical interventions [54]. Chalhoub (2016) likewise indicated that recruitment was challenging because the study relied on medical staff to determine whether patients met the inclusion criteria of the study, which involved identifying the medical outcomes of dental interventions [72].

A consistent theme among the studies was that recruiting older adults, whether in the community or nursing homes, poses a significant challenge for conducting research investigations. As a result, a pilot study should be conducted before the full scale of operations is conducted. This pilot study would be able to identify challenges for subject recruitment given the particular characteristics of the study. Most often, the challenges will include miscommunication due to sensory challenges, the use of technical terms in study brochures, or misconceptions about research, which can lead to a lack of participation by older adults in a study. However, providing adequate time for understanding the study and sending out simple but effective information to family or caregivers can help potential participants understand the aim and values of the study and, as a result, improve recruitment rates. Additionally, many older adults mistrust researchers or are unaware of studies going on in their communities. A good way to improve recruitment and raise awareness among community-based older adults is to maintain a good relationship with community advisory boards and establish their trust. These members can act as gatekeepers to their community and help research studies by hosting introductory meetings, educating their community members, and/or reassuring seniors [82].

11.3.5 Retention of the Sample Population

Of the 76 studies, 32 reported challenges in retaining study participants. These challenges included morbidity issues [17, 22, 64], residents leaving facility [22, 37], hospitalization [58, 72], and subjects being unwilling to continue with a long-term study [11, 37]. Some less common reasons for dropping out of the study include an unexpected adverse reaction (burning sensation in the mouth) [72], a participant taking a holiday [33], or loss of support from nursing staff and directors of residential homes [68].

Some issues, such as hospitalizations and deaths, cannot be addressed, but additional support and training for care staff in nursing homes can address some retention challenges. For example, recruiting research assistants (RAs) who can oversee the logistics of the study can reduce the workload for caregivers or nursing staff. This, in turn, can improve recruitment, retention, and adherence from them as well as from the participants. Hiring RAs will need to be included in the budgeting of the study at the start of the study.

Attrition rates are significantly greater for research with older adults than for the general population. These challenges need to be addressed at the start of the study when the sample size is being determined. Oversampling needs to be done so that the eventual attrition of the sample size can be absorbed without losing the power of the study.

11.3.6 Protocol Adherence

Of the 76 studies, 18 reported challenges associated with subjects failing to adhere to the research protocols. In some studies, participants refused oral care, were not able to follow instructions (e.g., forgot to use complete dentures for the prescribed hours), had mood changes that made it difficult for them to follow directions or were unavailable for examinations [22, 72]. Some caregivers also had difficulty adhering to the research protocols as a result of too much workload, the use of a new and unfamiliar electronic system for resident files, budget cuts, renovations and structural changes at nursing homes, and changes in the health system [35]. Additional adherence issues resulted from gaps in the instructions passed down to nursing staff and poor attitudes among caregivers. Kraft (2015) indicated that some patients refused to participate in the study, and adherence issues arose mostly during examinations and sampling of participants during their study [69]. Low adherence to exercise/training by patients was reported by Wakabayashi (2018) in his study [58]. Failure to prioritize the research, lack of caregiver time and support, cognitive challenges, and resistance to oral care were some reasons noted in the study [14].

Additionally, MacEntree (2007) reported that caregivers had poor attendance for educational seminars, and a labor dispute before the start of the study likely caused some adherence issues by diminishing staff and participant interest [17]. Fjeld (2018) reported that very few individuals received dental hygiene assistance but did not specify the reason [39, 40]. Lavigne et al. (2018) indicated that one potential explanation for poor adherence to protocols was the inability of the caregivers to deliver oral care to the residents of the nursing home [41]. Adherence issues among nursing home patients were principally due to resident or staff factors. Typically, when nursing home residents did not understand the personal benefit of the study or if they perceived the intervention as an invasion of privacy, adherence issues were often seen [83]. Additionally, nursing home staff, including caregivers, may have felt threatened that researchers could observe their routine care or add more work for them, e.g., record documentation, both of which lead to poor adherence. Some strategies recommended by Mody et al. (2008) to address these staff-related issues include meeting face-to-face with administrators and the Director of Nursing with informative brochures highlighting the study benefits and protocol and discussing financial costs and staff time to establish a positive working relationship between researchers and the nursing home [82]. Reimbursement for staff time and recognition of their efforts can also be attractive for caregivers. Also, periodic meetings with updates about the research project can improve nursing staff morale [82].

11.3.7 Consent Challenges

Three studies reported that securing informed consent was challenging. The challenges included time delays resulting from consulting with family members [72] and being unable to collect written consent from relatives [69]. According to Marchini et al. (2018), getting in touch with the guardians of nursing home residents for consent was difficult and often unsuccessful, and many guardians did not understand that enrolling their loved ones would be beneficial for the resident [19].

According to Mody et al. (2008), family or guardians of older adults often mistrust research personnel and feel as if they 'exploit' vulnerable populations [82]. Sometimes the nursing home staff voice their distrust and can discourage residents/guardians from enrolling in research projects. Clearly indicating the reasons for participating in the study to facility staff and family members with, for example, an eye-catching informative brochure with a simplified research protocol, the aims and benefits of the proposed study, a consent form, and some published research can increase their awareness of and consent to a research study [82]. If the facility is invested in the project, it can facilitate participation and help obtain consent for the study.

11.3.8 Cluster Randomization

Fourteen studies used cluster randomization in their methodology. Of these, 12 were based in nursing homes. One study based in a community setting had gender-based sample units, and one other hospital-based study had ward-based sample units. Cluster randomization is advantageous due to ease of administration, organization, and minimizing costs. With nursing home or community-based studies, there is less risk of contamination and possibly more adherence. However, one of the pitfalls of cluster randomization is that more individuals will need to be recruited for sound statistical analysis, and this is a serious drawback given that recruitment is challenging and drop-out rates are high in geriatric research. Insufficient randomization units may yield studies that do not have optimal power or inconclusive results.

Since cluster sampling includes individual institutions as a unit, more institutions—such as nursing homes, geriatric care facilities, and daycare homes—should be recruited at the start of the study. This ensures that the randomization units are sufficient even if facilities drop out during the study. To maximize participation in a nursing home, it is important to involve the administrators and staff in the study. Any financial costs or staff time commitments for the institution should be discussed beforehand, and reimbursement, if provided, needs to be clearly communicated. As above, a simple and informative brochure with study protocols that emphasize how study results enhance the care of older adults increases recruitment at nursing homes. Regular communication, feedback, and appreciation of the efforts of staff can help in retention and adherence within the facility.

11.3.9 Adherence to the Risk of Bias (ROB) Criteria

Bias refers to all those factors that systematically affect the observations and processes of a study and lead to erroneous or unjustified conclusions. Studies affected by bias can be inaccurate or under- or overestimate the outcome of interventions, which can, in turn, produce incorrect guidelines. Although it can be difficult to establish the precise extent to which bias affects a study, it is clear that certain flaws in the design, execution, and analysis of a randomized controlled trial can lead to bias. Thus, evaluating the methodology for the risk of bias results in more robust studies that are more likely to give valid and justifiable results. It is important to assess the risk of bias for each of the studies in this review, regardless of the results or validity of the studies [84]. The 76 articles (74 studies and 2 proposed study protocols) were subjected to the rigor of criteria for judging the risk of bias (ROB) adapted from the Cochrane Handbook of Systematic Reviews of Interventions [85–87]. The types of bias evaluated were (1) random sequence generation (selection bias); (2) allocation concealment (selection bias); (3) blinding of participants, personnel, and care providers (performance bias); (4) blinding of outcome assessor (detection bias); (5) incomplete outcome data (attrition bias); (6) selective reporting (reporting bias); and (7) other bias (bias not addressed elsewhere). Based on our assessment, the majority of the studies (>50%) had a low bias in random sequence, allocation concealment, blinding of the outcome assessor, incomplete outcome data, selective reporting, and other biases. Thirty-seven studies had a high risk of bias in the blinding of participants, personnel, or care providers. During cluster randomization, certain nursing homes indicated that they knew they were included in the intervention groups. Furthermore, for certain interventions in nursing homes, such as the use of electric versus manual toothbrushes and professional oral care versus routine care by caregivers, it is clear that both patients and caregivers were aware of the group to which they belonged. In many studies, it was noted that the intervention group included the application of preventive agents, and the control group consisted of routine care with no placebo agent application. Such a protocol would indicate to both patients and caregivers whether they belonged to the experimental group or not.

To overcome these limiting factors, future studies should plan procedures meticulously to reduce the risk of bias by blinding the participants and caregivers. For example, including a placebo when interventions include a preventive agent, having a protocol in place for the control group, staggering the intervention if participants share common premises/rooms/bathrooms, etc. can reduce the risk of bias. Furthermore, when research is being introduced to administrators of nursing homes, the need for randomization for research needs to be explained, and their acceptance of randomization should be included in the contract.

Table 11.3 provides a summary of the risk of bias in the reviewed articles.

Table 11.3 Risk of bias in the reviewed article recommendations

Random sequence generation (selection bias)	Allocation concealment (selection bias)	Blinding of participants and personnel/care providers (performance bias)	Blinding of the outcome assessor (detection bias)	Incomplete outcome data (attrition bias)	Selective reporting (reporting bias)	RoB-Other bias
High bias $N = 4$	High bias $N = 13$	High $N = 37$	High $N = 8$	High $N = 8$	High $N = 6$	High $N = 2$
Low bias $N = 46$	Low $N = 42$	Low $N = 26$	Low $N = 54$	Low $N = 63$	Low $N = 66$	Low $N = 62$
Unclear $N = 24$	Unclear $N = 21$	Unclear $N = 13$	Unclear $N = 14$	Unclear $N = 5$	Unclear $N = 4$	Unclear $N = 12$

11.4 Summary

As older adults retain more of their natural dentition and medical histories become more complex, the focus of geriatric dental research needs to expand to meet the oral health needs of this growing population of patients while addressing their medical and social complexities, aesthetic and functional demands, and quality of life. Overall, there is a need for high-quality RCTs particularly related to effective interventions for prevention and restoration of root caries; clinical and cost-effective alternative workforce models—such as caregivers providing oral hygiene in nursing homes; survival analysis of different restorative materials and techniques, including minimally invasive dentistry; replacement of missing dentition; and evaluations of improved oral health on systemic health and quality of life. Research is lacking in many other areas of oral care for older adults, such as endodontics, oral surgery, esthetic dentistry, orthodontics, teledentistry, and dental quality measures. There is also a significant workforce-related challenge in geriatric dentistry. Geriatric dentistry is not a recognized dental specialty in most countries and relies on pre-doctoral training and a few advanced education programs in the specialty. There is a shortage of oral health professionals with advanced training in geriatric dentistry who can provide clinical care and perform needed research in this field. More evidence-based clinical guidelines are needed to ensure that older adults receive the oral health care they need, and this is only possible if robust research is conducted.

11.5 Case Scenario Exercise

11.5.1 Case Scenario

The proposed study aimed to assess the clinical and microbiological effectiveness of a customized oral hygiene protocol. A convenience sample of 8 nursing facilities (NFs) was recruited, and each NF was assigned to one of three intervention groups: (1) control (current oral hygiene practice), (2) educational program only, and (3) educational program plus 1% chlorhexidine varnish monthly application. Demographic information, systemic health data, patient-centered data, oral health data, and microbiology samples will be collected at baseline and after 6 months.

Recruitment response rates were 21% for NFs and 23% for residents. A total of 81 residents were examined at baseline, and of those, 49 were examined at 6 months (39.5% attrition). Recruitment and retention posed a significant challenge to this trial, even with a relatively short observation period.

Questions

1. When planning a cluster-randomized clinical trial (the nursing home is the cluster unit), you find yourself with a reduced sample size after the initial recruitment. Although you were able to recruit a sufficient number of nursing homes, you were not able to recruit enough residents, as their significant others were not willing to give you the power of attorney for their loved ones to participate in the study. What could be the strategies to increase the sample size in this case?
2. What is a realistic attrition rate for a nursing home clinical trial lasting 1 year? How can you reduce your attrition rate and/or reduce the effect of your attrition rate on your final sample size?

Answers

1. Key approaches include early in-depth planning; minimizing exclusion criteria; securing cooperation from all interested parties; employing a full-time research coordinator, preferably with dental knowledge; using advisory boards, timely screening, identification, and approach of eligible patients; and carefully and thoroughly reviewing the benefits and risks with the participants and their family members/friends who have the power of attorney [19, 82].

2. A realistic attrition rate for a nursing home clinical trial lasting 1 year is 30–40% depending on the nature of the trial. One of the strategies to reduce the attrition rate is to request that the nursing facility provide written informed consent for the entire study and study period. To reduce the effect of attrition, consider the attrition rate in your sample size calculations during study planning [19].

Appendix. Criteria for Judging the Risk of Bias in the Reviewed Articles Recommendations

Random sequence generation (selection bias)	Allocation concealment (selection bias)	Blinding of participants and personnel/care providers (performance bias)	Blinding of the outcome assessor (detection bias)	Incomplete outcome data (attrition bias)	Selective reporting (reporting bias)	RoB-Other bias
High bias $N = 4$	High bias $N = 13$	High $N = 37$	High $N = 8$	High $N = 8$	High $N = 6$	High $N = 2$
Low bias $N = 46$	Low $N = 42$	Low $N = 26$	Low $N = 54$	Low $N = 63$	Low $N = 66$	Low $N = 62$
Unclear $N = 24$	Unclear $N = 21$	Unclear $N = 13$	Unclear $N = 14$	Unclear $N = 5$	Unclear $N = 4$	Unclear $N = 12$

References

1. Fact Sheet WHO. 2019. https://www.who.int/news-room/fact-sheets/detail/ageing-and-health (Accessed on 06/07/2021).
2. Disability impacts all of us. 2020. https://www.cdc.gov/ncbddd/disabilityandhealth/infographic-disability-impacts-all.html (Accessed on 06/07/2021).
3. Marchini L, Hartshorn JE, Cowen H, Dawson DV, Johnsen DC. A teaching tool for establishing risk of oral health deterioration in elderly patients: development, implementation, and evaluation at a U.S. Dental School. J Dent Educ. 2017;81(11):1283–90. https://doi.org/10.21815/JDE.017.086.
4. Yellowitz JA, Schneiderman MT. Elder's oral health crisis. J Evid Based Dent Pract. 2014;14:191–200. https://www.sciencedirect.com/science/article/pii/S153233821400075X
5. Abe S, Ishihara K, Adachi M, Sasaki H, Tanaka K, Okuda K. Professional oral care reduces influenza infection in elderly. Arch Gerontol Geriatr. 2006;43(2):157–64. https://www.sciencedirect.com/science/article/pii/S0167494305001330
6. Barbe AG, Kottmann HE, Derman SHM, Noack MJ. Efficacy of regular professional brushing by a dental nurse for 3 months in nursing home residents-a randomized, controlled clinical trial. Int J Dent Hyg. 2019;17(4):327–35. https://www.ncbi.nlm.nih.gov/pmc/articles/PMC6850188/pdf/IDH-17-327.pdf
7. Morino T, Ookawa K, Haruta N, Hagiwara Y, Seki M. Effects of professional oral health care on elderly: randomized trial. Int J Dent Hyg. 2014;12(4):291–7. https://doi.org/10.1111/idh.12068.
8. Beck AM, Damkjaer K, Beyer N. Multifaceted nutritional intervention among nursing-home residents has a positive influence on nutrition and function. Nutrition. 2008;24(11-12):1073–80. https://www.sciencedirect.com/science/article/pii/S0899900708002189
9. Beck AM, Damkjaer K, Sorbye LW. Physical and social functional abilities seem to be maintained by a multifaceted randomized controlled nutritional intervention among old (>65 years) Danish nursing home residents. Arch Gerontol Geriatr. 2010;50(3):351–5. https://www.sciencedirect.com/science/article/pii/S0167494309001411
10. Sumi Y, Ozawa N, Miura H, Michiwaki Y, Umemura O. Oral care help to maintain nutritional status in frail older people. Arch Gerontol Geriatr. 2010;51(2):125–8. https://www.sciencedirect.com/science/article/pii/S0167494309002386
11. Persson RE, Persson GR, Powell LV, Kiyak HA. Periodontal effects of a biobehavioral prevention program. J Clin Periodontol. 1998;25(4):322–9. https://doi.org/10.1111/j.1600-051X.1998.tb02448.x?sid=nlm%3Apubmed.
12. Powell LV, Persson RE, Kiyak HA, Hujoel PP. Caries prevention in a community-dwelling older population. Caries Res. 1999;33(5):333–9. https://www.karger.com/Article/Pdf/16531
13. De Visschere L, de Baat C, Schols JM, Deschepper E, Vanobbergen J. Evaluation of the implementation of an 'oral hygiene protocol' in nursing homes:

a 5-year longitudinal study. Community Dent Oral Epidemiol. 2011;39(5):416–25. https://doi.org/10.1111/j.1600-0528.2011.00610.x.

14. Seleskog B, Lindqvist L, Wardh I, Engstrom A, von Bultzingslowen I. Theoretical and hands-on guidance from dental hygienists promotes good oral health in elderly people living in nursing homes, a pilot study. Int J Dent Hyg. 2018;16(4):476–83. https://doi.org/10.1111/idh.12343.
15. Frenkel H, Harvey I, Newcombe RG. Improving oral health in institutionalised elderly people by educating caregivers: a randomised controlled trial. Community Dent Oral Epidemiol. 2001;29(4):289–97. https://doi.org/10.1034/j.1600-0528.2001.290408.x?sid=nlm%3Apubmed.
16. Yoneyama T, Yoshida M, Ohrui T, Mukaiyama H, Okamoto H, Hoshiba K, et al. Oral care reduces pneumonia in older patients in nursing homes. J Am Geriatr Soc. 2002;50(3):430–3. https://doi.org/10.1046/j.1532-5415.2002.50106.x?sid=nlm%3Apubmed.
17. MacEntee MI, Wyatt CC, Beattie BL, Paterson B, Levy-Milne R, McCandless L, et al. Provision of mouth-care in long-term care facilities: an educational trial. Community Dent Oral Epidemiol. 2007;35(1):25–34. https://doi.org/10.1111/j.1600-0528.2007.00318.x.
18. Zenthofer A, Dieke R, Dieke A, Wege KC, Rammelsberg P, Hassel AJ. Improving oral hygiene in the long-term care of the elderly—a RCT. Community Dent Oral Epidemiol. 2013;41(3):261–8. https://doi.org/10.1111/cdoe.12007.
19. Marchini L, Recker E, Hartshorn J, Cowen H, Lynch D, Drake D, et al. Iowa nursing facility oral hygiene (INFOH) intervention: a clinical and microbiological pilot randomized trial. Spec Care Dentist. 2018;38(6):345–55. https://www.ncbi.nlm.nih.gov/pmc/articles/PMC6246798/pdf/nihms-987235.pdf
20. De Visschere L, Schols J, van der Putten GJ, de Baat C, Vanobbergen J. Effect evaluation of a supervised versus non-supervised implementation of an oral health care guideline in nursing homes: a cluster randomised controlled clinical trial. Gerodontology. 2012;29(2):e96–106. https://doi.org/10.1111/j.1741-2358.2010.00418.x.
21. van der Putten GJ, Mulder J, de Baat C, De Visschere LM, Vanobbergen JN, Schols JM. Effectiveness of supervised implementation of an oral health care guideline in care homes; a single-blinded cluster randomized controlled trial. Clin Oral Investig. 2013;17(4):1143–53. https://doi.org/10.1007/s00784-012-0793-2.pdf.
22. Izumi M, Takeuchi K, Ganaha S, Akifusa S, Yamashita Y. Effects of oral care with tongue cleaning on coughing ability in geriatric care facilities: a randomised controlled trial. J Oral Rehabil. 2016;43(12):953–9. https://doi.org/10.1111/joor.12451.
23. Yonezawa H, Takasaki K, Teraoka K, Asaka T, Sato C, Tsuchiya K. Effects of tongue and oral mucosa cleaning on oral Candida species and production of volatile sulfur compounds in the elderly in a nursing home. J Med Dent Sci. 2003;50(1):1–8. (No digital copy)
24. Sato M, Yoshihara A, Miyazaki H. Preliminary study on the effect of oral care on recovery from surgery in elderly patients. J Oral Rehabil. 2006;33(11):820–6. https://doi.org/10.1111/j.1365-2842.2006.01634.x.
25. Ju LY, Weng SC, Chung YJ, Yang SH, Huang YH, Huang LG, et al. Effects of the bass brushing method on dental plaque and pneumonia in older adults hospitalized with pneumonia after discharge: a randomized controlled trial. Appl Nurs Res. 2019;46:1–7. https://www.sciencedirect.com/science/article/pii/S0897189718303574
26. Willumsen T, Solemdal K, Wenaasen M, Ogaard B. Stannous fluoride in dentifrice: an effective anti-plaque agent in the elderly? Gerodontology. 2007;24(4):239–43. https://doi.org/10.1111/j.1741-2358.2007.00161.x.
27. Zhang W, McGrath C, Lo EC, Li JY. Silver diamine fluoride and education to prevent and arrest root caries among community-dwelling elders. Caries Res. 2013;47(4):284–90. https://www.karger.com/Article/Pdf/346620
28. Leon S, Rivera M, Payero S, Correa-Beltran G, Hugo FN, Giacaman RA. Assessment of oral health-related quality of life as a function of non-invasive treatment with high-fluoride toothpastes for root caries lesions in community-dwelling elderly. Int Dent J. 2019;69(1):58–66. https://doi.org/10.1111/idj.12415.
29. Ekstrand KR, Poulsen JE, Hede B, Twetman S, Qvist V, Ellwood RP. A randomized clinical trial of the anti-caries efficacy of 5000 compared to 1450 ppm fluoridated toothpaste on root caries lesions in elderly disabled nursing home residents. Caries Res. 2013;47(5):391–8. https://www.karger.com/Article/Pdf/348581
30. Fure S, Gahnberg L, Birkhed D. A comparison of four home-care fluoride programs on the caries incidence in the elderly. Gerodontology. 1998;15(2):51–60. https://doi.org/10.1111/j.1741-2358.1998.00051.x?sid=nlm%3Apubmed.
31. Tan HP, Lo EC, Dyson JE, Luo Y, Corbet EF. A randomized trial on root caries prevention in elders. J Dent Res. 2010;89(10):1086–90. https://doi.org/10.1177/0022034510375825.
32. Simons D, Brailsford S, Kidd EA, Beighton D. The effect of chlorhexidine acetate/xylitol chewing gum on the plaque and gingival indices of elderly occupants in residential homes. J Clin Periodontol. 2001;28(11):1010–5. https://doi.org/10.1111/j.1600-051X.2001.281104.x?sid=nlm%3Apubmed.
33. Clavero J, Baca P, Junco P, Gonzalez MP. Effects of 0.2% chlorhexidine spray applied once or twice daily on plaque accumulation and gingival inflammation in a geriatric population. J Clin Periodontol. 2003;30(9):773–7. https://doi.org/10.1034/j.1600-051X.2003.00365.x?sid=nlm%3Apubmed.
34. Hollaar VRY, van der Putten GJ, van der Maarel-Wierink CD, Bronkhorst EM, de Swart BJM,

Creugers NHJ. The effect of a daily application of a 0.05% chlorhexidine oral rinse solution on the incidence of aspiration pneumonia in nursing home residents: a multicenter study. BMC Geriatr. 2017;17(1):128. https://www.ncbi.nlm.nih.gov/pmc/articles/PMC5477106/pdf/12877_2017_Article_519.pdf
35. Weitz M, Brownstein C, Deasy M. Effect of a twice daily 0.12% chlorhexidine rinse on the oral health of a geriatric population. Clin Prev Dent. 1992;14(3):9–13. https://pubmed.ncbi.nlm.nih.gov/1499250/
36. Sharif-Abdullah SS, Chong MC, Surindar-Kaur SS, Kamaruzzaman SB, Ng KH. The effect of chlorhexidine in reducing oral colonisation in geriatric patients: a randomised controlled trial. Singap Med J. 2016;57(5):262–6. https://pubmed.ncbi.nlm.nih.gov/27211885/
37. Baca P, Clavero J, Baca AP, Gonzalez-Rodriguez MP, Bravo M, Valderrama MJ. Effect of chlorhexidine-thymol varnish on root caries in a geriatric population: a randomized double-blind clinical trial. J Dent. 2009;37(9):679–85. https://www.sciencedirect.com/science/article/pii/S0300571209000979
38. Brailsford SR, Fiske J, Gilbert S, Clark D, Beighton D. The effects of the combination of chlorhexidine/thymol- and fluoride-containing varnishes on the severity of root caries lesions in frail institutionalised elderly people. J Dent. 2002;30(7-8):319–24. https://www.sciencedirect.com/science/article/pii/S0300571202000453
39. Fjeld KG, Eide H, Mowe M, Sandvik L, Willumsen T. A 1-year follow-up of a randomized clinical trial with focus on manual and electric toothbrushes' effect on dental hygiene in nursing homes. Acta Odontol Scand. 2018;76(4):257–61. https://doi.org/10.1080/00016357.2017.1416166?needAccess=true&.
40. Fjeld KG, Mowe M, Eide H, Willumsen T. Effect of electric toothbrush on residents' oral hygiene: a randomized clinical trial in nursing homes. Eur J Oral Sci. 2014;122(2):142–8. https://doi.org/10.1111/eos.12113.
41. Lavigne SE, Doupe MB, Iacopino AM, Mahmud SM. The effects of power toothbrushing on C-reactive protein levels in nursing home residents: a randomized controlled trial. Can J Dent Hyg. 2018;52(1):20–7. https://go.gale.com/ps/retrieve.do?tabID=Magazines&resultListType=RESULT_LIST&searchResultsType=MultiTab&hitCount=1&searchType=AdvancedSearchForm&currentPosition=1&docId=GALE%7CA541288160&docType=Report&sort=Relevance&contentSegment=ZHRC-MOD1&prodId=HWRC&pageNum=1&contentSet=GALE%7CA541288160&searchId=R1&userGroupName=uiowa_main&inPS=true
42. Tawse-Smith A, Duncan WJ, Payne AG, Thomson WM, Wennstrom JL. Relative effectiveness of powered and manual toothbrushes in elderly patients with implant-supported mandibular overdentures. J Clin Periodontol. 2002;29(4):275–80. https://doi.org/10.1034/j.1600-051X.2002.290401.x?sid=nlm%3Apubmed.
43. da Mata C, Allen PF, McKenna G, Cronin M, O'Mahony D, Woods N. Two-year survival of ART restorations placed in elderly patients: a randomised controlled clinical trial. J Dent. 2015;43(4):405–11. https://www.sciencedirect.com/science/article/pii/S0300571215000160
44. Lo EC, Luo Y, Tan HP, Dyson JE, Corbet EF. ART and conventional root restorations in elders after 12 months. J Dent Res. 2006;85(10):929–32. https://doi.org/10.1177/154405910608501011.
45. Gil-Montoya JA, Mateos-Palacios R, Bravo M, Gonzalez-Moles MA, Pulgar R. Atraumatic restorative treatment and Carisolv use for root caries in the elderly: 2-year follow-up randomized clinical trial. Clin Oral Investig. 2014;18(4):1089–95. https://doi.org/10.1007/s00784-013-1087-z.pdf.
46. da Mata C, Cronin M, O'Mahony D, McKenna G, Woods N, Allen PF. Subjective impact of minimally invasive dentistry in the oral health of older patients. Clin Oral Investig. 2015;19(3):681–7. https://doi.org/10.1007/s00784-014-1290-6.pdf.
47. da Mata C, Allen PF, Cronin M, O'Mahony D, McKenna G, Woods N. Cost-effectiveness of ART restorations in elderly adults: a randomized clinical trial. Community Dent Oral Epidemiol. 2014;42(1):79–87. https://doi.org/10.1111/cdoe.12066.
48. McKenna G, Allen F, Woods N, O'Mahony D, Cronin M, DaMata C, et al. Cost-effectiveness of tooth replacement strategies for partially dentate elderly: a randomized controlled clinical trial. Community Dent Oral Epidemiol. 2014;42(4):366–74. https://doi.org/10.1111/cdoe.12085.
49. McKenna G, Allen PF, Flynn A, O'Mahony D, DaMata C, Cronin M, et al. Impact of tooth replacement strategies on the nutritional status of partially-dentate elders. Gerodontology. 2012;29(2):e883–90. https://doi.org/10.1111/j.1741-2358.2011.00579.x.
50. McKenna G, Allen PF, O'Mahony D, Cronin M, DaMata C, Woods N. The impact of rehabilitation using removable partial dentures and functionally orientated treatment on oral health-related quality of life: a randomised controlled clinical trial. J Dent. 2015;43(1):66–71. https://www.sciencedirect.com/science/article/pii/S0300571214001882
51. McKenna G, Allen PF, O'Mahony D, Flynn A, Cronin M, DaMata C, et al. Comparison of functionally orientated tooth replacement and removable partial dentures on the nutritional status of partially dentate older patients: a randomised controlled clinical trial. J Dent. 2014;42(6):653–9. https://www.sciencedirect.com/science/article/pii/S0300571214000864
52. McKenna G, Allen PF, Woods N, O'Mahony D, DaMata C, Cronin M, et al. A preliminary report of the cost-effectiveness of tooth replacement strategies for partially dentate elders. Gerodontology. 2013;30(3):207–13. https://doi.org/10.1111/j.1741-2358.2012.00665.x.
53. Michaud PL, de Grandmont P, Feine JS, Emami E. Measuring patient-based outcomes: is treatment satisfaction associated with oral health-related quality of

life? J Dent. 2012;40(8):624–31. https://www.sciencedirect.com/science/article/pii/S0300571212000905

54. Muller F, Duvernay E, Loup A, Vazquez L, Herrmann FR, Schimmel M. Implant-supported mandibular overdentures in very old adults: a randomized controlled trial. J Dent Res. 2013;92(Suppl. 12):154s–60s. https://www.ncbi.nlm.nih.gov/pmc/articles/PMC3860063/pdf/10.1177_0022034513509630.pdf
55. Passia N, Abou-Ayash S, Reissmann DR, Fritzer E, Kappel S, Konstantinidis I, et al. Single mandibular implant study (SMIS)—masticatory performance—results from a randomized clinical trial using two different loading protocols. J Dent. 2017;65:64–9. https://www.sciencedirect.com/science/article/pii/S0300571217301719
56. Watando A, Ebihara S, Ebihara T, Okazaki T, Takahashi H, Asada M, et al. Daily oral care and cough reflex sensitivity in elderly nursing home patients. Chest. 2004;126(4):1066–70. https://www.sciencedirect.com/science/article/pii/S0012369215312794
57. Juthani-Mehta M, Van Ness PH, McGloin J, Argraves S, Chen S, Charpentier P, et al. A cluster-randomized controlled trial of a multicomponent intervention protocol for pneumonia prevention among nursing home elders. Clin Infect Dis. 2015;60(6):849–57. https://www.ncbi.nlm.nih.gov/pmc/articles/PMC4415071/pdf/ciu935.pdf
58. Wakabayashi H, Matsushima M, Momosaki R, Yoshida S, Mutai R, Yodoshi T, et al. The effects of resistance training of swallowing muscles on dysphagia in older people: a cluster, randomized, controlled trial. Nutrition. 2018;48:111–6. https://www.sciencedirect.com/science/article/pii/S0899900717302599
59. Komulainen K, Ylostalo P, Syrjala AM, Ruoppi P, Knuuttila M, Sulkava R, et al. Oral health intervention among community-dwelling older people: a randomised 2-year intervention study. Gerodontology. 2015;32(1):62–72. https://doi.org/10.1111/ger.12067.
60. van der Putten GJ, De Visschere L, Schols J, de Baat C, Vanobbergen J. Supervised versus non-supervised implementation of an oral health care guideline in residential care homes: a cluster randomized controlled clinical trial. BMC Oral Health. 2010;10:17. https://www.ncbi.nlm.nih.gov/pmc/articles/PMC2912776/pdf/1472-6831-10-17.pdf (Protocol only)
61. Bellomo F, de Preux F, Chung JP, Julien N, Budtz-Jorgensen E, Muller F. The advantages of occupational therapy in oral hygiene measures for institutionalised elderly adults. Gerodontology. 2005;22(1):24–31. https://doi.org/10.1111/j.1741-2358.2004.00047.x?sid=nlm%3Apubmed.
62. Jablonski RA, Kolanowski AM, Azuero A, Winstead V, Jones-Townsend C, Geisinger ML. Randomised clinical trial: efficacy of strategies to provide oral hygiene activities to nursing home residents with dementia who resist mouth care. Gerodontology. 2018;35(4):365–75. https://www.ncbi.nlm.nih.gov/pmc/articles/PMC6289838/pdf/nihms974533.pdf
63. Kikutani T, Enomoto R, Tamura F, Oyaizu K, Suzuki A, Inaba S. Effects of oral functional training for nutritional improvement in Japanese older people requiring long-term care. Gerodontology. 2006;23(2):93–8. https://doi.org/10.1111/j.1741-2358.2006.00104.x.
64. Peltola P, Vehkalahti MM, Simoila R. Effects of 11-month interventions on oral cleanliness among the long-term hospitalised elderly. Gerodontology. 2007;24(1):14–21. https://doi.org/10.1111/j.1741-2358.2007.00147.x.
65. Morita Y, Ishikawa K, Nakano M, Wakabayashi H, Yamauchi K, Abe F, et al. Effects of lactoferrin and lactoperoxidase-containing food on the oral hygiene status of older individuals: a randomized, double blinded, placebo-controlled clinical trial. Geriatr Gerontol Int. 2017;17(5):714–21. https://doi.org/10.1111/ggi.12776.
66. Nakano M, Wakabayashi H, Sugahara H, Odamaki T, Yamauchi K, Abe F, et al. Effects of lactoferrin and lactoperoxidase-containing food on the oral microbiota of older individuals. Microbiol Immunol. 2017;61(10):416–26. https://doi.org/10.1111/1348-0421.12537.
67. Gil-Montoya JA, Guardia-Lopez I, Gonzalez-Moles MA. Evaluation of the clinical efficacy of a mouthwash and oral gel containing the antimicrobial proteins lactoperoxidase, lysozyme and lactoferrin in elderly patients with dry mouth—a pilot study. Gerodontology. 2008;25(1):3–9. https://doi.org/10.1111/j.1741-2358.2007.00197.x.
68. Simons D, Brailsford SR, Kidd EA, Beighton D. The effect of medicated chewing gums on oral health in frail older people: a 1-year clinical trial. J Am Geriatr Soc. 2002;50(8):1348–53. https://doi.org/10.1046/j.1532-5415.2002.50355.x?sid=nlm%3Apubmed.
69. Kraft-Bodi E, Jorgensen MR, Keller MK, Kragelund C, Twetman S. Effect of probiotic bacteria on oral candida in frail elderly. J Dent Res. 2015;94(Suppl. 9):181s–6s. https://doi.org/10.1177/0022034515595950.
70. Kobayashi K, Ryu M, Izumi S, Ueda T, Sakurai K. Effect of oral cleaning using mouthwash and a mouth moisturizing gel on bacterial number and moisture level of the tongue surface of older adults requiring nursing care. Geriatr Gerontol Int. 2017;17(1):116–21. https://doi.org/10.1111/ggi.12684.
71. Takeuchi S, Motohashi J, Kimori H, Nakagawa Y, Tsurumoto A. Effects of oral moisturising gel containing egg yolk antibodies against Candida albicans in older people. Gerodontology. 2016;33(1):128–34. https://doi.org/10.1111/ger.12139.
72. Chalhoub E, Emami E, Freije M, Kandelman D, Campese M, St-Georges A, et al. Effectiveness of an alcohol-free essential oil-containing mouthwash in institutionalised elders receiving long-term care: a feasibility study. Gerodontology. 2016;33(1):69–78. https://doi.org/10.1111/ger.12119.
73. Higashiguchi T, Ohara H, Kamakura Y, Kikutani T, Kuzuya M, Enoki H, et al. Efficacy of a new post-mouthwash intervention (wiping plus oral nutritional supplements) for preventing aspiration pneumonia

in elderly people: a multicenter, randomized, comparative trial. Ann Nutr Metab. 2017;71(3-4):253–60. https://www.karger.com/Article/Pdf/485044
74. Yamaoka M, Uematsu T, Shiba T, Matsuura T, Ono Y, Ishizuka M, et al. Effect of inorganic polyphosphate in periodontitis in the elderly. Gerodontology. 2008;25(1):10–7. https://doi.org/10.1111/j.1741-2358.2007.00185.x.
75. Simons D, Kidd EA, Beighton D, Jones B. The effect of chlorhexidine/xylitol chewing-gum on cariogenic salivary microflora: a clinical trial in elderly patients. Caries Res. 1997;31(2):91–6. https://www.karger.com/Article/Abstract/262382
76. Mitchell C, Gross AJ, Milgrom P, Mancl L, Prince DB. Silver diamine fluoride treatment of active root caries lesions in older adults: a case series. J Dent. 2021;105:103561. https://www.sciencedirect.com/science/article/pii/S0300571220303092?via%3Dihub
77. Nair R, Chiu SE, Chua YK, Dhillon IK, Li J, Yee Ting Fai R. Should short-term use of alcohol-containing mouthrinse be avoided for fear of worsening xerostomia? J Oral Rehabil. 2018;45(2):140–6. https://doi.org/10.1111/joor.12587.
78. Pearson NK, Gibson BJ, Davis DM, Gelbier S, Robinson PG. The effect of a domiciliary denture service on oral health related quality of life: a randomised controlled trial. Br Dent J. 2007;203(2):E3. discussion 100-1. https://www.nature.com/articles/bdj.2007.569.pdf
79. Emami E, Lavigne G, de Grandmont P, Rompre PH, Feine JS. Perceived sleep quality among edentulous elders. Gerodontology. 2012;29(2):e128–34. https://doi.org/10.1111/j.1741-2358.2010.00426.x.
80. Lowe C, Blinkhorn AS, Worthington HV, Craven R. Testing the effect of including oral health in general health checks for elderly patients in medical practice—a randomized controlled trial. Community Dent Oral Epidemiol. 2007;35(1):12–7. https://doi.org/10.1111/j.1600-0528.2007.00360.x.
81. Weijenberg RA, Lobbezoo F, Knol DL, Tomassen J, Scherder EJ. Increased masticatory activity and quality of life in elderly persons with dementia—a longitudinal matched cluster randomized single-blind multicenter intervention study. BMC Neurol. 2013;13:26. https://www.ncbi.nlm.nih.gov/pmc/articles/PMC3615955/pdf/1471-2377-13-26.pdf (Protocol only)
82. Mody L, Miller DK, McGloin JM, Freeman M, Marcantonio ER, Magaziner J, Studenski S. Recruitment and retention of older adults in aging research. J Am Geriatr Soc. 2008;56(12):2340–8. https://www.ncbi.nlm.nih.gov/pmc/articles/PMC2695395/
83. Lam HR, Chow S, Taylor K, Chow R, Lam H, Bonin K, Rowbottom L, Herrmann N. Challenges of conducting research in long-term care facilities: a systematic review. BioMed Central Geriatr. 2018;18(1):242. https://doi.org/10.1186/s12877-018-0934-9.
84. Higgins JPT, Thomas J, Chandler J, Cumpston M, Li T, Page MJ, Welch VA, editors. Cochrane handbook for systematic reviews of interventions version 6.2 (updated February 2021). Cochrane, https://training.cochrane.org/handbook; 2021.
85. van Tulder M, Furlan A, Bombardier C, Bouter L, Editorial Board of the Cochrane Collaboration Back Review Group. Updated method guidelines for systematic reviews in the cochrane collaboration back review group. Spine (Phila Pa 1976). 2003;28(12):1290–9. https://journals.lww.com/spinejournal/Fulltext/2003/06150/Updated_Method_Guidelines_for_Systematic_Reviews.14.aspx
86. Boutron I, Moher D, Tugwell P, Giraudeau B, Poiraudeau S, Nizard R, et al. A checklist to evaluate a report of a non pharmacological trial (CLEAR NPT) was developed using consensus. J Clin Epidemiol. 2005;58:1233–40. https://www.sciencedirect.com/science/article/pii/S0895435605002118?via%3Dihub
87. Julian P. T. Higgins, Sally Green Cochrane handbook of systematic reviews of interventions, Chapter 8 (Version 5.1, updated March 2011). 2011. https://back.cochrane.org/sites/back.cochrane.org/files/public/uploads/PDF/ROB%20criteria_Aug2011.pdf.

12 Randomized Controlled Trials Related to Behavioral Interventions in Dentistry

Tamanna Tiwari, Nayanjot Rai, and Judith Albino

12.1 Defining Behavioral Interventions

Oral health depends on initiating and sustaining behaviors that directly promote positive oral health outcomes, including the prevention of disease [1]. Whether the focus is establishing or improving oral hygiene practices, reducing intake of a cariogenic diet, or utilizing professional dental healthcare, what we are trying to achieve can be described as changing the behavior of individuals [1, 2]. Empowering people to adopt healthy behaviors should be a part of the treatment plan for all dental diseases. Whatever its specific form, this empowerment reflects behavioral strategy, and just as any other new treatment should be carefully tested before being recommended for use, behavioral strategies also need to be proven. Clinicians have long relied on RCTs as the gold standard for proof of the effectiveness of treatments, and it is increasingly understood that this must also be the case for behavioral strategies—whether those strategies are used in support of clinical treatment or as primary prevention efforts themselves [3].

As we have suggested, behavioral oral health interventions are tested as either: (1) direct, or "standalone," interventions expected to directly impact oral health outcomes; or (2) "supportive" interventions designed to ensure the use of, or maximize the oral health outcomes of, clinical interventions. Direct behavioral interventions are intended to reduce dental caries, periodontal disease, or other oral diseases by working with or influencing the behaviors in which individuals engage, including brushing, flossing, and other self-care behaviors. Supportive behavioral interventions may include approaches similar to those of direct interventions but are intended to ensure the use of clinical strategies, or are viewed as supplemental strategies. The clinical approaches employed may include drugs or devices, such as fluoride varnish or chlorhexidine mouthwash, or participation in sealant programs, with the ultimate result of a combined behavioral/clinical effect on oral health outcomes. Both direct and supportive behavioral interventions impact oral health through mechanisms of action that may include skills training, strategies aimed at improving knowledge or changing beliefs and attitudes, or motivational strategies focused on practical aspects of changing behavior patterns. In well-designed clinical trials, the specific mechanisms employed are determined by the

T. Tiwari (✉) · N. Rai
University of Colorado School of Dental Medicine, Aurora, CO, USA
e-mail: tamanna.tiwari@cuanschutz.edu; nayanjot.rai@cuanschutz.edu

J. Albino
University of Colorado School of Dental Medicine, Aurora, CO, USA

Colorado School of Public Health, Aurora, CO, USA
e-mail: judith.albino@cuanschutz.edu

R. Kohli et al. (eds.), *Randomized Controlled Trials in Evidence-Based Dentistry*,
https://doi.org/10.1007/978-3-031-47651-8_12

theoretical model of behavior change chosen to address the needs of a specific population group.

As our review reflects, most studies have looked at behavioral interventions as supportive rather than direct approaches to influencing oral health outcomes. Moreover, the distinction between a direct and a supportive behavioral strategy is rarely made clear in RCTs.

There are at least two important reasons for this: first, most trials are designed in such a way that the entire program—including both behavioral and clinical components—is considered to be the intervention, making it impossible to determine the effects that can be attributed to the behavioral component of the intervention, the clinical component, or to the combination. However, in many RCTs, changes in knowledge, beliefs or attitudes, and even behaviors are measured and used, along with clinical status, and are often considered to be secondary outcomes. The appropriateness of this approach, of course, depends on the theoretical model driving the study design. Second, behavioral interventions have also been used to test strategies for reducing fear and anxiety in patients utilizing dental care. Interestingly in these cases, we are more likely to see direct use of behavioral strategies—presumably because the outcome is usually behavior, also (e.g., experience and actions related to fear or anxiety), rather than clinical status. RCT formats have been used only rarely to test these interventions, however; so fear/anxiety studies are not the focus of this review [4].

In this chapter, we will review behavioral RCTs that were both direct behavioral interventions and supportive behavioral interventions that maximize the prevention—or limit the increase—of dental diseases. However, to provide an overarching view of the behavioral strategies studied, we will group these studies according to theoretical or conceptual approaches used, rather than the more narrowly descriptive labels of direct or supportive interventions. In all cases, we will report these theories and approaches, as well as the trial designs used and the reported changes in oral health outcomes. We also will review what these behavioral interventions have contributed to the literature and the gaps in the literature that need to be filled. Finally, we will discuss the logistics of implementation of behavioral RCTs, and real-world challenges and solutions.

12.2 Review of Behavioral RCTs

Over the past 10 years, RCTs focused on behavioral interventions have been used to improve oral health outcomes, including avoiding or limiting dental caries in children, improving periodontal health outcomes, and increasing access to dental care. Most RCT behavioral studies base their interventions on a theoretical model or behavior change theory or approach—Motivational Interviewing (MI), the Theory of Planned Behavior (TPB), salutogenic theory or Sense of Coherence (SOC), Social Competence, Self-Determination Theory (SDT), Social Cognitive Theory (SCT), or others [2]. These theories help define expectations for how the interventions work and establish the tools for measuring behavioral outcomes, usually in addition to the clinical outcomes that are measured by dental screenings or examinations. Several researchers have pointed out that using psychological/behavioral strategies will increase the efficacy of interventions and potentially motivate patients to use their knowledge to change existing oral health behaviors or to establish new behaviors [5]. The following sections describe theoretical approaches to influencing behaviors that have been used in recent RCTs, as well as examples of studies.

12.2.1 Motivational Interviewing

At a personally meaningful level, patients need understanding about the etiology and prevention of oral disease—preferably provided by healthcare professionals. Although common, highly directive approaches, where health professionals instruct patients to follow recommended oral health behaviors, may not be the best approach to instilling these behaviors [6]. Interventions that support patients in minimizing risk behaviors, or promoting protective behaviors through education or coaching generally are more helpful. MI—first used in the treatment of addiction—has been used to elicit behavior change for oral health and has been readily accepted in some communities [6]. MI employs a coaching strategy that provides supportive guidance for choosing behavioral goals and strategies, rather than directing those choices. The approach is designed to be respectful and non-confrontational toward participants and to help individuals resolve discrepancies between their values and their behaviors [7]. An early study of MI with mothers of infants 6–18 months old found that the caries increment was significantly lower for those who participated in the MI program, although it has been difficult to replicate this result in clinical trials or over longer periods of time [6].

Although not originally based on a specific theory of behavior change, the extensive use of MI has given rise to a theoretical rationale based on its relational and technical components [7]. In practice, MI shares some assumptions with social determination and social cognitive theories, as well as others. It has been recommended for use in clinical settings for a number of years. The first controlled studies showed mixed results, and the approach continues to be challenging because it is time-consuming and requires training, as well as continued monitoring to avoid drift or loss of fidelity in implementation and measurement. Moreover, the approach needs to be adapted to meet the specific needs of various group characteristics, including careful attention to cultural practices and concerns. Indeed, MI is being used as an approach to prevent dental diseases throughout the world and has generated perhaps the largest number of behavioral RCTs in recent years. The studies described here demonstrate increasing sophistication in the application of the theory behind MI, and its popularity based on success in other fields has warranted the more rigorous test that RCTs can provide.

Two RCTs that used the MI approach were recently and concurrently completed [8, 9]. The studies included large samples and used comparable MI interventions and questionnaires to assess oral health knowledge and behavior. The clinical examiners collecting the primary outcome data for each study used the same inclusion criteria, methods, and calibration procedures. Both trials were well controlled with high fidelity and good participant retention, and both used community-based participatory research methodology to generate the study design and implementation process:

Direct Intervention in Indian Country. This RCT was conducted in an American Indian (AI) population living on a Northern Plains Indian Reservation [10] to determine whether using MI with AI in new mothers will result in more limited caries experience in children younger than 3 years old. This study focused on a direct behavioral intervention, in that no additional clinical approaches were used, and the focus was on supporting individual parents in implementing recommended home oral healthcare for their infant children. A total of 600 mothers were enrolled in this RCT, with the control group for this intervention defined in terms of enhanced community services. These included providing oral health supplies for the child and immediate family members, informational handouts with culturally specific artwork and designs, public service announcements in the local newspaper and the tribal radio, and billboards placed in strategic locations on the reservation focusing on key Early Childhood Caries (ECC) risk factors. The MI intervention consisted of four visits, the first shortly after childbirth, and the next three at 6, 12, and 18 months of age. MI was delivered by tribal laypersons who received intensive MI training, as well as instruction in oral health and hygiene. At each of the four MI visits, each AI mother selected two topics to address from a list of eight options. Stratified blocked randomization was developed using a random number generator. Randomly selected block sizes of 2 and 4 were used, and blocked randomization of randomly selected sizes was used to prevent field staff from knowing during recruitment what treatment assignment the next participant would receive. The intervention providers and participants could not be masked in this study; however, the licensed dental professionals who performed the annual oral health screenings were blinded to group assignment. Data analysis was based on intention-to-treat (ITT). There were no statistically significant differences in changes in decayed, missing, filled surfaces (DMFS) over time or in time-averaged DMFS levels between the two groups. Oral health knowledge in primary caregivers was significantly higher in the MI group at 12 months and 24 months, but the groups no longer significantly differed at 36 months.

Supportive Intervention in a Boston Housing Project. The second trial was a cluster RCT to test the effect of MI on caries increments for children living in public housing in the greater Boston area [9]. This study comprised a supportive MI intervention; additional clinical approaches in the form of fluoride varnish application for the children were also provided. The main goal of this study—with 1065 mother-child dyads enrolled—was to limit new dental caries in participating children. The unit of randomization was the public housing development (PHD). The statistician stratified the 26 PHDs based on size and racial/ethnic composition. Within the six strata, housing sites were block randomized to the intervention groups via a computerized random number generator. The participants, interventionists, and field staff collecting questionnaire data could not be blinded, but the dental professionals conducting the clinical exam were blinded to group assignment. The control group (686 participants) received a dental exam measured by DMFs, fluoride varnish, toothbrush, toothpaste, and a handout on caries prevention. Although the behavioral strategy was the same as in the AI study described above, this RCT also included a clinical intervention in the form of fluoride varnish applications applied four times a year. The intervention group (379 participants) received everything that the control received, plus quarterly MI counseling; nine MI counseling sessions were given to participants in their homes over the 2-year study period. The MI intervention was delivered by trained laypersons to the primary caregivers. Participating primary caregivers were presented with a menu of ECC prevention strategies and asked to choose a topic. The primary outcome measure was an increment in DMFs over 2 years. Data analysis was based on the ITT principle. No significant difference was seen in caries increments between the control and intervention groups, but a statistically significant group × time interaction effect (primary test of intervention effects) was seen in the oral health knowledge of primary caregivers.

Direct MI Intervention in Hong Kong. A single-blinded RCT was conducted to evaluate the direct effectiveness of three intervention schemes—prevailing health education (PE), MI, and MI + RA (risk assessment)—to enhance adolescents' oral health self-efficacy, change their oral health behaviors, and prevent dental caries [11]. An RA using a Cariogram is valid among adolescents; the Cariogram displays participants' caries risk via a pie diagram where risk is quantified into various aspects, including diet and oral hygiene. The RA facilitates MI in several ways, including helping participants with self-reflection, finding direction, and exploring possible health gains resulting from behavior changes. To facilitate the dental counseling process, an interactive dental caries RA program was used. Fifteen schools were recruited from three main districts in Hong Kong; schools in each district were randomly assigned to the three intervention groups: 1–PE, 2–MI, and 3–MI + RA. A total of 512 participants were enrolled in the study; at baseline, Group 1 (n = 161) participants received a 30-minute oral health talk by a dental hygienist and three pamphlets, namely "Cleaning teeth properly—you can do it," "How to use dental floss" and "Healthy diet, healthy teeth." Group 2 (n = 163) participants joined a 15- to 30-minute one-on-one, face-to-face MI session. Standard MI approaches were followed, including the four spirits (evocation, compassion, acceptance, and collaboration), four processes (engaging, focusing, eliciting, and planning), and four skills (open questions, affirmation, reflection, and summary) [6]. Group 3 (n = 188) participants received MI sessions with the inclusion of an interactive RA program at different stages of MI, as appropriate to facilitate the counseling process. Five telephone calls were made in both the MI groups at 2 weeks, 1 month, 2 months, 4 months, and 6 months after initial counseling to facilitate the start of behavior change, maintain it, and avoid the relapse. Participants were followed at 6 and 12 months. A questionnaire was completed by the participants at baseline, and after 6 and 12 months, to gather information on their demographic and socioeconomic background, oral health self-efficacy, and oral health behaviors. Oral hygiene and tooth status were evaluated. At the 6- and 12-month points, both the MI groups showed more favorable self-efficacy and behaviors compared to the PE group ($p < 0.001$). Also at the 6- and 12-month points, the plaque score reduction was greater in the MI + RA group compared to the two other groups. The caries increment was lower in the MI + RA group at 12 months, compared to the PE group. Both the MI group and the MI + RA group were more likely to increase their tooth brushing frequency after 12 months. MI was more effective than PE in eliciting positive changes in adolescent oral health behaviors.

Supporting MI Intervention for Australian Aboriginals. A large-scale RCT focused on MI was conducted to test its supportive effectiveness in reducing ECC in Aboriginal Australian communities [12]. This study used a supportive behavioral intervention with a clinical component, with the primary outcome of reduction in dental caries. This single-blind, parallel-arm trial tested an intervention that included MI delivered in conjunction with anticipatory guidance for 448 new mothers. The intervention also included the provision of dental care to mothers during pregnancy and the application of fluoride varnish to children at ages 6, 12, and 18 months. The randomization was accomplished via a computerized random number generator, and random block sizes of 4, 6, and 8. MI intervention was provided by a trained layperson with mothers during pregnancy, and when children were ages 6, 12, and 18 months. The primary outcome measure was an increment in decayed teeth (DT) measured at 24 months. Data analysis was based on the ITT principle. The mean number of DT at age 2 was significantly lower in the intervention group than in the control group.

Supporting MI Intervention in the United Kingdom. A large-scale, two-arm multicenter RCT with blinded outcome assessment was conducted in the UK to determine the efficacy of a dental nurse-delivered MI intervention—the Dental RECUR Brief Negotiated Interview for Oral Health (DR-BNI) to reduce the recurrence of dental caries in children with a primary tooth extraction [13]. The DR-BNI "talking intervention" was a 30-minute therapeutic conversation informed by MI with a focus on dental caries prevention. A clinical health psychologist developed the intervention based on the MI approach. Participants in the study comprised 241 children (5–7 years old) who were scheduled to have one primary tooth extraction. The intervention group (n = 119) of parents received DR-BNI and appointments were made with the child's dental practitioner to treat the child as being high risk. The control group included 122 parents who talked with the nurses about their child's future tooth eruption and were advised about visiting a general dentist. Mean DMF scores were calculated at baseline and 2 years after the intervention for both groups. Sixty-two percent of the children developed caries in the control group compared to 44% in the intervention group. There was a 29% decrease in the relative risk of new caries experience in the DR-BNI group as compared with the control; also, the odds of new caries experience were reduced in the intervention group participants compared to those in the control condition.

Direct MI Intervention in Iran. Finally, a two-arm, cluster RCT was conducted in Hamadan, western Iran, to evaluate changes in mothers' cognitive predictors, as well as reported behavior of teeth cleaning of their children (ages 1–2 years old) [14]. This study used a direct behavioral intervention with no clinical component, focusing on the primary outcome of changing maternal oral hygiene behaviors for their children. Ten daycare centers were randomly selected and allocated to two groups: an intervention group (five centers, 45 mothers) and a control group (5 centers, 45 mothers). The intervention was based on the TPB theoretical model but used a standard MI intervention approach: express empathy, develop discrepancy, roll with resistance, support self-efficacy and avoid argumentation; three MI sessions were conducted with the participants. TPB is a social cognitive model of attitude and behavior relationship that is mediated by intentions [15]; it assumes that the predictors of behavior are a person's intention to perform that behavior and Perceived Behavioral Control (PBC)—that is, a person's perception of the ease or difficulty of performing a given behavior. According to TPB, intention influences behavior and is predicted by attitude, PBC, and subjective norms [15, 16]. Although some researchers have used TPB-based interventions in non-RCT studies, their use in RCTs has been limited [4, 17]. Based on the TPB model, the behavior change technique addressed knowledge, attitude, and PBC in mothers. The intervention consisted of three sessions at daycare, a booklet, and text message reminders for all five centers in the intervention group. The mothers received a booklet at the start of the second session targeting knowledge and PBC and encouraging action through self-monitoring and goal-setting. Additionally, the intervention group mothers received eight different text messages, 45 days after the last session. A 25-item questionnaire was developed, and variables were measured before receiving the intervention—10 days after the intervention and 3 months after follow-up. The primary outcome was a change in oral hygiene behavior; secondary outcome measures were changes in knowledge and cognitions of TPB. Significant differences in knowledge, attitude, PBC, and cleaning of children's teeth were reported by mothers in the intervention group at 10-day and 3-month assessments. Also, the attitude and PBC scores of the intervention group improved over the assessment period. This intervention moderately improved the mothers' cognitions and self-reported cleaning of their children's teeth.

12.2.2 Self-Determination Theory

SDT underscores the importance of individual engagement and responsibility in undertaking change. It suggests that health behavior change is most effectively achieved in autonomy-supportive contexts, in which "significant others offer choice, provide a meaningful rationale, minimize pressure, and acknowledge the target individual's feelings and perspectives" [18]. The principle of self-determination can be seen in the previously described MI strategy, but a self-determination approach lacks the carefully prescribed steps and other MI components.

Direct Self-Determination Intervention in Iowa. A comparison of the autonomy-supportive psychoeducational videotaped message, informed by SDT, to a neutral message delivered by brochure was the approach of an RCT designed to measure changes in mothers' behaviors concerning their children's oral health [19]. Four hundred fifteen mother-child dyads were randomly assigned to intervention (n = 283) and control groups (n = 132). The intervention group mothers were provided with a 15-minute videotaped oral health message informed by SDT, covering a variety of oral health topics—including the process of tooth decay, oral hygiene practices, dietary habits affecting caries susceptibility, checking a child's teeth for early sign of cavities and bacterial transmission from mother to child. The control group mothers received the educational component using a neutral style through a brochure containing the same information provided in the videotaped message of the SDT intervention. The paper brochure was selected for the control group as it is considered to be the standard dental education delivery tool in many women, infants, and children (WIC) and dental clinics. SDT proposes that, if the mother has internalized the message, the changes should be evident within a short period of time. The study also employed a series of questions at baseline, one- and 6-month follow-ups to collect demographic information and assess any changes in mothers' self-reported oral health behaviors regarding their children's oral health; dental plaque and caries status were also recorded at baseline and 6-month follow-ups. Positive changes were observed for dietary/oral hygiene behaviors among the intervention group at 1- and 6-month follow-ups compared to the control group. A significantly greater proportion of mothers in the intervention group checked for white spot lesions at 6 months, compared to baseline. The SDT videotaped message was more effective in changing mothers' behaviors concerning their children's oral health compared to the brochure.

12.2.3 Salutogenic Theory

Direct Salutogenic Intervention in Thailand. One method for examining underlying causes of behavior is via salutogenic factors that seek to explain why some individuals who live in adverse conditions and are surrounded by stressful environments can maintain and improve their health. The central concept of salutogenesis is SOC, described as a "global orientation for viewing life in coherent, manageable and meaningful ways [20]"; based on Aaron Antonovsky's salutogenesis model, SOC is a psychosocial attribute that reflects the degree to which individuals perceive their life challenges to be meaningful, as well as the degree to which they can understand and manage challenges, such as oral health problems [21]. A systematic review concluded that salutogenic factors—such as higher maternal SOC, positive coping strategies, resiliency, internal locus of control, and other protective psychosocial factors—are associated with "adherent" oral health behavior [22]. According to salutogenic theory, protective psychosocial factors help in buffering stresses of daily life and provide higher problem-solving capacity. Thus, these individuals have a better orientation towards adopting positive oral health behaviors and movement in an oral health-promoting direction.

A school-based cluster randomized trial was conducted in Thailand testing the effect of an intervention to enhance SOC in children aged 10–12 years old [23]. The unit of randomization was the school; 12 schools were selected and randomly assigned to the intervention (133 children) or control group (128 children). Group allocation used block permutation to balance the number of schools/participants in each group. The schools were listed, and a random sequence of blocks of four was created. The RCT did not demonstrate a difference in caries increments (DMFs) between the intervention and control groups. However, the intervention increased the SOC scores and improved oral health quality of life in children who participated in the trial. The intervention was child-centered, and child participation and empowerment were demonstrated in most oral health education sessions. For example, after the intervention was over, the children decided that sweetened foods would not be sold in the schools and that the schools would provide toothbrushes and fluoridated toothpaste to all students. These decisions intended to create healthy environments wherein students could adopt desired behaviors and enhance components of SOC.

12.2.4 Social Competence Model

Direct Intervention Using Storytelling in Hong Kong. This trial operationalized a Social Competence model in the form of social stories used to illustrate the importance of positive oral health practices. A 24-month, two-arm RCT was conducted to assess the efficacy of a social story-based intervention to promote oral health status among preschool children with special healthcare needs [24]. The intervention included educational training for 306 children, 2–6 years old, with moderate to severe disabilities. All the participants received standardized toothbrush training and oral health education materials. In the intervention group (156 children), the children were told social stories while the control group children (150 children) received standard leaflets. Social stories have been successfully used in the past to promote social behaviors in children. These stories are written from a child's perspective with visual depictions of the behaviors that are targeted in the stories. Pre- and post-intervention child oral health status and oral health-related behaviors were assessed. Dental examinations were performed at baseline and Phase 3 (24-month follow-up) using DMF primary teeth. Oral hygiene and gingival status indices were measured at baseline and each follow-up visit; tooth brushing performance was also measured. No significant difference in the caries experience was found between the groups. However, children in the intervention group showed better oral hygiene status and tooth brushing performance and were more likely to visit a dentist. The investigators concluded that social stories could be used to improve oral health-related behaviors among children with special healthcare needs.

12.2.5 Social Cognitive Theory

SCT addresses individuals' learning that occurs by observing others and understanding one's own behavior in the context of social interactions, experiences, and outside media influences [25]. SCT also emphasizes that for individuals to change their behavior, they need appropriate levels of knowledge, self-efficacy, and self-control over behaviors and outcome expectations, such as health consequences.

Social Cognitive Direct Intervention in Australia. An RCT was conducted for an indigenous adult population in a community-based setting in South Australia to determine the direct effects of a behavioral intervention on oral health literacy-related outcomes [26]. The oral health literacy intervention was based on SCT, which suggests that individuals will not change their behaviors unless they have appropriate levels of knowledge and self-efficacy. The intervention, developed with two indigenous researchers, comprised interactive contextually relevant oral health workshops with the following topics: information about dental disease processes, accessing dental services, and becoming familiar with the dental clinic. The themes for the workshop were oral health-related self-efficacy, oral health-related fatalism, oral health knowledge, access to dental care, and rights as a patient. In total, 400 adults—203 in the intervention group and 197 in the control group—were enrolled in the trial. The primary outcome was oral health literacy as assessed by the 14-item Health Literacy Dental Scale (HeLD-14) instrument. Oral health literacy partially improved in the intervention group versus the control group. Oral health literacy improved when assessed under some scenarios. Improvement was seen in perceptions of control, oral health-related fatalism, and perceived stress.

12.2.6 Personalized and Community Teaching Strategies

Several RCTs characterized as studies of behavioral strategies have not referenced specific theoretical models, but rather have used traditional teaching strategies—such as information-based oral hygiene instruction for parents and children, and oral health education and promotion. Some of these interventions employ personalized approaches adapted to ensure cultural sensitivity. In addition, these interventions often use lay people from the community to deliver oral health promotion and disease prevention activities.

Supporting Intervention Using Instruction by Navajo Tribal Members. A reservation-based, 3-year cluster-randomized clinical trial was conducted for Navajo children attending 52 Head Starts (26 intervention and 26 usual care), which delivered an Oral Health Promotion (OHP) intervention, with outcomes measured as relative caries increments [27]. In total, 1016 mother-child dyads (518 in the intervention group and 498 in the control group) were enrolled in the RCT. The behavioral intervention included a set of five child OHP interventions and four caregiver OHP interventions, along with the delivery of four fluoride applications in Head Starts from 2011 to 2012 and 2012 to 2013. The defining aspect of the intervention was that it was delivered exclusively by tribal members who received a one-week training every year in oral health and hygiene, as well as instructional approaches. The intervention was manualized, and it described the intervention in detail sufficient for reproduction and assurance of fidelity. The unit of randomization for this study was the Head Start Center (HSC); HSCs were randomly assigned to the intervention or the usual-care groups using a random number generator. The usual care group did not receive any intervention but did receive toothbrushes and toothpaste for their families. The impact of the intervention was evaluated using an index of DMF tooth surfaces and compared to the usual care group. An increase in DMFs was seen in both the intervention and usual care groups after 3 years, with the DMFs' increment being smaller for the HSCs receiving the intervention than for those assigned to usual care [28]. Caries prevalence also increased in the caregiver-child dyads receiving 1 year of intervention in both groups. The study concluded that the prevalence and severity of dental diseases were extremely high in the Navajo population assessed, and it was recommended that more highly personalized intervention approaches be developed that could be shaped by cultural perspectives attentive to social determinants of health. Parents often did not attend the oral health sessions due to such factors as their living mostly in remote areas, having very low incomes, and facing several other challenges, like lack of transportation. But the importance of parental engagement cannot be emphasized enough, because when parents did participate, there were positive results in terms of behavior change [29].

Supporting Instructional Intervention in California. A large-scale RCT was conducted in a low-income Hispanic population of 361 California mother-child dyads. Several strategies were used, including a chlorhexidine mouth rinse regimen for mothers postpartum, oral health counseling, and fluoride varnish applications for children every 6 months from ages 12 to 36 months old [30]. Mothers and their infants were randomly assigned using computer-generated blocks. The intervention used a *promotora* approach, in which mothers received one-on-one oral health counseling in Spanish or English, guided by a culturally suitable script from trained community health workers. The topics of discussion with the mothers by the *promotoras* were age-specific for the child and included oral hygiene, diet, and nutrition, the role of sugar in dental caries, appropriate fluoride use, appropriate pacifier use, the appropriate time for nursing bottle use, and injury prevention. Clinical exams were conducted for both the mother and the child by calibrated dental examiners. Despite this strong combination of potentially effective clinical and behavioral intervention strategies, however, no reduction in caries was seen in the primary dentition of participants. Although there were no differences between the control and intervention groups, participants had one-half the ECC prevalence and lower caries severity compared with their community's historical data. The trial concluded that these interventions may need to be combined with additional or longer-term therapies to significantly reduce ECC in high-risk populations.

Supporting Instructional Intervention in Australia. A 2-year, prospective, cluster-randomized, concurrently controlled open trial using a Community-Based Participatory Research (CBPR) model involved 666 Australian Aboriginal children, aged 18–47 months old. The randomization design allocated communities at random to either the intervention group (344 children) or the control group (322 children), such that all children within a given community received the same intervention. The intervention was delivered by Aboriginal health workers who provided fluoride varnish applications and engaged parents and families during dental screenings and varnish applications at children's playgroups, preschool and community councils, and other community events. Advice to parents was given in two settings: one was during a fluoride varnish application where a clinician provided information on dental caries prevention; the other was at children's preschool, where non-healthcare providers gave similar information. Health promotion information was also provided to community leaders to promote a community-wide oral health promotion campaign. Face painting was used alongside fluoride varnish applications to increase the acceptability of the varnish in children. Significantly lower decayed surface increments were seen over 2 years when those receiving the intervention were compared with children in control communities [31]. This resource-intensive intervention reduced the dental caries increment by 2.3–3.5 surfaces per child, which is 24–36% fewer tooth surfaces per child that developed dental caries over 2 years. Still, it was discouraging that 89% of children in the intervention group developed caries during the 2 years.

Supporting Instructional Intervention in Greece. A double-blind RCT with two parallel arms was conducted in schools in medium and low socioeconomic areas of Athens, Greece [32]. Children (n = 328) were stratified according to caries risk before the randomization so that a similar number of high- and low-risk caries children were present in each group. A child was considered at high risk if there was at least one carious lesion and/or presence of mutants streptococci in a microbiological test. Random blocks of size eight were used and the randomization lists were produced with computer software. The intervention used twice-yearly fluoride varnish applications, along with oral hygiene instructions, daily supervised tooth brushing with fluoridated toothpaste, and a few other oral health promotion activities conducted at school. Oral hygiene and dietary advice were given in a classroom setting by dental professionals. Dental caries increments after 2 years did not lower for the intervention group compared to the control group. The children in the study were aged 2–5 years old and had been identified as high caries risk, with 37% of them having experienced caries at baseline. The school setting encouraged compliance and participation by the students in the daily oral health activities and facilitated the fluoride varnish applications.

12.3 Technical and Logistical Considerations in RCT Implementation

Once the trial design has been finalized and all approvals have been received, the implementation of a behavioral RCT has its own set of guidelines and common challenges faced during implementation. These usually include the following issues:

Summary of Supportive Interventions

Supportive behavioral interventions supported clinical approaches, such as fluoride varnish, chlorhexidine mouthwash and other chemical approaches, and also produced mixed results.

Although clinically change is visible in supporting interventions, such as reduction in dental caries, it becomes difficult to distinguish the impact of the behavioral intervention from the clinical intervention in such studies. Thus, these studies do not capture the effectiveness of behavioral interventions.

Summary of Direct Interventions

The direct MI intervention provided a mixed result. It is possible, of course, that these results reflect dose problems—that is, that the intervention needed to be more intense or involve more intervention sessions to result in more positive outcomes. It should be noted, however, that the interventions in these studies may have varied considerably in their adherence to standard MI approaches, with the two U.S. studies and the Australian study descriptions suggesting the strictest adherence to the model.

Other Direct intervention were also based on Salutogenic, Social and Cognitive theories. These studies demonstrated promise in behavior change, including an increase in the capacity of the individuals to take ownership of the behavior change, which could be related to improving oral hygiene or reducing cariogenic diet.

Changes at clinical level, such as reduction in dental caries level were either rarely seen or not captured in these studies. One of the main reasons is that clinical changes are seen after a longer duration of behavior change, and most behavioral RCTs do not run for a long enough period of time to capture the clinical change.

12.3.1 Conceptual Framework

The articulation of a conceptual framework for a behavioral trial provides a structure for systematically thinking about factors that need to be considered in developing meaningful interventions. By clarifying the theory behind the intervention, it suggests the mechanisms by which change can be achieved and increases the capacity for reproducing the study and its results.

The Center for Native Oral Health Research (CNOHR), funded by the National Institutes of Dental and Craniofacial Research and directed by Dr. Judith Albino, conducted two behavioral interventions with reservation-based AI populations that were among the studies described here. CNOHR used a CBPR methodology to design and implement the RCTs [33]. The conceptual model (Fig. 12.1) used by CNOHR emphasized the importance of early environments and social context, including stressors related to race and socioeconomic status, but with adaptations reflecting the context of oral health issues and concerns. Developed with AI community input, the framework identified a series of factors—demographic, behavioral, psychological, health, and others, as well as intervention factors—that may contribute differentially both to oral health and to responses to an oral health intervention. The framework begins with factors that affect oral health at the macro level but are largely outside the influence of the intervention. The mediators/moderators in the second column may provide a greater understanding of responses to interventions, thereby suggesting valuable strategies for developing maximally effective interventions. Oral health outcomes reflected the complexity of the oral health system that the intervention could influence. The developmental dimensions that influenced the elements of the intervention and potential outcomes were also noted in the conceptual model. Both oral health problems themselves and the best strategies for intervention were influenced by age, life context, and the concerns of different developmental stages, as indicated in the conceptual framework.

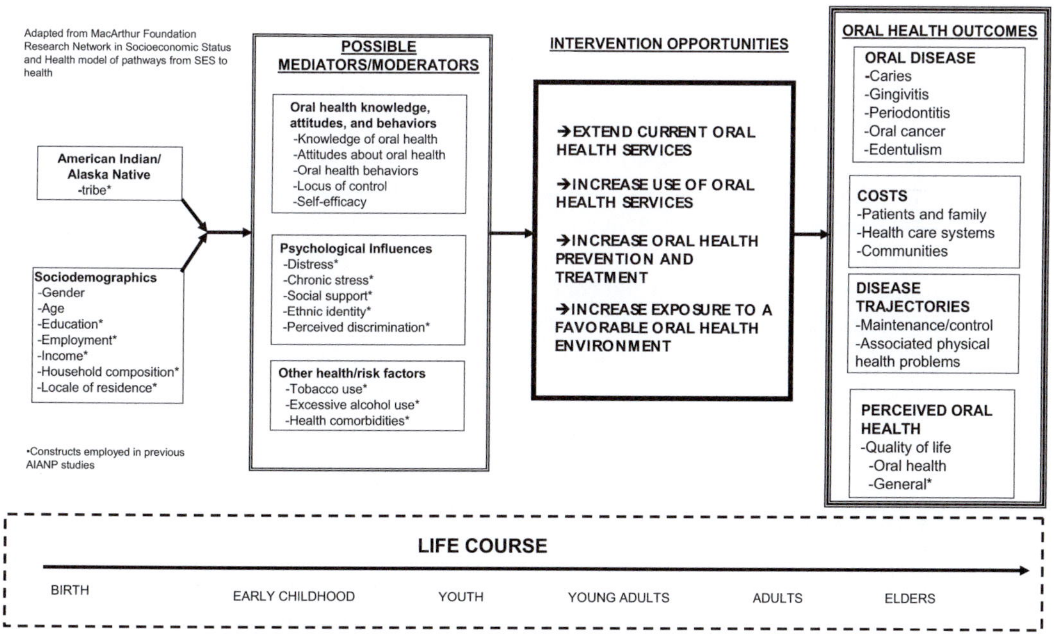

Fig. 12.1 Conceptual framework for center for native oral health research

12.3.2 Community-Based Approaches in Behavioral Trials

CBPR is an effective model for achieving success in RCTs, especially within ethnic minority communities in which cultural perspectives may differ from those within the larger society. CBPR principles require "recognition of a community as a unit of identity; facilitate collaborative, equitable partnership in all phases of the research, achievement of a balance between knowledge generation and intervention for the mutual benefit of all partners, capacity building among all partners and long term sustainability" [34].

Most behavioral RCTs—even those not labeled here as Personalized/Culturally Specific Models, used laypersons to engage the community, recruit and retain study participants, and implement the intervention. This, of course, is consistent with CBPR standards and has been one of the key factors in the successful implementation of behavioral RCTs—particularly when conducted with minority racial and ethnic group populations. Using laypeople as healthcare workers has several advantages, including building trust with the community, facilitating recruitment and retention of study participants, and—above all—providing a sustainable resource for the community [35]. It is not surprising that many recent RCTs take this approach since most such work with behavioral strategies is conducted within the context of large community-based interventions. These approaches are both expected by the communities where participation is sought, or they are simply important strategies that rely on understanding the motivations and understanding of participants' life situations and social contexts.

12.3.3 Manual of Procedures

As is the case for all randomized clinical trials in the United States, regulations exist regarding all aspects of planning, implementation, and reporting. The Food and Drug Administration Amendments Act of 2007 (FDAAA) is the basis for most of these today. Trials funded by the National Institutes of Health (NIH) institutes or centers, including the National Institute of Dental and Craniofacial Research (NIDCR), are generally expected to comply with all FDAAA regulations and are monitored carefully in that regard by the funding agencies. In the United Kingdom and Wales, the National Institute for Health and Clinical Excellence (NICE) provides guidelines for trials funded through the National Health Service (NHS). The European Medicines Agency (EMA) in the European Union and the Department of Health (DOH) in Australia—as well as similar agencies in other countries—assume similar roles. While all of the regulations for clinical trials of drugs and devices may not seem relevant to behavioral trials, the governing agencies ordinarily expect them to be followed.

Among the expectations for clinical trials in the United States—which have been described elsewhere in this volume—is the Manual of Procedures (MOP). Given the unexpected nature of human behavior, interventions to test behavioral interventions can especially benefit from a detailed and well-written MOP. A strong MOP, followed rigorously during pilot tests, can ensure the identification of unforeseen problems, and thereby greatly improve procedures and add value in the implementation of the final trial. Moreover, it provides specific information about the implementation of design and potential variations necessary in real-world situations and challenges. The MOP can define a balance between the extreme rigidity of behavioral interventions and the necessary flexibility that may be needed for the implementation of behavioral interventions. Finally, the MOP is a significant document, not only to direct the original implementation of a study but also to guide the efforts of researchers who may want to replicate the study. It provides an essential understanding of how the intervention was designed and how it evolved during the implementation phase without jeopardizing the fidelity of the intervention.

12.3.4 Ethical Considerations and Approvals

As in all other RCTs, behavioral RCTs require ethical approvals from their institutional review boards before study recruitment or implementation in the field. It also may be necessary to seek ethical approvals from the community where the study is to be conducted. It is always advisable to develop a strong understanding and acceptance of a study within a community, regardless of formal requirements for approval. It is important to find out the guidelines and processes involved in receiving ethical approvals from community review boards and incorporate the time needed and expenses required to fulfill them before research activities start in the field. Some communities—including AI tribes—may have well-developed structures for review and approval of research, and their rules will often override concerns of institutional review boards. Ensuring that multiple sets of requirements are met may mean going back and forth between boards.

For example, CNOHR sought and received ethical approvals from the tribal institutional review boards and from the area Indian Health Service, as well as from the university institutional review board. AI communities strongly recommend the use of CBPR methodologies in research and clinical trials conducted on reservations. In addition to research review boards, RCTs may have community advisory boards and other structures for community participation in research design, approvals, and implementation. CNOHR worked with the tribes to set up planning meetings that involved tribal governance and other AI community members and representatives, health board representatives, and education board representatives, and also consulted with Indian Health Service representatives before submitting the grant application [10, 27]. If one board asked for some consideration that had not been approved by the other board, this meant going back to the first board; obviously, negotiations were important in how these matters would be handled. Moreover, after final approvals were achieved, a Community Advisory Committee (CAC) that provided input on all CNOHR research activities and Community Advisory Boards (CABs) that provided input on each of the two clinical trials were formed to consult on the project throughout the trials.

12.3.5 Hiring and Training of Staff

There were several lessons learned by CNOHR staff and faculty in our work to receive cooperation and approvals from the communities within which we worked. Above all, these are time-consuming processes. Community review boards have their protocols, meeting times, and communication methodologies, as well as their specific concerns that may seem to have little relationship to the goals of the research, but that nonetheless must influence the conduct of the trial. Thus, RCTs using CBPR approaches should include extra time within their framework and great flexibility in accommodating the needs of community review boards and advisory groups. Second, it is important to build trust with the community before seeking approval. A good approach is to include on the team an investigator, or a key staff member, from the community. Third, many communities consider it a sign of respect if the principal investigator or senior leader from the team is present during the review board meetings to describe the study and answer questions that may concern review board members. The research review board of a Southwestern reservation with which we worked stipulated that the principal investigator should be present at all review board meetings, despite the fact that traveling to these meetings from the university required a flight and a four-hour drive—sometimes only to discover that the review group did not have a quorum and, therefore, could not take action; the location of another review board with which we worked required a 12-hour drive. In both cases, substantial commitments of time and budget were required to accommodate working in these communities.

One of the most difficult challenges faced by any RCT is hiring and retaining the staff who implement the trial in the field. Most behavioral RCTs hire people from the community and train them to implement the study, which helps reduce turnover.

The Early Childhood Caries Collaborating Centers (EC4) included the Center to Address. Disparities in Children's Oral Health at the University of California San Francisco (UCSF), the Center for Research to Evaluate and Eliminate Dental Disparities at Boston University (BU), and the Center for Native Oral Health Research at the University of Colorado Denver (UCD). The EC4 has reported extensively on the hiring and training of staff. Although the three centers involved worked with different populations and in different areas of the United States, they faced similar challenges in retaining study staff. One of the common methods used by all three centers was to engage the study staff frequently with the principal and contributing investigators for the RCTs [36]. Several strategies used in behavioral trials conducted in the Aboriginal community in Australia, First Nations people in Canada, and the Maori community in New Zealand have been reported, as well [37–39]. Investigators in all these RCTs spent considerable time listening to the concerns of study staff, motivating them, and, most importantly, acknowledging their accomplishments. All these trials hired staff from the communities where they were implementing the research. This not only reduced turnover, but also helped to build trust with the communities and retain study participants.

12.3.6 Instrument Development for Data Collection

Measurement in behavioral trials is perhaps even more important in the design of a study than in trials focused on a drug or device. The defined outcomes—both primary and secondary—must be carefully considered and measured; usually, it is also important to consider moderating and/or mediating variables that may influence response to the intervention and to ensure that they are properly measured. Even the intervention itself must be carefully measured—often in terms of duration or other variables, and also in terms of fidelity to the defined procedures for implementation.

Clinical data are collected to measure the effect of clinical outcomes, of course, and there are usually standard approaches to these types of assessments. However, it is important to consider the use of the data, the primary concern being whether the measure chosen will allow us to identify group differences in the way and at the level required for a clinical trial. More specific to behavioral trials are concerns related to the theoretical model guiding the research; measures of attitudes, beliefs, and/or behaviors, as well as some sociodemographic or social determinants, may be needed—either to assess their moderating or mediating effects on outcomes or to determine the effect of the intervention directly on these variables, which may be used as outcomes (usually secondary). For these purposes, behavioral RCTs are well-advised to use validated surveys and tools already available; or to build into their study the necessary procedures not only for developing their own tools but also for assessing the reliability and validity of these instruments. The latter approach is time-consuming and requires a team of experts who know the theoretical background for the intervention have specific assessment expertise, and possess the requisite biostatistical skills.

In the context of their series of coordinated behavioral trials, the EC4 developed a comprehensive assessment instrument, the Basic Research Factors Questionnaire (BRFQ); more than 50 national experts were involved in the development of the BRFQ [40]. A systematic, multi-step process in selecting and defining measures was used. Working groups were assembled, comprising experts from all of the behavioral, social, psychological, and demographic areas covered by the questionnaire. These groups developed questions or used existing questions under the domains that were then included in the survey. The EC4 published the development process of the BRFQ, as well as the questions so that others who want to use the survey or develop their own will have guidance for doing so.

Investigators planning behavioral RCTs may not have the extensive resources needed to develop measurement tools, and the use of previously developed and validated tools provides an efficient and effective approach to moving a trial forward. Moreover, previously validated instruments may increase confidence in the trial, even if some adjustments are needed to adapt an established instrument to suit the population participating in the trial.

12.3.7 Reporting Behavioral Trials

Most—if not all—RCTs use the Consolidated Standards of Reporting Trials (CONSORT) criteria for reporting their methods and results. Several journals require RCTs to follow the CONSORT guidelines, including them in the electronic submission format [41]. Registered clinical trials of behavioral interventions, as well as other treatments, also must track and record adverse events—especially if the trials used a device/drug in conjunction with the behavioral intervention [32, 42]. The EC4 group mentioned above developed a common approach to these requirements; although all three centers implemented behavioral RCTs, they reported the incidence of adverse events related to fluoride varnish treatment in three clinical trials on the prevention of ECC. Children who participated in these three trials received a cumulative total of 10,249 fluoride varnish treatments; on average, each child received 4.2 fluoride varnish treatments. No fluoride varnish-related adverse events were found in more than 10,000 applications, nor were there any reported adverse events as the result of behavioral strategies used [42].

12.3.8 Recruitment, Retention, and Engagement of the Population

Like most other RCTs, behavioral RCTs face challenges related to the recruitment and retention of study participants. Although most institutional review boards will take an interest in—and may require changes in—procedures related to recruitment and retention of subjects, these are nonetheless issues that investigators need to think through carefully themselves to ensure the integrity of the research. Researchers who evaluated retention and recruitment efforts in dental trials in the United Kingdom and Australia reported that RCTs require participants to take part in the intervention, which can involve multiple, time-consuming sessions, as well as the completion of long and cumbersome surveys [43].

Improved strategies for recruitment of participants may be key to ensuring that participants stay engaged in the intervention, complete the study for longer, and don't compromise data by becoming fatigued in the process [36]. It is important to be clear and transparent with study participants regarding study expectations and time commitment. Although this step can lead to participants' declining participation, it is better to lose them before enrollment rather than after the study has begun, which may negatively impact results and incur unnecessary costs.

Respondent, or participant, compensation is a critical element of recruiting that needs special attention. Participants should be paid reasonably for their time, yet payment should not be so generous as to become a coercive factor—or one that invites misrepresentation on the part of potential participants. These are always considerations in the approval of studies by institutional review boards, although compensation may be decided based on guidelines provided by either the institutional review board or the community review board. In making decisions about appropriate payment, however, the specific social and economic characteristics of the community from which the participants are drawn need to be taken into consideration, and it may be up to the investigators to provide review boards with this information and an appropriate interpretation. Respondent fatigue can also be reduced by providing surveys on tablets or computers, reducing the chance of missing survey questions. Surveys can be administered using software that can read the questions aloud to participants, perhaps in a language of their choosing; this can provide important assistance for participants who may have issues with reading and literacy.

The retention of participants can be another challenge with the potential loss of follow-up data in longitudinal trials [44]. If the trial is CBPR-guided, the investigators should keep the established community advisory board informed about the recruitment and retention numbers. Community members are always the best resource to discuss strategies related to recruitment and retention; they know best what works in their community, and can help the investigators who may be "outsiders" to understand the culture of the community and to keep participants retained. A trial conducted in Wales vested extensive time in recruitment and retention efforts of a community-based trial. They reported that recruitment was one of the most challenging parts of the trial, although—once recruited—only 11.6% of participants dropped out of the trial [45]. The trial also reported extensive efforts to retain participants, including up to 15 home visits for some children. The EC4 provided several approaches used in the RCTs that improved retention; some of these were paying for transportation costs or meeting people at their homes. They also learned to collect alternative phone numbers at enrollment in order to contact the participants, should they move or disconnect a phone line. It is good practice to learn participants' preferred methods for being contacted; depending on circumstances, telephone, texting and even social media may be preferred.

12.3.9 Fidelity

Although the concept of treatment fidelity had been discussed over a number of years, it received greater emphasis after the 1999 establishment of the NIH Behavior Change Consortium intended to provide best practices for methodological strategies to monitor and enhance the reliability and validity of behavioral interventions [46]. The Consortium has defined methods to assess fidelity based on five key components: study design, training providers, delivery of treatment, receipt of treatment, and enactment of treatment skills [47, 48]. Addressing fidelity in all these areas can improve scientific confidence in a study, and reduce threats to the study's internal and external validity, thereby enabling researchers to draw more accurate conclusions. Recently, behavioral RCTs in oral health have published independent fidelity reports to provide in-depth assessments of the process and impact of fidelity on trial outcomes [48, 49].

Fidelity in data collection is usually discussed in terms of reliability and validity of measurement. Examiner or rater calibration is essential to ensure this quality and, in most cases, data from these calibrations and later checks on reliability are reported along with the results of the trial. Several studies reported here have included fidelity monitoring in their protocols, and some funding agencies in the United States, including the NIDCR, require that fidelity monitoring be included in the grant application process of an RCT. Two of the MI-focused RCTs described above were involved in the development of detailed common procedures and gold standards for clinical data collection.

Although the examples provided for RCTs applied different theoretical models and approaches, some made fidelity to the intervention an important component of their work. Publications describing the process of fidelity followed in the trial [48, 49] are proving especially valuable as resources for the development of new trials. Multiple investigators and research staff are involved in the implementation of large-scale trials, making it especially important to ensure the reliability of the approach, including avoidance of intervention "drift" over time. An example of best practice with respect to fidelity is demonstrated in MI studies that have used MITI—a coding system designed to measure treatment fidelity for MI clinical trials, providing structured, formal feedback about improving practice [50]. Several behavioral RCTs have manualized their interventions to improve reproducibility. Although following a fidelity process improves confidence, reliability, and validity, it may also reduce flexibility for implementation of the behavioral intervention in the field. The temptation to give in to the desire to modify an intervention in the midst of a trial is more easily resisted when interventions have been thoroughly pilot-tested and manualized in great detail, and the circumstances that might provoke a need for such flexibility have been thought through and discussed with those responsible for implementation.

12.4 Gap Analysis for Behavioral Trials

Today, we know far more about the role of behavior in oral health than a decade or two ago, in large part due to efforts made to conduct clinical trials focused on behavioral strategies to improve health. Standard controls on clinical trials provide some guidance and commonality of structure that ensures confidence in results and lends legitimacy to outcomes. Nonetheless, this framework has not served the development of behavioral strategies at nearly the level we have seen for clinical treatments or biochemical approaches to prevention. We can attribute this fact to where we currently stand in our conceptual knowledge of behavioral strategies, and how they can or should be used to improve oral health.

Likely the greatest gap in our knowledge about RCTs in testing behavioral strategies in the context of oral health is reflected by the limited number of theoretical approaches that have been submitted to this most rigorous test of efficacy. We believe this challenge emerges from our failure to distinguish and account for the role of behavioral strategies—as discussed in our description of direct and supportive uses of behavioral interventions—and a resulting lack of confidence in the promise of behavioral strategies. Unlike in the case of medical problems, such as diabetes or even some areas of cardiovascular disease, we have yet to develop the depth of understanding that says oral disease is a problem that must be addressed *primarily* in terms of behavioral approaches. We seem reluctant to say that oral disease—even caries in children—is *best* prevented by behavioral steps, such as diet control and oral hygiene practices. As such, when allowed to use scarce funds to conduct an expensive RCT, we are unwilling to go the distance to test the efficacy of a standalone behavioral strategy. In all likelihood, this is because it just seems too expensive when we believe—albeit not always correctly—that we have greater evidence for biochemical methods of prevention or surgical approaches to repair. This thinking seems misguided at best and gets in the way of developing the complete knowledge base needed on the role of behavior in oral health.

Perhaps the lack of confidence in behavioral strategies stems from the fact that these approaches simply are not well understood. Even our efforts to describe them are admittedly less than precise, and the almost haphazard way in which they have been combined with other strategies, including clinical approaches, can render the trial design inappropriate for addressing the question being posed. Further complicating matters, many studies do not even attempt to describe the mechanisms whereby a behavioral strategy might be expected to achieve a specific change or outcome. Indeed, our own attempt to categorize the kinds of behavioral trials that have been conducted was often frustrating as the information provided in reporting these trials lacks consistency or a common language. None of this is entirely surprising, of course, since the methodology of clinical trials has been honed and refined in the study of pharmaceuticals—a model that does not easily translate to human behavior and all its vicissitudes. Although the basic clinical trial design can serve us well in studying the effectiveness of behavioral strategies, the fit is not always perfect. The behavior of human beings is over-determined, and we may never be able to achieve the degree of control that might be possible in delivering and examining the effects of specific chemical treatments, for example. Nonetheless, we must attempt to do just that.

Two basic kinds of information are needed to move forward our progress in conducting clinical trials of behavioral strategies for improving oral health. The first is conceptual knowledge, as mentioned above; the second is more knowledge about research methods and designs that are appropriate for conducting behavioral trials.

1. Conceptual knowledge. We must thoroughly understand the various behavioral models used so that we are not dependent on the brief descriptions and loose interpretations often found in protocols for clinical trials. In clinical and research literature, we need theoretical analyses of these models and how the strategies based on these models would be operationalized in the oral health setting. This means translating the behavioral strategy from psychological literature into the specific applied context, with projections about what we might expect to see. This should include translations, also from basic psychological science, about expected mediators and moderators of behavior in the oral health setting. Only with this background can we design

studies that allow us to test the efficacy of the behavioral intervention, or—as is often the case—the behavioral *component* of the intervention.
2. Methodological knowledge. In this chapter, we discussed a number of challenges in conducting clinical trials of behavioral strategies, and we identified some successful approaches to addressing those challenges. Unfortunately, to do so, we most often had to draw on our own work or studies of colleagues whose work we know well because it has not been the convention in this area of research to publish protocols with details related to design and implementation—or even to publish data on such elements of the research as fidelity to intervention. It is only through this kind of rigorous attention to all aspects of the research process, however, that the conduct of these behavioral trials will contribute to a coherent picture of the efficacy of behavioral strategies for improving oral health.

If we could fully commit to exploring behavioral strategies for oral health through the RCT methodology, by seeking the kind of information described here, we would have the foundational knowledge that permits moving toward identifying not only strategies that are sometimes effective, but the standard application of those strategies. Moreover, we could compare various strategies—cognitive-behavioral strategies with MI, for example. We could test culturally specific interventions with more generic approaches. And, perhaps most important, we could know whether the behavioral strategy is as effective as the clinical one, whether it boosts the clinical one, and where and when those various choices could be applied. Our ability to credibly test such questions depends on our developing and sharing the two kinds of knowledge described above. Those tasks themselves are formidable, but the payoff could be enormous—not only in terms of knowledge gained but also in future improvements in oral health.

12.5 Conclusion

Clinical trials of behavioral interventions in dentistry point toward an understanding of the value of these approaches and underscore their role in improving oral health. These trials bring a rigor that provides confidence in standard results. A number of the studies described in this chapter are outstanding examples of superbly conducted studies of complex approaches in situations where it may be difficult to provide true controls or to follow up in standardized ways. We are learning from these trials, yet enormous conceptual and methodological challenges remain. Consequently, even in the few areas where results from multiple trials exist, we rarely can make general or definitive statements about the efficacy of the approaches. That must be seen not as a failure of the strategies themselves, however, but rather as a function of the stage of development of this field of research.

As we observed at the beginning of this chapter, clinical trials of behavioral strategies are often conducted using designs that position the behavioral approach as an adjunct to a clinical approach. The decision to construct a study in this way is understandable in the context of dental care and oral health. We have often observed that—no matter how effective the clinical or biochemical strategy may be—its implementation requires human behavior, whether to use the product or to keep the appointment; and many clinical approaches require considerable effort in adhering to regimens or otherwise following through with professional recommendations. This pairing of behavioral strategies with clinical strategies, however, means that we cannot always separate the effects of the two approaches. And, not surprisingly, our clinical trials may demonstrate different outcomes for what would seem to be tests of the same behavioral strategy. We do not yet seem to be at a point in the evolution of clinical trials of behavioral interventions in dentistry that we are willing to invest in the development of the strategies themselves—even comparing "doses," for example, or carefully analyzing behaviors that are possible to achieve, or the mediating and moderating factors that may enhance or impede desired behavior. Rather, with a sense of urgency about going to the ultimate test, we are pressed to make our "best guesses" about too many elements related to the application of the intervention. With this in mind, we humbly suggest that some clinical trials conducted—perhaps including our own—should not have been clinical trials (not that they did not embody good questions and good designs, but rather that they were not yet ready for clinical trials because more preliminary work needed to be done). Yet there is always pressure to move to the "gold standard" of the clinical trial. As researchers, as funders, and as advisors to research funding agencies, we must always keep this question in mind. Clinical trials are not the only way to learn about behavioral strategies. Just as laboratory studies are important in developing basic biological and chemical knowledge, and translational studies may represent a step before clinical trials, we need to think about behavioral science in the same way.

This situation is exacerbated by the fact that the conduct of RCTs of behavioral interventions is especially expensive. Usually, these trials must be conducted with large numbers of participants in field settings. They are resource-intensive in every respect, requiring substantial human and financial resources to implement interventions. This may account to some degree for the relatively small number of such trials conducted—which, in turn, increases competition among applicants responding to clinical trial funding opportunities.

Resources for oral health research are limited and behavioral research may not receive a high priority compared to trials focused on biochemical approaches, devices, or surgical treatments. In our gap analysis, we identified a lack of understanding of the role of behavior in oral health as the underlying cause. That said, several behavioral trials have been conducted in several countries around the world in the last 10 years, adding significant knowledge to the literature related to the importance of behavior change in improving oral health outcomes. The field is an exciting one, albeit a still nascent one. Oral health and behavior are inseparable, and the behavioral side deserves our best efforts—including completion of the foundational and translational work that will create better RCTs of behavioral interventions in the future.

12.6 Case Scenario Exercise

12.6.1 Case Scenario

Description of the case: An oral health disparities research center focusing on early childhood caries prevention in a low-income, rural Hispanic community is implementing a Randomized Controlled Trial (RCT) to test the efficacy of MI on behavior change in young mothers. The study participants are recruited at community clinics and community events. The MI intervention is delivered at 6, 12, and 18 months, with an additional follow-up period of 2 years. You are part of a Community Advisory Board (CAB) that advocates for the community and advises study investigators on recruitment and retention strategies, and other study procedures.

Situation: During a CAB meeting with the study investigators and the research team, the team describes the challenges in recruiting and retaining participants in the study.

Challenges Faced in the Implementation of the RCT

Recruitment

- Participants who miss their initial study enrollment appointments cause delays in completing recruitment for the study.
- Lack of reliable transportation and/or disconnected phone service cause delays in contacting potential participants.

Retention

- *Missed appointment*: Parents miss scheduled appointments for a variety of reasons, including conflicting work schedules, lack of childcare for other children, or providing care for other children in the family.
- *Transience*: Participants move frequently, making it difficult for staff to keep track of them over time.
- *Disconnected/nonfunctioning phone service*: Many participants do not have landline service, relying instead on prepaid cellular service which often changes or becomes disconnected.
- *Transportation*: Although the study provides respondent compensation for participation, three participants this past week expressed difficulties getting to the field office for the study visit because of a lack of reliable transportation.
- *Staff retention*: There is high turnover in field study staff, which results in time and effort spent training new staff, rather than on recruitment and retention efforts and data collection.

Questions

1. Discuss the strategies that might be used to improve retention and recruitment in this behavioral RCT.

Answers

1. The recruitment and retention strategies are discussed in Sect. 12.3.8 of this chapter. Respondent, or participant, compensation is a critical element of recruiting that needs special attention. Participants should be paid reasonably for their time, yet payment should not be so generous as to become a coercive factor—or one that invites misrepresentation on the part of potential participants. In making decisions about appropriate payment, however, the specific social and economic characteristics of the community from which the participants are drawn need to be taken into consideration, and it may be up to the investigators to provide review boards with this information and an appropriate interpretation. Respondent fatigue can also be reduced by providing surveys on tablets or computers, reducing the chance of missing survey questions.

The retention of participants can be another challenge with the potential loss of follow-up data in longitudinal trials. The investigators should keep the established community advisory board informed about recruitment and retention numbers. Community members are always the best resource for discussing strategies related to recruitment and retention; they know best what works in their community and can help investigators who may be "outsiders" understand the culture of the community and retain participants. The EC4 provided several approaches used in the RCTs that improved retention; some of these were paying for transportation costs or meeting people at their homes. They also learned to collect alternative phone numbers at enrollment in order to contact the participants, should they move or disconnect a phone line. It is good practice to learn participants' preferred methods for being contacted; depending on circumstances, telephone, texting and even social media may be preferred.

References

1. Albino J, Tiwari T. Behavior change for caries prevention: understanding inconsistent results. JDR Clin Transl Res. 2020;5(1):6–9.
2. Albino J, Tiwari T. Preventing childhood caries: a review of recent behavioral research. J Dent Res. 2016;95(1):35–42.
3. Hariton E, Locascio JJ. Randomised controlled trials—The gold standard for effectiveness research. BJOG. 2018;125(13):1716.
4. Kvale G, Berggren U, Milgrom P. Dental fear in adults: a meta-analysis of behavioral interventions. Community Dent Oral Epidemiol. 2004;32(4):250–64.
5. Twetman S. Prevention of Early Childhood Caries (ECC) review of literature published 1998–2007. Eur Arch Paediatr Dent. 2008;9(1):12–8.
6. Miller WR, Rollnick S. Motivational interviewing: helping people change. Guilford Press; 2012.
7. Miller WR, Rose GS. Toward a theory of motivational interviewing. Am Psychol. 2009;64(6):527.
8. Batliner TS, Tiwari T, Henderson WG, Wilson AR, Gregorich SE, Fehringer KA, et al. Randomized trial of motivational interviewing to prevent early childhood caries in American Indian Children. JDR Clin Transl Res. 2018;3(4):366–75.
9. Henshaw M, Borrelli B, Gregorich S, Heaton B, Tooley E, Santo W, et al. Randomized trial of motivational interviewing to prevent early childhood caries in public housing. JDR Clin Transl Res. 2018;3(4):353–65.
10. Batliner T, Fehringer KA, Tiwari T, Henderson WG, Wilson A, Brega AG, et al. Motivational interviewing with American Indian mothers to prevent early childhood caries: study design and methodology of a randomized control trial. Trials. 2014;15:125.
11. Wu L, Gao X, Lo EC, Ho SM, McGrath C, Wong MC. Motivational interviewing to promote oral health in adolescents. J Adolesc Health. 2017;61(3):378–84.
12. Jamieson L, Smithers L, Hedges J, Parker E, Mills H, Kapellas K, et al. Dental disease outcomes following a 2-year oral health promotion program for Australian Aboriginal children and their families: a 2-arm parallel, single-blind, randomised controlled trial. EClinicalMedicine. 2018;1:43–50.
13. Pine C, Adair P, Burnside G, Brennan L, Sutton L, Edwards RT, et al. Dental RECUR randomized trial to prevent caries recurrence in children. J Dent Res. 2020;99(2):168–74.
14. Makvandi Z, Karimi-Shahanjarini A, Faradmal J, Bashirian S. Evaluation of an oral health intervention among mothers of young children: a clustered randomized trial. J Res Health Sci. 2015;15(2):88–93.
15. Ajzen I. The theory of planned behavior. Organ Behav Hum Decis Process. 1991;50(2):179–211.
16. Armitage CJ, Conner M. Efficacy of the theory of planned behaviour: a meta-analytic review. Br J Soc Psychol. 2001;40(4):471–99.
17. Amin M, Elyasi M, Bohlouli B, ElSalhy M. Application of the theory of planned behavior to predict dental attendance and caries experience among children of newcomers. Int J Environ Res Public Health. 2019;16(19):3661.
18. Deci EL, Ryan RM. The" what" and" why" of goal pursuits: Human needs and the self-determination of behavior. Psychol Inq. 2000;11(4):227–68.
19. Weber-Gasparoni K, Warren JJ, Reeve J, Drake DR, Kramer KW, Marshall TA, et al. An effective psychoeducational intervention for early childhood caries prevention: Part II. Pediatr Dent. 2013;35(3):247–51.
20. Antonovsky A. The structure and properties of the sense of coherence scale. Soc Sci Med. 1993;36(6):725–33.
21. Antonovsky A. Unraveling the mystery of health: how people manage stress and stay well. Jossey-Bass; 1987.
22. Silva AN, Alvares De Lima ST, Vettore MV. Protective psychosocial factors and dental caries in children and adolescents: a systematic review and meta-analysis. Int J Paediatr Dent. 2018;28(5):443–58.
23. Nammontri O, Robinson PG, Baker SR. Enhancing oral health via sense of coherence: a cluster-randomized trial. J Dent Res. 2013;92(1):26–31.
24. Zhou N, Wong HM, McGrath C. Social story-based oral health promotion for preschool children with special healthcare needs: a 24-month randomized controlled trial. Community Dent Oral Epidemiol. 2020 Oct;48(5):415–22.
25. Bandura A. Health promotion from the perspective of social cognitive theory. Psychol Health. 1998;13:623–49.
26. Ju X, Brennan D, Parker E, Mills H, Kapellas K, Jamieson L. Efficacy of an oral health literacy intervention among Indigenous Australian adults. Community Dent Oral Epidemiol. 2017;45(5):413–26.
27. Quissell DO, Bryant LL, Braun PA, Cudeii D, Johs N, Smith VL, et al. Preventing caries in preschoolers: successful initiation of an innovative community-based clinical trial in Navajo Nation Head Start. Contemp Clin Trials. 2014;37(2):242–51.
28. Braun PA, Quissell DO, Henderson WG, Bryant LL, Gregorich SE, George C, et al. A cluster-randomized, community-based, tribally delivered oral health promotion trial in Navajo Head Start Children. J Dent Res. 2016;95(11):1237–44.
29. Bryant LL, Quissell DO, Braun PA, Henderson WG, Johs N, George C, et al. A community-based oral health intervention in Navajo Nation Head Start: participation factors and contextual challenges. J Community Health. 2016;41(2):340–53.

30. Ramos-Gomez FJ, Gansky SA, Featherstone JD, Jue B, Gonzalez-Beristain R, Santo W, et al. Mother and youth access (MAYA) maternal chlorhexidine, counselling and paediatric fluoride varnish randomized clinical trial to prevent early childhood caries. Int J Paediatr Dent. 2012;22(3):169–79.
31. Slade GD, Bailie RS, Roberts-Thomson K, Leach AJ, Raye I, Endean C, et al. Effect of health promotion and fluoride varnish on dental caries among Australian Aboriginal children: results from a community-randomized controlled trial. Community Dent Oral Epidemiol. 2011;39(1):29–43.
32. Agouropoulos A, Twetman S, Pandis N, Kavvadia K, Papagiannoulis L. Caries-preventive effectiveness of fluoride varnish as adjunct to oral health promotion and supervised tooth brushing in preschool children: a double-blind randomized controlled trial. J Dent. 2014;42(10):1277–83.
33. Tiwari T, Sharma T, Harper M, Zacher T, Roan R, George C, et al. Community based participatory research to reduce oral health disparities in American Indian Children. J Family Med. 2015;2(3):1028.
34. Israel BA, Schulz AJ, Parker EA, Becker AB, Allen AJ, Guzman JR, et al. Critical issues in developing and following CBPR principles. In: Minkler M, Wallerstein N, editors. Community-based participatory research for health: advancing social and health equity. San Francisco, CA: Jossey-Bass; 2017. p. 31–46.
35. Berkman LF. The role of social relations in health promotion. Psychosom Med. 1995;57(3):245–54.
36. Tiwari T, Casciello A, Gansky SA, Henshaw M, Ramos-Gomez F, Rasmussen M, et al. Recruitment for health disparities preventive intervention trials: the early childhood caries collaborating centers. Prev Chronic Dis. 2014;11:E133.
37. Tiwari T, Jamieson L, Broughton J, Lawrence HP, Batliner TS, Arantes R, et al. Reducing indigenous oral health inequalities: a review from 5 nations. J Dent Res. 2018;97(8):869–77.
38. Merrick J, Chong A, Parker E, Roberts-Thomson K, Misan G, Spencer J, et al. Reducing disease burden and health inequalities arising from chronic disease among Indigenous children: an early childhood caries intervention. BMC Public Health. 2012;12(1):323.
39. Broughton JR, Maipi JTH, Person M, Thomson WM, Morgaine KC, Tiakiwai SJ, et al. Reducing disease burden and health inequalities arising from chronic disease among indigenous children: an early childhood caries intervention in Aotearoa/New Zealand. BMC Public Health. 2013;13(1):1177.
40. Albino J, Tiwari T, Gansky SA, Henshaw MM, Barker JC, Brega AG, et al. The basic research factors questionnaire for studying early childhood caries. BMC Oral Health. 2017;17(1):83.
41. Needleman I, Worthington H, Moher D, Schulz K, Altman DG. Improving the completeness and transparency of reports of randomized trials in oral health: the CONSORT statement. Am J Dent. 2008;21(1):7.
42. Garcia RI, Gregorich SE, Ramos-Gomez F, Braun PA, Wilson A, Albino J, et al. Absence of fluoride Varnish-related adverse events in caries prevention trials in young children, United States. Prev Chronic Dis. 2017;14:E17.
43. Martin-Kerry JM, Lamont T, Keightley A, Calache H, Martin R, Floate R, et al. Practical considerations for conducting dental clinical trials in primary care. Br Dent J. 2015;218(11):629–34.
44. Garcia RI, Tiwari T, Ramos-Gomez F, Heaton B, Orozco M, Rasmussen M, et al. Retention strategies for health disparities preventive trials: findings from the Early Childhood Caries Collaborating Centers. J Public Health Dent. 2017;77(1):63–77.
45. Chadwick BL, Treasure ET, Playle RA. A randomised controlled trial to determine the effectiveness of glass ionomer sealants in pre-school children. Caries Res. 2005;39(1):34–40.
46. Borrelli B, Sepinwall D, Ernst D, Bellg AJ, Czajkowski S, Breger R, et al. A new tool to assess treatment fidelity and evaluation of treatment fidelity across 10 years of health behavior research. J Consult Clin Psychol. 2005;73(5):852.
47. Bellg AJ, Borrelli B, Resnick B, Hecht J, Minicucci DS, Ory M, et al. Enhancing treatment fidelity in health behavior change studies: best practices and recommendations from the NIH Behavior Change Consortium. Health Psychol. 2004;23(5):443.
48. Jamieson L, Bradshaw J, Lawrence H, Broughton J, Venner K. Fidelity of motivational interviewing in an early childhood caries intervention involving indigenous Australian mothers. J Health Care Poor Underserved. 2016;27(1):125–38.
49. Wilson AR, Fehringer KA, Henderson WG, Venner K, Thomas J, Harper MM, et al. fidelity of motivational interviewing in an American Indian oral health intervention. Community Dent Oral Epidemiol. 2018;46(3):310–6.
50. Moyers T, Martin T, Manuel J, Miller W, Ernst D. Revised global scales: motivational interviewing treatment integrity 3.1. 1 (MITI 3.1. 1). Unpublished manuscript. Albuquerque, NM: University of New Mexico; 2010.

Index

R. Kohli et al. (eds.), *Randomized Controlled Trials in Evidence-Based Dentistry*,
https://doi.org/10.1007/978-3-031-47651-8

MIX
Papier aus verantwortungsvollen Quellen
Paper from responsible sources
FSC® C105338

If you have any concerns about our products,
you can contact us on
ProductSafety@springernature.com

In case Publisher is established outside the EU,
the EU authorized representative is:
Springer Nature Customer Service Center GmbH
Europaplatz 3, 69115 Heidelberg, Germany

Printed by Libri Plureos GmbH
in Hamburg, Germany